D0742023

Color Atlas of

Respiratory Diseases

Second Edition

D. Geraint James
MA, MD(Cantab.), FRCP(London), FACP(Hon) LLD(Hon)

Visiting Professor of Medicine
Royal Free Hospital School of Medicine, Hampstead NW3
University of London, England
Adjunct Professor, Departments of Medicine and Epidemiology,
University of Miami School of Medicine, Miami, Florida

Peter R. Studdy
MD, FRCP, FDS(Eng)

Physician, Harefield Hospital, Middlesex and Watford General Hospital, Hertfordshire

With a substantial contribution by Dr Basil Strickland
FRCR, FRCP, FACR(Hon)

Consultant Radiologist
Royal Brompton Hospital
London

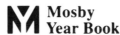

Mosby Year Book

St. Louis   Baltimore   Boston   Chicago   London   Philadelphia   Sydney   Toronto

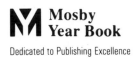

Mosby
Year Book

Dedicated to Publishing Excellence

Mosby-Year Book, Inc.
11830 Westline Drive
St Louis, MO 631146

ISBN 0–8151–4845–3

English First edition published in 1981 by Wolfe Publishing, an imprint of
Mosby-Year Book Europe Limited, 2–16 Torrington Place, London WC1E 7LT, UK.
Second edition published 1992.

Library of Congress Cataloging-in-Publication Data

James. D. Geraint (David Geraint)
    A colour atlas of respiratory diseases / D. Geraint James, Peter
R. Studdy. – 2nd ed.
        p.   cm.
    Includes index.
    ISBN 0–8151–4845–3
    1. Respiratory organs–Diseases–Atlases. I. Studdy, Peter R.
II. Title.
    [DNLM: 1. Respiratory Tract Diseases–atlases. WF 17 J27c]
RC711.J35 1992
616.2'0022'2–dc20
DNLM/DLC
for Library of Congress   92-24902
                                                                  CIP

Contents

Preface to the second edition

The aims and structure remain the same as in the previous edition, but the whole text has been reviewed and updated. Chapters have been added on HIV and immunocompromised respiratory disease, parasitic diseases of the lung and pulmonary vascular disease and sections added to illustrate lung imaging, pneumonia, sleep apnœa and malignant disease.

There has been revision and expansion elsewhere, notably the use of many new pictures to take into account computerised tomography, a valuable diagnostic technique which is now widely available. Dr Basil Strickland, Consultant Radiologist at the Royal Brompton Hospital, London, pioneered High Resolution CT scanning of the chest and has generously provided some 55 scans to illustrate this edition. We are especially pleased to acknowledge this contribution.

Other friends across the world have sent in radiographs, pathology specimens, and other photographs to maintain the zest and liveliness of the first edition. We have added new figures and line drawings to help candidates for the MRCP, Boards and other higher examinations, and also to help medical students to obtain honours in their finals.

This edition has been designed to provide a visual supplement to the many standard text books on respiratory medicine, to which the reader should refer for detailed discussion on up-to-date therapy of lung diseases.

Preface to the first edition

This book is designed to complement the bedside studies of medical students, postgraduates working for higher degrees, nurses, and the most helpful growing army of paramedical personnel who are shouldering an increasing and responsible role in the care of patients around the world. Whichever he or she may be, the diagnostician must obtain an adequate history of the disorder and relate it to the abnormal physical signs noted on examination. The next steps in the clinical examination are to link these symptoms and signs with the chest radiograph.

Abnormalities encountered in the chest x-ray are described in Chapters 1 to 14. Each chapter has a brief, comprehensive description of all abnormalities that may be encountered together with radio-graphic examples. The student will never regret mastering these abnormal radio-graphic patterns, because they keep recurring throughout the working life of the doctor and radiologist. However, being a bedside radiologist is not enough. He must integrate the clinical and radiographic abnormalities into a pattern of disease. Thus the chest x-ray abnormality becomes transformed into the sick patient who may need further investigations before he can be treated accurately. Chapters 15 to 28 correlate these patterns of respiratory disease with the histology or other definitive abnormalities. The respiratory component is often just an incident in a wider multisystem pattern of disease. We have tried to illustrate these multisystem patterns.

This book is a visual representation of Respiratory Diseases. It will be a pictorial supplement to the numerous textbooks on the subject.

Acknowledgements

We gratefully acknowledge the generosity of friends and colleagues who have allowed us to reproduce slides from their collections or helped us in many other ways.

Dr B Afzelius
Dr D J Atherton
Dr Judy Ball
Dr Françoisc Basset
The late Mr M Bates
Dr Eve Blenkinsopp
Dr K Blenkinsopp
Mr T E Bucknall
Dr Margaret Burke
The late Dr L Capel
Dr M Caplin
Dr L S Carstairs
Miss Pat Chapman
Dr P D B Davies
Dr R J Davies
Dr Roy Davies
Dr R Dick
Dr Jennifer Dyson
Dr H E Einstein
Dr A M Emmerson
Dr D J Evans
Mr W Fountain
Mr A I Friedmann
Dr I Kelsey Fry
Dr C N Gamble
Mr G Glover
Dr I Gordon
Dr J Govan
Dr W Gross
Dr C Hardy
Dr P Haslam
Dr C W Havard
Dr C J Heather
Miss Susan Hunt
Dr I M James
Dr W Jones Williams
Dr C Lai

Dr R G Levitt
Mr O Maiwand
Professor T Marshall
Professor E Florence McKeown
Mr M. McKinnon
Dr J B Mitchell
Dr M Moulsdale
Dr I Nakla
Dr A Nath
Dr A Newman-Taylor
Dr L A Phillips
Dr Melanie Powell
The Editor of *Radiology*
Dr P Richman
Professor Gianfranco Rizzato
Dr F C Rodgers
Dr F Clifford Rose
Dr A Sakula
Dr A M Salzberg
Mr M Sanders
Mr R Sandon
Professor P Scheuer
Dr R Seal
Dr O P Sharma
Professor Dame Sheila Sherlock
The late Dr L E Siltzbach
Dr G Sinha
Dr Monica Spiteri
Dr S Steel
Dr P Stradling
Miss B E Stryjak
Dr A G Taylor
Dr A Tookman
Dr F R Vicary
Wellcome Museum of Medical Science
Dr J W Wilson
Dr R A Womersley

1 Anatomy of the lung and thorax

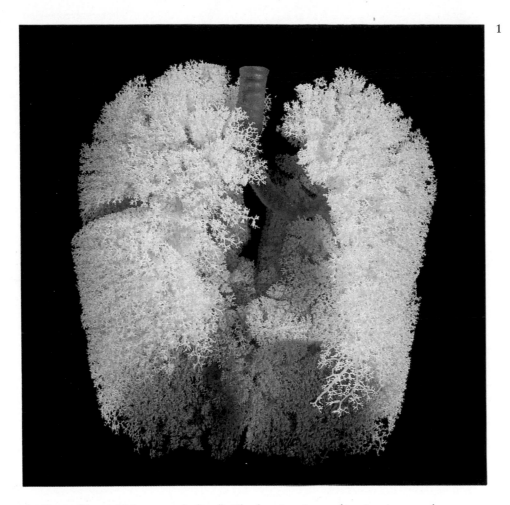

1 Cast of bronchial tree and alveoli. The lung's primary function is to exchange gas between circulating blood and alveolar air. To perform this function the normal adult lung possesses at least 300 million thin-walled distensible air sacs – the alveoli. The alveolar surface area available for gas exchange in the average adult male is estimated at 70–85m^2. At birth, the immature lung possesses 20 million alveoli; growth is rapid and the adult number of alveoli is reached at about 8 years of age.

From the trachea to the alveoli there are between 8 and 23 generations (divisions) of airways. All but the last 1 cm of the breathing passages is made up of purely conductive airways, the bronchi and non-respiratory bronchioles. The respiratory zone lying beyond the terminal bronchioles consists of respiratory bronchioles, alveolar ducts, and alveolar sacs leading to the alveoli.

The gas exchanging ability of the lung can be assessed by measuring the arterial oxygen (PaO_2) and carbon dioxide ($PaCO_2$) tensions. Successful gas exchange depends not only upon normal airways and pulmonary vasculature, but also upon intact neuromuscular and cardiac function.

Some naturally circulating substances are metabolised as they pass through the pulmonary capillary bed. Bradykinin, 5-hydroxytryptamine, and some prostaglandins are inactivated, while angiotensin I is converted into the pressor substance angiotensin II. Some drugs are also metabolised.

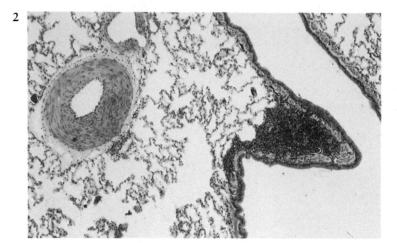

2 Normal adult lung. Histological appearance after pressure fixation with formal saline. The larger air spaces are alveolar ducts, with intact alveoli opening into them.

The normal alveolus is lined by a layer of attenuated epithelial tissue, continuous with the lining epithelium of the alveolar ducts and bronchioles.

Two types of alveolar epithelial cells (pneumatocytes) are described; the flattened plate-like surface, lining alveolar epithelial cells (type 1 pneumatocytes) and the rounded, granular, alveolar epithelial cells (type 2 pneumatocytes) that may produce surfactant.

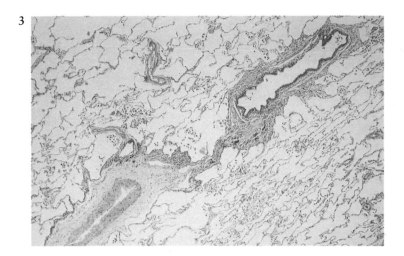

3 Normal adult lung. Functional area between the conductive airways and the respiratory portion of the lung. The terminal (non-respiratory) bronchiole is lined with a continuous cuboidal epithelium. The alveoli open off the respiratory bronchiole. (H & E.)

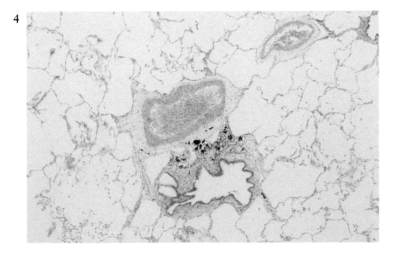

4 Normal adult lung. Bronchiole (below) and muscular artery (above) in the centre surrounded by normal patent alveoli. (Histological section H & E.)

External anatomy

5–7 External anatomy. The diagrams show usual limits of the pleural reflections and the positions of the principal fissures. The oblique fissure lies beneath a line joining the second thoracic spine posteriorly to the sixth costochondral junction anteriorly (line 1). The right horizontal fissure follows the fourth intercostal space anteriorly to meet the oblique fissure at the fifth rib in the mid-axillary line (line 2).

The position of the nipple varies considerably in the female, but in the male usually lies in the fourth intercostal space.

The dark stippled areas indicate the inferior pleural recess where parietal surfaces are in contact and only separated by lung on full inspiration. (A = D₂ spine, B = fourth costal cartilage, C = sixth costal cartilage.)

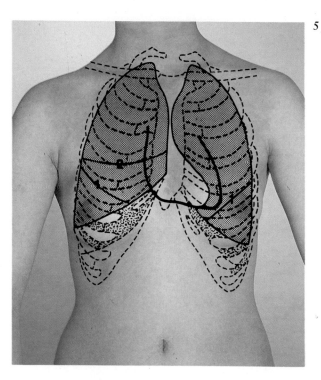

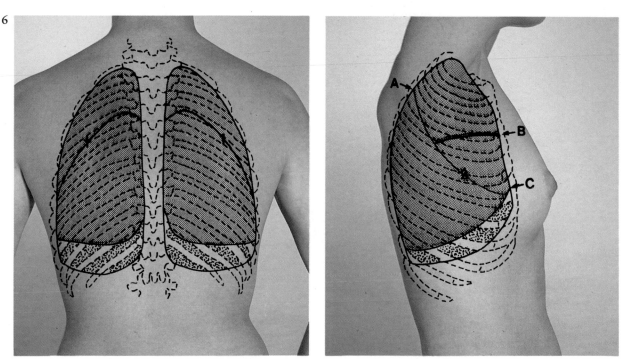

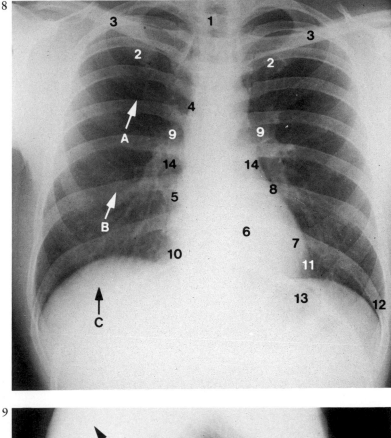

Radiology

8 Posteroanterior view of thorax.
Arrows indicate:
(A) second costal cartilage
(B) fourth costal cartilage
(C) sixth rib in mid-clavicular line

1 Trachea
2 First rib
3 Clavicles
4 Superior vena cava
5 Right atrium
6 Right ventricle
7 Left ventricle
8 Left atrium (auricular appendage)
9 Pulmonary artery
10 Inferior vena cava
11 Left cardiophrenic angle
12 Left costophrenic angle
13 Gas in fundus of stomach
14 Pulmonary veins

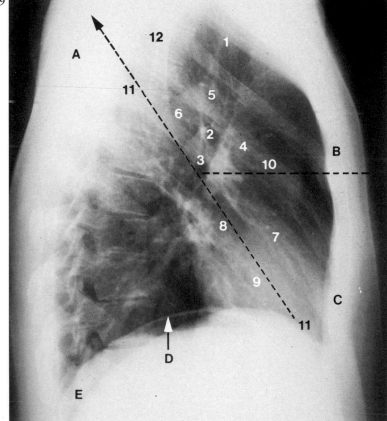

9 Lateral view of thorax.
Arrows indicate:
(A) second thoracic spine
(B) fourth costal cartilage
(C) sixth costal
(D) eighth rib in mid-axillary line
(E) tenth spine

1 Trachea
2 Left main bronchus
3 Right main bronchus
4 Ascending thoracic aorta
5 Aortic arch
6 Descending thoracic aorta
7 Right ventricle
8 Left atrium
9 Left ventricle
10 Horizontal fissure
11 Oblique fissure
12 Scapula

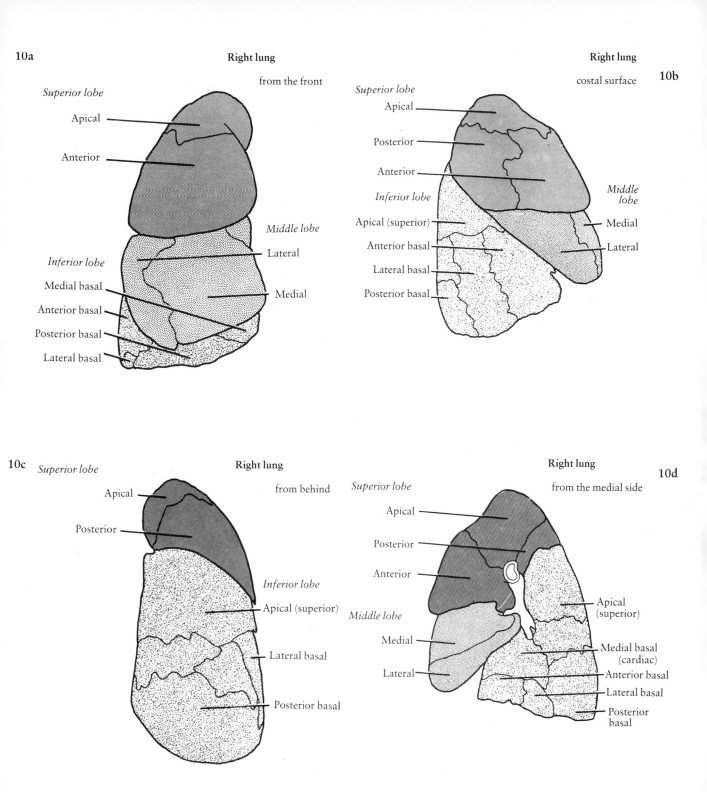

Right lung

from the front

Superior lobe

Apical

Anterior

Middle lobe

Lateral

Inferior lobe

Medial

Medial basal

Anterior basal

Posterior basal

Lateral basal

Right lung

costal surface

Superior lobe

Apical

Posterior

Anterior

Inferior lobe

Apical (superior)

Anterior basal

Lateral basal

Posterior basal

Middle lobe

Medial

Lateral

Superior lobe

Right lung

from behind

Apical

Posterior

Inferior lobe

Apical (superior)

Lateral basal

Posterior basal

Right lung

from the medial side

Superior lobe

Apical

Posterior

Anterior

Middle lobe

Medial

Lateral

Apical (superior)

Medial basal (cardiac)

Anterior basal

Lateral basal

Posterior basal

10 (a)–(d)   Bronchopulmonary segments of the right lung.

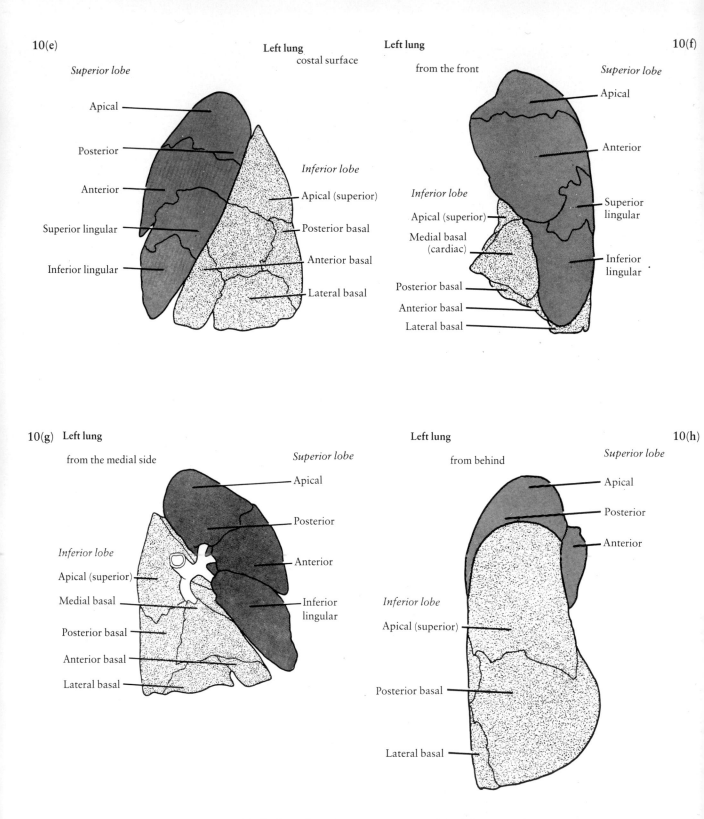

10(e)

Superior lobe

Left lung
costal surface

Apical

Posterior

Anterior

Inferior lobe

Superior lingular

Apical (superior)

Posterior basal

Inferior lingular

Anterior basal

Lateral basal

Left lung
from the front

10(f)

Superior lobe

Apical

Anterior

Superior
lingular

Inferior lobe

Apical (superior)

Medial basal
(cardiac)

Inferior
lingular

Posterior basal

Anterior basal

Lateral basal

10(g) Left lung

from the medial side

Superior lobe

Apical

Posterior

Inferior lobe

Apical (superior)

Anterior

Medial basal

Posterior basal

Inferior
lingular

Anterior basal

Lateral basal

Left lung

from behind

10(h)

Superior lobe

Apical

Posterior

Anterior

Inferior lobe

Apical (superior)

Posterior basal

Lateral basal

10 (e)–(h) Bronchopulmonary segments of the left lung.

14

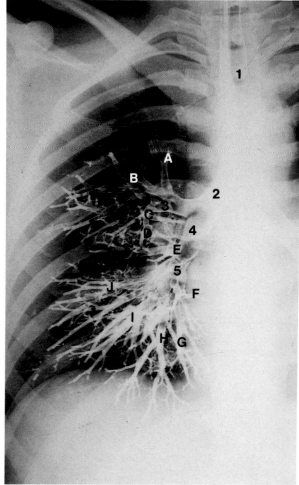

11 Posteroanterior bronchogram of right lung. The right lung is divided into three lobes, the upper, middle and lower, which are further subdivided into broncho-pulmonary segments.

1 Trachea
2 Right main bronchus
3 Right upper lobe bronchus dividing into
  (A) apical segment
  (B) posterior segment
  (C) anterior segment
4 Middle lobe bronchus dividing into
  (D) lateral segment
  (E) medial segment
5 Right lower lobe bronchus
  (F) apical segment
  (G) medial basal segment
  (H) anterior basal segment
  (I) posterior basal segment
  (J) lateral basal segment

12 Lateral bronchogram of right lung.

1 Trachea
2 Right main bronchus
3 Right upper lobe bronchus dividing into
  (A) apical segment
  (B) posterior segment
  (C) anterior segment
4 Middle lobe bronchus dividing into
  (D) lateral segment
  (E) medial segment
5 Right lower lobe bronchus
  (F) apical segment of lower lobe
  (G) medial basal segment
  (H) anterior basal segment
  (I) lateral basal segment
  (J) posterior basal segment

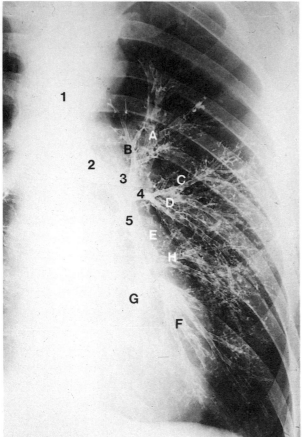

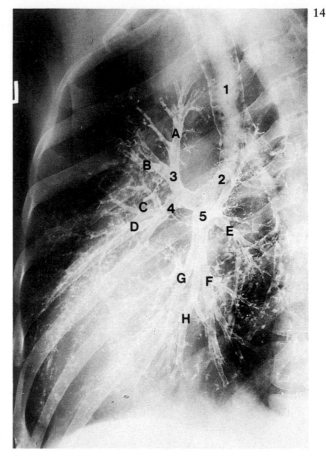

13 Posteroanterior bronchogram of left lung. The left lung is divided into two major lobes by the oblique fissure. The upper lobe and lingula lie above the fissure; the lower lobe lies below.

1 Trachea
2 Left main bronchus
3 Left upper lobe bronchus dividing into
  (A) apicoposterior segment
  (B) anterior segment
4 Lingular lobe bronchus dividing into
  (C) superior segment
  (D) inferior segment
5 Left lower lobe bronchus
  (E) apical segment
  (F) posterior basal segment
  (G) anterior basal segment
  (H) lateral basal segment

14 Lateral bronchogram of left lung. Lateral oblique bronchogram of left lung.

1 Trachea
2 Left main bronchus
3 Left upper lobe bronchus dividing into
  (A) apicoposterior segment
  (B) anterior segment
4 Lingular lobe bronchus dividing into
  (C) superior segment
  (D) inferior segment
5 Left lower lobe bronchus dividing into
  (E) apical segment
  (F) posterior basal segment
  (G) anterior basal segment
  (H) lateral basal segment

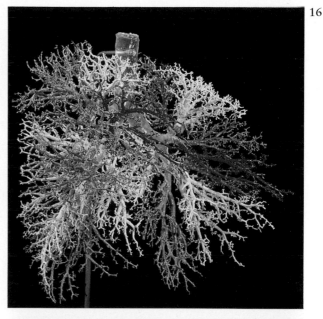

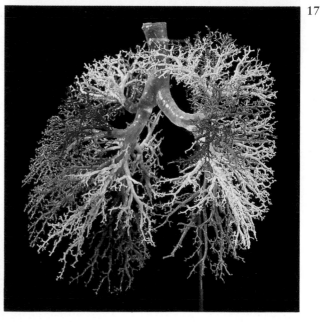

15–17 Casts of bronchial tree showing the different bronchopulmonary segments as outlined in the preceding bronchograms.

Lobar bronchi arise from the right or left main bronchi and divide repeatedly into smaller bronchi; after about 10 divisions they give off bronchioles which in turn divide about five times before the terminal bronchioles are reached. The terminal bronchioles are characterised by an absence of supporting cartilage.

The terminal bronchioles then split into respiratory bronchioles and these finally divide into the alveolar ducts, sacs and alveoli.

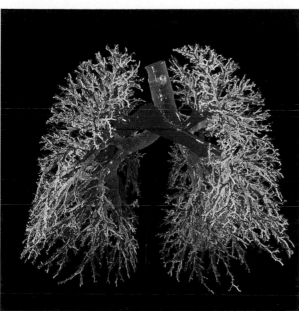

18 Casts of bronchial tree and pulmonary artery. The right and left pulmonary arteries divide in the same manner as the bronchi which they accompany down to the level of the terminal or respiratory bronchioles.

The terminal ramifications of the pulmonary artery do not follow each alveolar duct directly, but drain into the distensible alveolar wall capillary network and then on to the pulmonary veins which lie separately in the periphery of the lung.

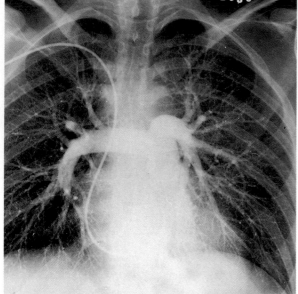

19 Pulmonary angiogram, arterial phase. Normal appearances. The catheter tip has slipped back into the right ventricle. The arterial tree is outlined down to the fourth division. This appearance virtually excludes an embolus if carried out shortly after its suspected occurrence.

Note the higher 'take off' of the left pulmonary artery. This accounts for the higher position of the left hilum on the chest radiograph in 95% of normal people. The left hilum is rarely lower than the right hilum in the normal.

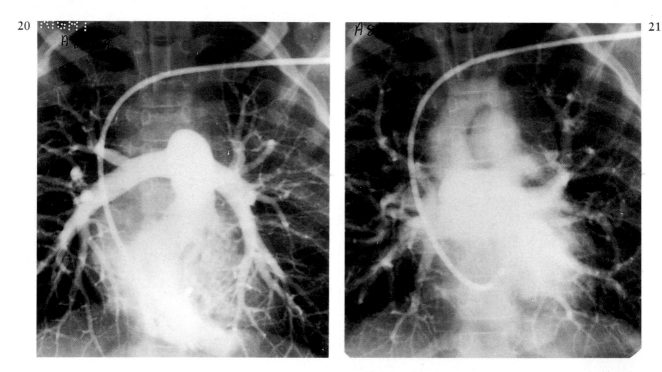

20, 21 Angiocardiogram. Catheter in the right ventricle (RV). In the arterial phase (**20**) the right ventricle is outlined. The interventricular septum causes a concave impression on the cavity of the RV. The main pulmonary artery (PA), right and left branches and subdivisions are clearly seen. The course of the arterial branches to the upper lobe is more vertical on the left. This is normal.

In the venous phase (**21**) the pulmonary veins enter the left atrium at a level well below the pulmonary artery. The left atrium, left ventricle and aorta are clearly seen as well as the left atrial appendage (a small amount of contrast medium outlines the main PA indicating the presence of a minor left to right shunt at ventricular level).

Radioisotope lung imaging

Valuable information which may show local abnormalities of perfusion or ventilation can be obtained by radioisotope lung scanning.

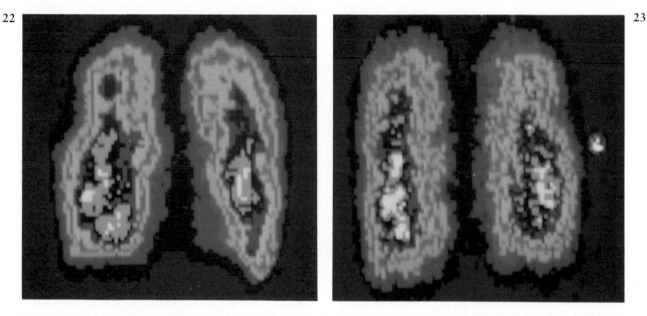

22, 23 Normal regional perfusion scan of the lung: anterior view (**22**), posterior view (**23**). Technetium-99m (^{99m}Tc) labelled albumin microspheres are injected intravenously. The particles range in size between 15 and 70 μm and impact in the pulmonary circulation.

The distribution of gamma ray emission from the ^{99m}Tc labelling is proportional to regional perfusion. A normal perfusion scan provides firm evidence against a diagnosis of pulmonary embolism.

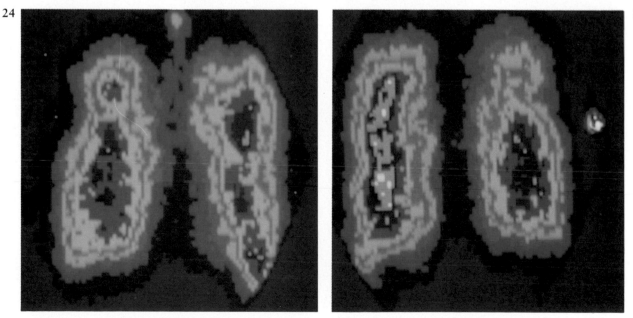

24, 25 Normal regional ventilation scan of the lung: anterior view (**24**), posterior view (**25**). Krypton-81 m has a half life of 13 seconds and gives emissions suitable for high resolution gamma camera images.

The gamma emission in any part of the lung at one time relates to the regional ventilation and provides supplementary information to link with the perfusion scan. Ventilation and perfusion are well matched in normal lungs.

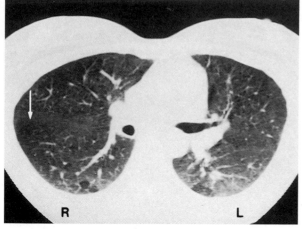

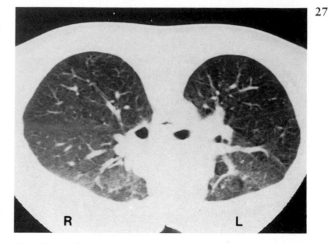

26   **Normal scan – supine position.** The areas of density posteriorly are due to vascular distension in dependent lung parenchyma and are removed by repeating the scan in the prone position (27). On the right, the fissure is visible as a band of increased density within a broad area of relative avascularity (arrowed).

27   **Normal scan, prone position** (same patient as in 26). The areas of density have moved to the anterior portions of the lung, revealing normal parenchyma posteriorly.

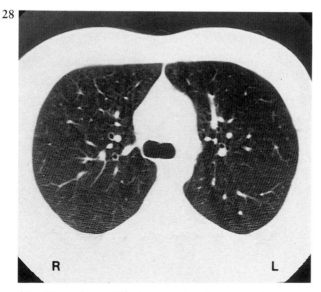

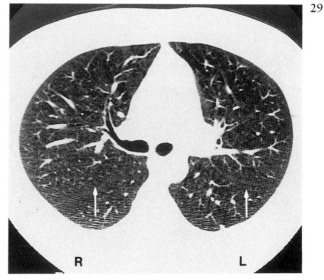

28   **Normal scan.** The bronchi lie adjacent to the arteries and are all of approximately similar size in cross section. The vessels appear dense and rounded in cross section, and branched in the plane of the section. A few thin lines reach the pleura and these represent interlobular septa.

29   **Normal scan.** In the plane of the section the bronchi appear as slightly converging double lines, and the vessels as dots in cross section and branched in the plane of the section. The fissure on the right forms a faint broad curved band of density (arrowed). On the left, the fissure is seen as a thin curved line extending from mediastinum to pleura (arrowed).

Magnetic resonance imaging

30–32 Magnetic resonance imaging (MRI) of thorax: normal appearances in coronal (**30**), sagittal (**31**) and transverse axial planes (**32**). MRI may be carried out in any plane without moving the patient's position. The mediastinal structures are well delineated by the mediastinal fat (which appears white), but ventricular muscle and wall thickness is also well demonstrated as well as the cardiac chambers and great vessels. MRI is of little value for demonstrating the lung parenchyma. In non-cardiac thoracic disease, MRI should be used to complement CT where this is indicated, i.e. mediastinal tumours, invasion of bone, the presence of fat, etc. Calcification cannot be seen on MRI.

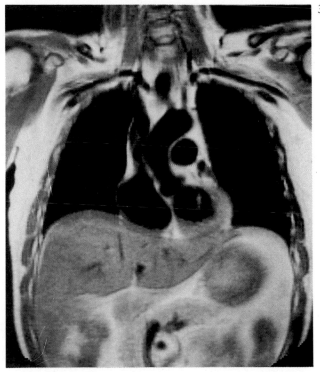

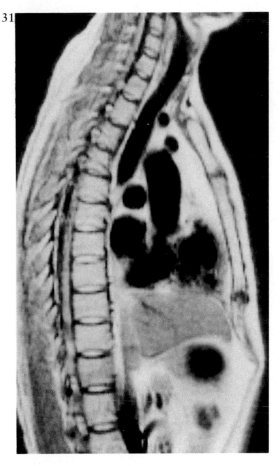

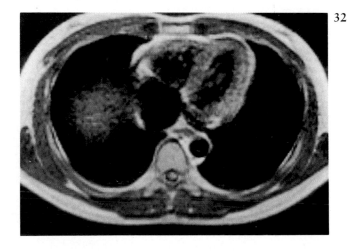

Shape and symmetry of the chest

The external shape of the chest varies widely with body build, but some appearances are characteristic of respiratory conditions.

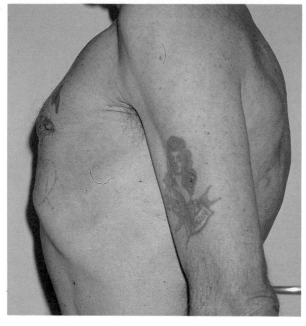

33 Barrel-shaped chest with increase in anteroposterior diameter is frequently caused by hyperinflation and is seen with emphysema or asthma.

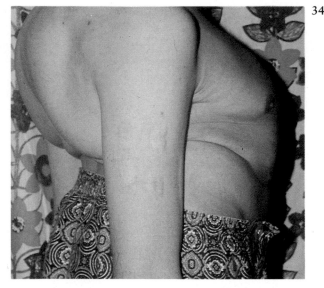

34 Severe kyphoscoliosis. There is an increased anterior convexity, exaggerated lumbar lordosis, and moderate lateral deviation producing a secondary rotation of the rib cage. Causes include spinal tuberculosis or infection, trauma, poliomyelitis or congenital spinal abnormalities. In most cases the aetiology is uncertain.

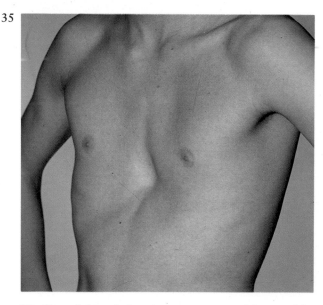

35 Funnel-shaped chest (pectus excavatum) is caused by depression of the lower end of the sternum narrowing the anteroposterior diameter of the thorax. This congenital abnormality is seldom of physiological significance. The heart may be displaced to the left. Surgical correction of the cosmetic deformity may be necessary.

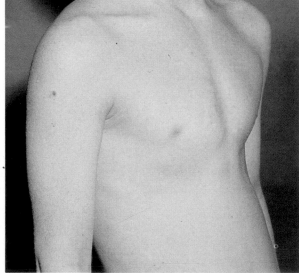

36 Pigeon chest caused by prominence of the upper sternum may be congenital or follow severe persistent overinflation from childhood asthma.

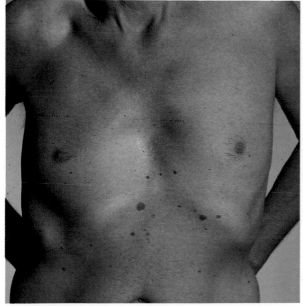

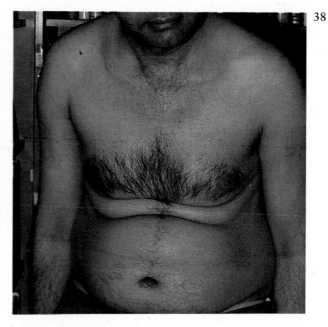

37 Flattening of right upper anterior chest as a consequence of loss of volume of the underlying lung, due to fibrosis secondary to chronic tuberculous infection. The trachea and mediastinum are deviated to the right.

38 Ankylosing spondylitis ('Poker back'). The back forms a continuous curve from the base of the skull to the sternum, the abdomen is protuberant and the chest is 'fixed' with very reduced expansion and upper anterior flattening.

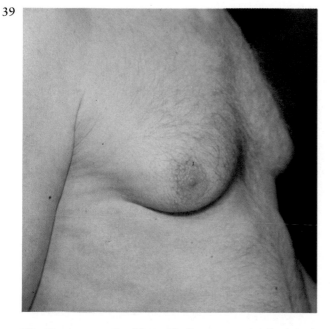

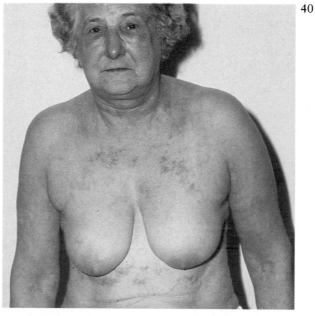

39 Gynaecomastia. The male breast may be feminised by oestrogen or oestrogen-like substances. Endogenous oestrogen from tumours or secreted at puberty may be responsible, as may exogenous oestrogen or drugs with an oestrogen-like structure, such as digitalis, spironolactone and the phenothiazines.

40 Superior vena cava obstruction. The distended veins over the lower chest, non–pulsatile elevation of the jugular venous pressure, swollen arms and bloated face are characteristic.

2 Pleural effusions

In health the visceral and parietal layers of the pleura are separated by a thin layer of fluid, present in the pleural space. Excess fluid may accumulate by transudation or exudation in a wide variety of conditions. A small effusion may be undetectable, but if 500 ml or more of fluid are present, chest wall movement is diminished, percussion note breath sounds and vocal resonance are reduced, and vocal fremitus is absent.

Breathlessness is a common clinical feature with large effusions, and pleurisy is a common feature of pleural inflammation.

The effusion may be:

- Massive with mediastinal shift.
- Moderate in size. Whatever the aetiology, pleural fluid often presents the familiar radiographic appearance of a homogenous opacity with a concave upper border that is higher laterally than medially – the so-called pleural meniscus. Actually, there is nothing in the pleural sac of this shape. If it were possible to solidify the fluid, the lung would be found encased in a cup-shaped cast, thick at the base and tapering to a fine edge at the top. The meniscus is a tangential radiographic projection of the lateral side of this cast.
- Minimal. The costophrenic angle may either be obliterated or be visible only posteriorly in the lateral film. A lateral decubitus film may help to distinguish free fluid from thickened pleura.
- Loculated. This may be interlobar, parietal, perilobar or subperilobar, or subpulmonary.

Examination of pleural fluid

The fluid to be examined (**Table 1**) may be blood, lymph, pus, transudate (protein content <30 g/l) or an exudate (protein content >30 g/l). The nature of the fluid can only be determined by visual and laboratory inspection of an aspirated specimen, which should be obtained in all cases of pleural effusion except those that are obviously cardiac in origin.

Table 1. Examination of pleural fluid.

Protein content	>30 g/l exudate
	<30 g/l transudate
Cytology	Polymorphs – Infection
	Lymphocytes – Tuberculosis, sarcoidosis, malignancy
	Eosinophils – Parasites, bleeding, collagen vascular disorders
	Mesothelial cells
	Malignant cells
	Red blood cells – malignancy, pulmonary embolus
Glucose	<2 mmol/l – Rheumatoid arthritis
Amylase	Pancreatitis
Lactic dehydrogenase	>200 IU/l in exudates
Chylomicrons	Chylothorax
Bacterial culture	Common pathogens
	Smear/culture for acid-fast bacilli
Pleural biopsy	

Transudates are caused by systemic conditions, which alter the hydrostatic pressures or osmotic forces across the pleural membrane. Usually bilateral, although often asymmetrical, they may appear on one side of the chest before the other. If the cause is corrected, the fluid is quickly reabsorbed and resolution is complete, leaving no scarring.

The most common causes are cardiac failure, hepatic cirrhosis and renal failure. Rare causes include myxoedema, pulmonary emboli, and Meig's syndrome due to ovarian fibroma. The diaphragmatic lymphatic plexus is better developed on the right, which may account for the higher incidence of right-sided effusions.

Exudates are commonly unilateral and are due to local disease, causing increased capillary permeability or lymphatic obstruction. The protein content of the pleural fluid is increased, resolution is slow, and healing may leave pleural thickening and adhesions. Exudates may be associated with acute bacterial pneumonia, tuberculosis, or subphrenic abscess. Malignant effusions are usually caused by bronchial carcinoma and less often by alveolar cell carcinoma, metastases, primary pleural tumours, mesothelioma, lymphoma or multiple myeloma. Exudates may also be a feature of rheumatoid arthritis, systemic lupus erythematosus, pulmonary infarction, sarcoidosis, asbestos exposure, and chronic idiopathic lymphoedema (yellow nail syndrome).

Exudates usually have a protein content of >30 g/l, high specific gravity and a lactic dehydrogenase (LDH) activity of >200 IU/l.

Haemothorax is caused by trauma, surgery, pulmonary infarction, rupture of an aneurysm or adhesions from a spontaneous pneumothorax, anticoagulant therapy or a coagulation disorder.

Chylothorax, a rare phenomenon due to the leakage of lymph from the thoracic duct, is caused by trauma, thoracic surgery or mediastinal malignancy. The condition is rarely spontaneous.

Clinical appearances of aspirated pleural fluid

41

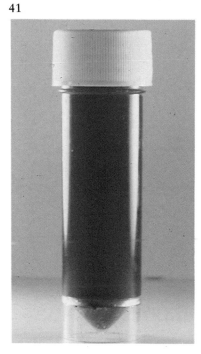

42

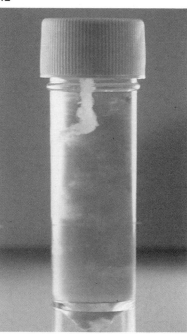

43

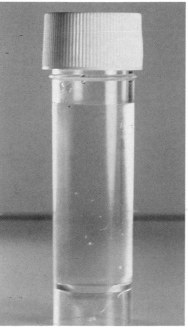

41 Blood-stained pleural effusion. This is commonly found with pulmonary infarction or malignancy and occasionally with tuberculous effusions.

42 Proteinaceous exudate. A yellow turbid aspirate with a high protein content (>30 g/l) and a high specific gravity (>1.015). The proteinaceous clot floating in the fluid is characteristic of an exudate.

43 Clear transudate with a low protein content (<30 g/l) and low specific gravity (<1.015).

Radiographic appearances of pleural effusion

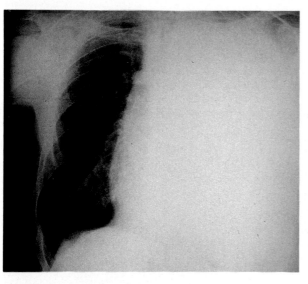

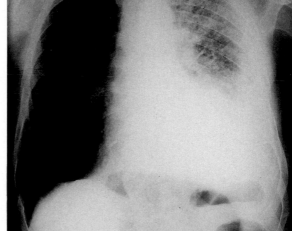

44 Massive malignant pleural effusion. The mediastinum is deviated to the right and the diaphragm depressed by the weight of fluid. Tuberculosis or haemothorax may result in similar massive effusions.

45 Massive malignant pleural effusion. Five litres of fluid were aspirated with considerable relief of symptoms. The mediastinum is now central and the gastric air bubble is visible. The upper border of the fluid appears concave.

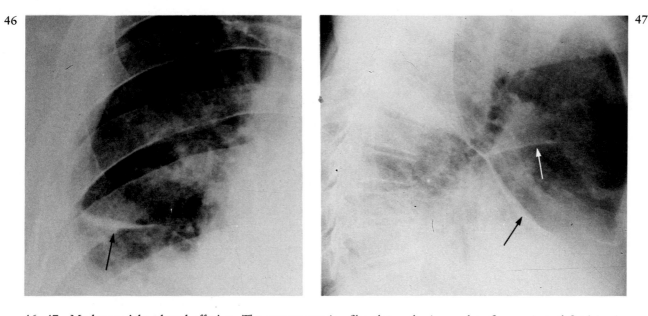

46, 47 Moderate right pleural effusion. The posteroanterior film shows the incomplete fissure sign of fluid in the oblique fissure. The curvilinear edge on the posterioanterior film (arrowed) is formed by fluid in the oblique fissure which is incomplete medially. The lateral film (**47**) shows fluid in the oblique and horizontal fissure (arrows).

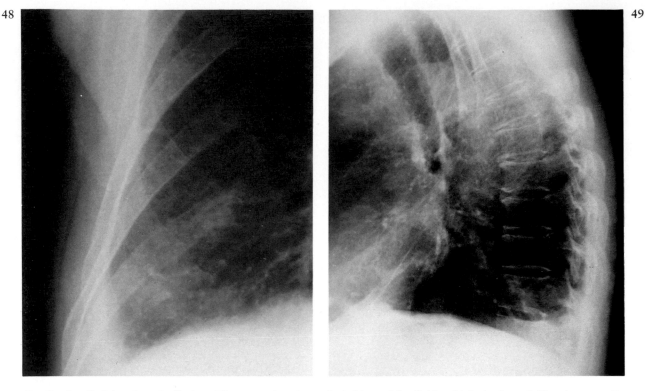

48, 49 Small right pleural effusion. The costophrenic angle is blunted by fluid, which the lateral film shows to lie posteriorly.

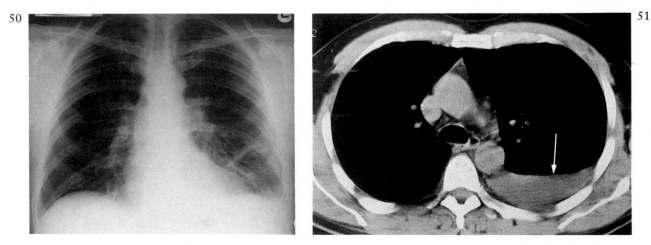

50, 51 Left subpulmonary effusion. Note the slight elevation of the left diaphragm and costophrenic angle pleural reaction. The CT scan (**51**), taken with patient supine, disclosed an unexpectedly large left pleural effusion. Aspiration revealed malignant cells. (Upper border of effusion shown by arrow.)

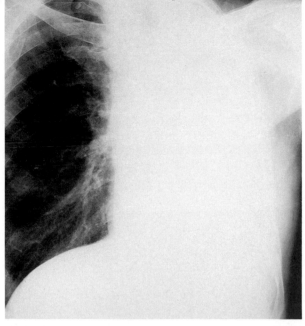

52 Postpneumonic pleural effusion. The pleural cavity normally fills with fluid after pneumonectomy. The mediastinum and heart are deviated to the left, the operated side.

53 Postpneumonectomy pleural effusion. Bronchopleural fistula. The x-ray was taken after the patient had expectorated 3 litres of straw-coloured fluid. The fluid level indicates that air has entered the chest cavity. The bronchial stump may be eroded by infection, or, as in this case, by recurrent malignancy 8 months after pneumonectomy.

The yellow nail syndrome

The basic defect is hypoplasia of the lymphatic system, resulting in impaired lymphatic drainage. Patients present with exudative pleural effusions, lymphoedema of the lower limbs and thickened dystrophic yellow nails. Sinusitis, protein-losing enteropathy and bronchiectasis can occur. The three main features of the syndrome may develop at widely different times. Development of lymphoedema and pleural effusions does not occur in some patients unless the lymphatic system is stressed by infection.

Effusions may be bilateral and can be massive. Aspiration reveals a clear exudate in which lymphocytes predominate. There is no specific treatment and the fluid recurs after tapping. Pleurodesis is sometimes helpful.

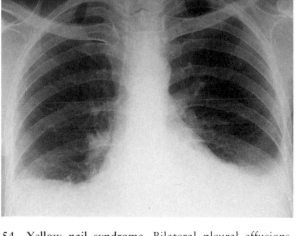

54 Yellow nail syndrome. Bilateral pleural effusions. A dramatic improvement in breathing followed bilateral pleurocentesis and pleurodesis.

55

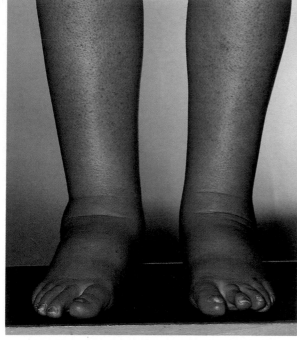

56

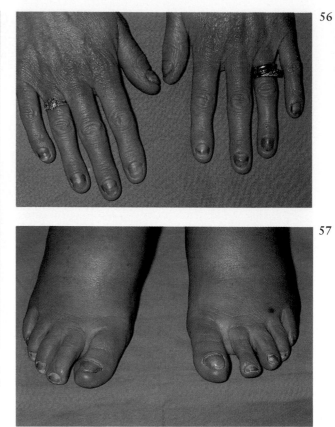

57

55–57 Yellow nail syndrome. Primary lymphoedema of the legs (55) and yellow discoloration of dystrophic fingernails (56) and toenails (57).

3 Pneumothorax and mediastinal emphysema

A pneumothorax develops when air escapes into the pleural cavity, allowing separation of the visceral and parietal layers of the pleura and collapse of the underlying lung.

Four different types of pneumothorax are described:

1 Primary spontaneous pneumothorax. Around 85% of cases occur in males, most commonly between 20 and 40 years of age and of ectomorphic physique. The recurrence rate is 20% after the first episode, and 50% if two episodes of pneumothorax have occurred. Primary spontaneous pneumothorax is usually caused by rupture of small subpleural bullae, 1–2 cm in diameter at the lung apex. It is also a common complication of histiocytosis X and connective tissue disorders such as Marfan's syndrome.

2 Secondary pneumothorax is common in chronic bronchitis and in emphysema caused by rupture of subpleural bullae. It may complicate pneumonia, lung abscess, tuberculosis, asthma, cystic fibrosis or bronchial carcinoma.

3 Traumatic pneumothorax from penetrating injuries of the chest wall.

4 Artificial or induced pneumothorax.

The mechanical problems caused by a pneumothorax may be considered as:

- Closed pneumothorax. The hole in the visceral pleura closes spontaneously. Irrespective of the cause, a pneumothorax slowly decreases in size when the air leak seals. If the lung and pleura are healthy, a 50% pneumothorax takes about 40 days to be fully reabsorbed.
- Open pneumothorax. Air leaks through the visceral pleura preventing re-expansion of the lung.
- Tension pneumothorax. A valvular mechanism at the site of pleural air leak allows a progressive increase in intrapleural pressure, which compresses the affected lung and the mediastinal structures against the contralateral lung. This is potentially a fatal condition.

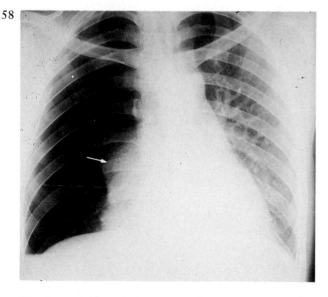

58 **Spontaneous tension pneumothorax** presenting with acute pleuritic pain and severe dyspnoea. Pleural air is seen as a radiolucent crescent devoid of lung markings, bounded by the edge of the lung (arrowed) and chest wall.

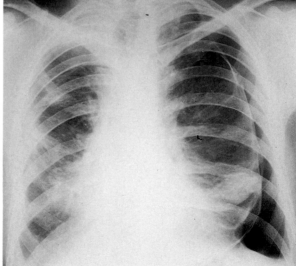

59 **Artificial induced pneumothorax.** Collapse therapy for cavitating apical pulmonary tuberculosis in the pretuberculous chemotherapy era.

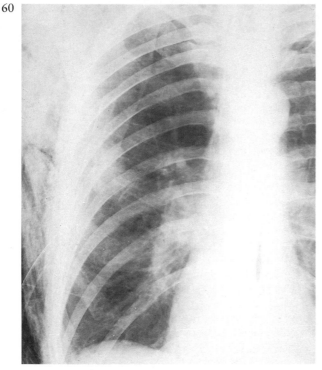

60 Secondary pneumothorax with surgical emphysema of the chest wall. Air has tracked past the intercostal drainage tube into the chest wall tissues to outline the pectoral muscles. On clinical examination, a characteristic 'crackling' sensation can be elicited on palpation of the chest wall.

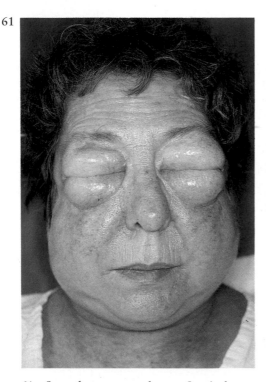

61 Secondary pneumothorax. Surgical emphysema of the face. Gross surgical emphysema of the chest wall, neck and face as a consequence of air leaking through an open pneumothorax.

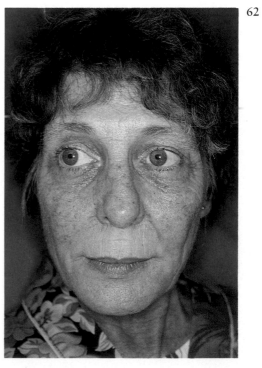

62 Secondary pneumothorax. Surgical emphysema. The same patient as in **61**, showing complete resolution of the surgical emphysema.

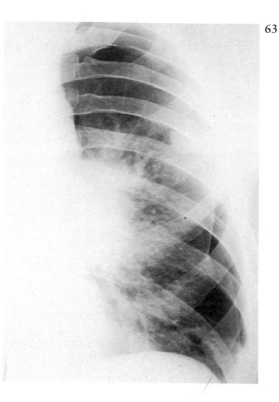

63 Traumatic left pneumothorax following needle biopsy of a peripheral lesion. An enlarged hilum caused by oat-cell carcinoma is also visible. Small pneumothoraces commonly occur after aspiration needle biopsy, but they seldom cause symptoms or require drainage.

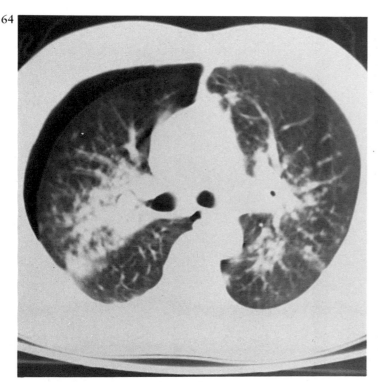

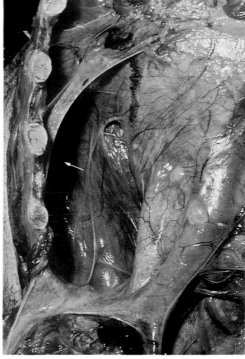

64 Traumatic pneumothorax following transbronchial lung biopsy. CT scan showing a shallow right pneumothorax and pulmonary infiltration due to sarcoidosis. The post-bronchoscopy chest x-ray failed to show any evidence of pneumothorax, a common occurrence when there is a shallow pneumothorax.

65 Fatal tension pneumothorax. Necropsy specimen after removal of anterior ribs and sternum showing collapsed lung and large pleural space (arrowed).

Mediastinal emphysema

Air may enter the mediastinum directly from a ruptured bronchus or oesophagus, or indirectly along the pulmonary vessels after rupture of the alveoli.

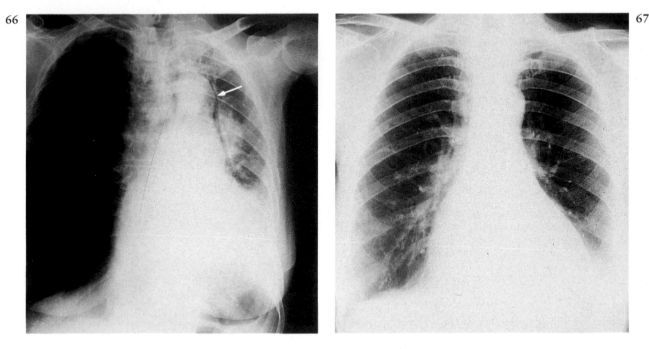

66 & 67   Mediastinal emphysema. In **66** the left lung is partially collapsed and the trachea deviated to the left. Air in the mediastinum appears as a narrow translucent halo outlining the heart and aortic arch (arrowed). The left main bronchus was occluded by a tenacious mucus plug in this asthmatic patient. The left lung re-expanded when the mucus plug was aspirated (**67**).

4 The diaphragm

The diaphragm (**68**) is the most important respiratory muscle. In normal quiet breathing it is responsible for three-quarters of the inhaled total volume. The intercostal muscles contribute the remaining quarter. Unilateral paralysis reduces the ventilating capacity by some 20%, but is well tolerated unless the lungs are diseased. Even total bilateral diaphragmatic paralysis is compatible with life, because of partial compensation by other muscles of respiration. The arched musculotendinous division between the thorax and the abdomen has its origin in vertebral, costal and spinal attachments, from which muscular fibres curve inwards and upwards from the periphery to be inserted into the fibrous sheet called the central tendon.

The largest portion originates from the fourth mesodermal somite, bringing innervation from C4 with minor contributions from C3 and C5 via the phrenic nerve. Development is completed around the twelfth week of foetal life.

The diaphragm is rarely affected by intrinsic disease, but because of its complex embryological development, it is subject to a number of congenital abnormalities. Failure of fusion allows the gut to lie in the thorax and critically impede development of the bronchial tree, which is only completed at 16 weeks of intrauterine life. Normal diaphragms have a characteristic humped shape on the x-ray and are well defined. Flattening is usually caused by hyperinflation, and loss of outline indicates adjacent pleural or pulmonary disease.

The diaphragm may be elevated or depressed by disease above or below it; it may be paralysed by phrenic nerve involvement or it may be the site of congenital or traumatic herniation.

68

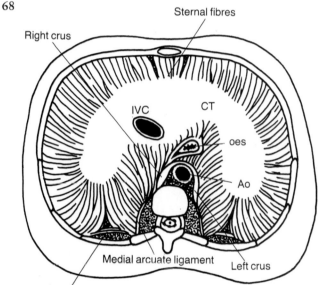

68 The diaphragm viewed from below (CT, central tendon of the diaphragm; IVC, opening for inferior vena cava; Ao, aorta; and oes, oesophagus). There is considerable individual variation in the arrangement of muscle fibres. Usually the oesophageal opening is invested in fibres derived from the right crus.

Table 2. Causes of abnormal position of the diaphragm.

Unilateral elevation	Phrenic nerve paralysis
	Pulmonary embolus
	Basal/diaphragmatic pleurisy
	Viral infections:
	Herpes zoster, poliomyelitis, Coxsackie
	Pulmonary resection
	Atelectasis
	Subphrenic abscess
Eventration }	partial right-sided complete left-sided
False elevation }	subpulmonary effusion chest mass
Bilateral elevation	Neurological disease:
	motor neurone disease
	multiple sclerosis
	Guillain–Barré
	Muscle disease:
	dystrophia myotonica
	Subdiaphragmatic:
	pregnancy
	paralytic ileus
	ascites
Unilateral depression	Pneumothorax
	Basal lung cyst with air trapping
Bilateral depression	Emphysema
	Acute severe asthma
	Carcinoma of the trachea

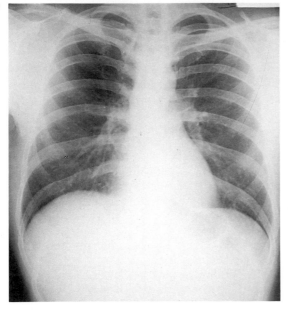

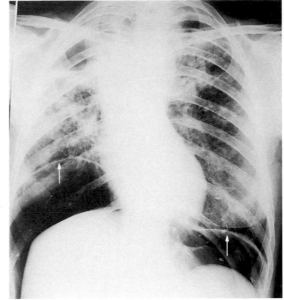

69 Normal appearance of the diaphragm. The right hemidiaphragm is normally higher than the left; the common explanation is that the underlying liver elevates the diaphragm. However, studies of isolated dextrocardia show that the position of the diaphragm is influenced most by the mass of the overlying heart.

70 Bilateral elevation of the diaphragm. Therapeutic pneumoperitoneum induced as treatment for active cavitating pulmonary tuberculosis in the pre-antibiotic era. The very high position of the right diaphragm is caused by a right phrenic nerve section. The thin diaphragm muscle is clearly seen (arrowed).

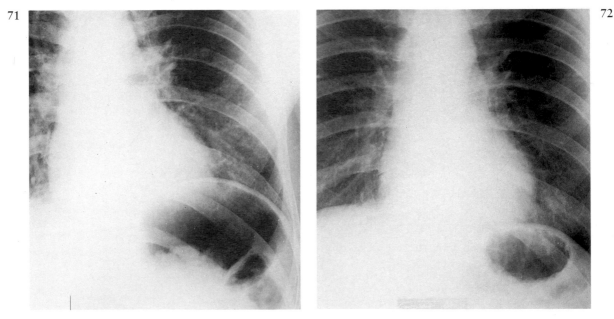

71 Elevated left diaphragm. Considerable gaseous distension of the stomach has caused a physiological elevation of the left diaphragm.

72 Elevated left diaphragm (same patient as in **71**). A repeat film shows less gas and a normal position of the diaphragm.

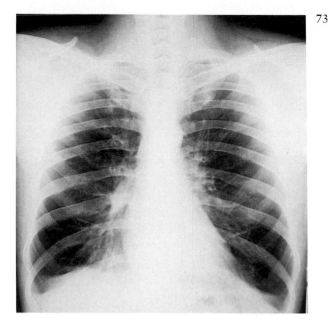

73 Bilateral descent of the diaphragm. Scalloping of the diaphragm occurred during an acute attack of asthma. The costal attachments become visible when hyperinflation depresses the diaphragm muscle.

Diaphragmatic hernias

Congenital or acquired defects of the diaphragm may allow the abdominal contents to herniate into the thorax. Large congenital hernias are rare but, when present, cause respiratory embarrassment in infancy. At least three-quarters of diaphragmatic hernias occur through the oesophageal hiatus, usually are acquired, and present with symptoms from middle age onwards.

Three main types of oesophageal hiatus hernias are shown in **74–76**.

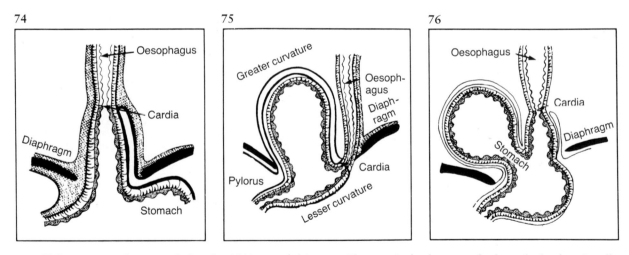

74 Sliding or oesophagogastric hernia. 90% are of this type. The gastric fundus ascends through the functionally incompetent hiatal orifice into the posterior mediastinum. Symptoms are variable and caused by reflux.

75 Rolling or paraoesophageal hernia. The gastric cardia is normally placed, but the greater curvature or, rarely, the whole stomach ascends into the posterior mediastinum. Symptoms are from recurrent gastric volvulus rather than reflux.

76 Mixed hiatus hernia: a combination of oesophagogastric and paraoesophageal.

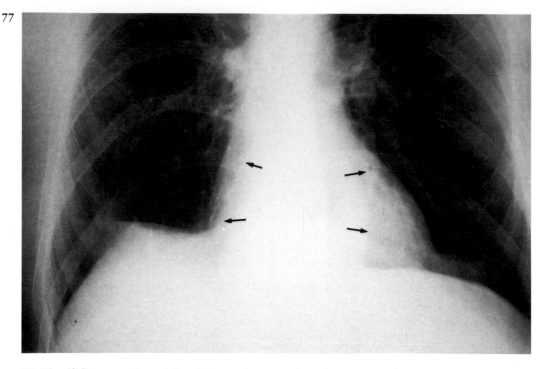

77–79 Sliding oesophageal hernia (oesophagogastric). The portion of stomach lying above the diaphragm is seen as a radiolucency lying behind the heart in the posterior mediastinum (77, 78). Fluid levels may be seen on occasion. The barium meal investigation (79) outlines the portion of stomach lying above the diaphragm in the sliding hernia. More than 90% of all diaphragmatic hernias occur through the oesophageal hiatus.

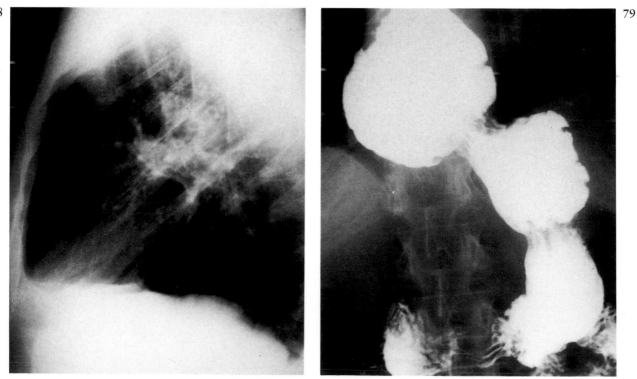

78

79

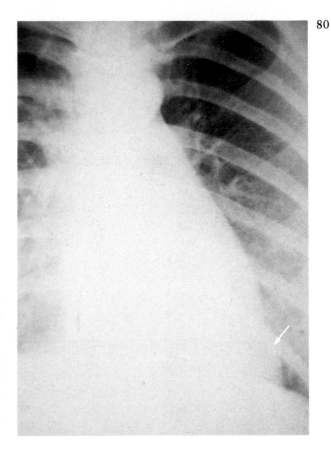

80–82 Hernia of Bochdalek (posterolateral). The posterior mass lying above the diaphragm (**80, 81**) is shown by intravenous urogram (**82**) to be the left kidney. The diaphragm closes at the twelfth week of foetal life. Failure of fusion of lateral segments of the fourth mesodermal somite may leave an unclosed diaphragmatic pleuroperitoneal canal. This defect most commonly involves the left diaphragm and allows the abdominal organs to move freely into the chest cavity. Severe respiratory embarrassment in the neonate may draw attention to the diaphragmatic defect.

81

82

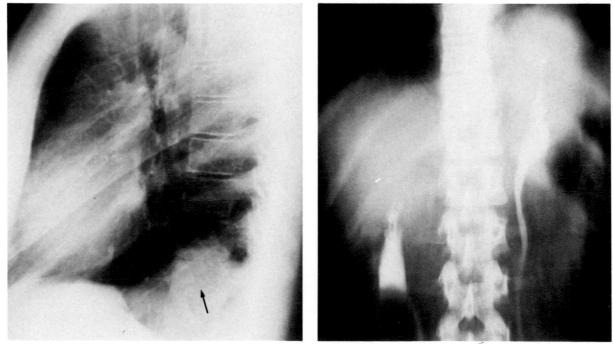

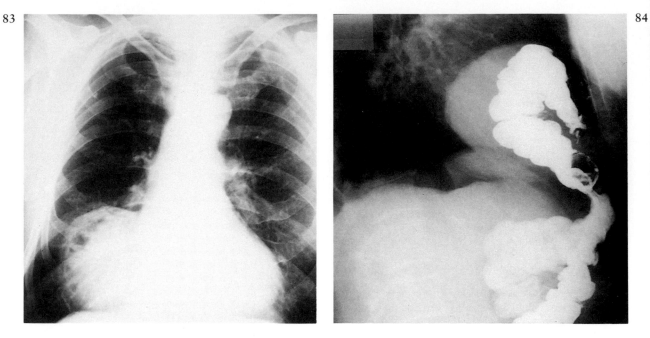

83, 84 Foramen of Morgagni hernia (anterior). The defect lies between the sternal and costal attachments of the diaphragm; it is more common on the right side. These hernias are seldom as extensive as the posterolateral type and rarely cause respiratory embarrassment. Omental fat or intestine may herniate through the foramen.

This example shows small bowel containing barium and air-filled large bowel. Posteroanterior chest radiograph (**83**); and barium small bowel study, lateral view (**84**).

5 Hilar adenopathy

The hilar shadows

The normal radiographic appearance of the hilar shadows is composed of the pulmonary arteries and their main branches, the upper lobe pulmonary veins, the major bronchi and the lymph glands (85). The bronchi contribute little to the hilar shadows because they are filled with air, and normal lymph nodes are too small to add size or density. It is important to distinguish enlarged vascular shadows from lymphadenopathy; this is usually evident in the lateral film. There are significant differences between the causes of unilateral and bilateral hilar enlargement, so it is important to establish the extent of involvement, if necessary by CT scanning or, exceptionally, by angiography. Causes of unilateral and bilateral hilar enlargement are summarised in **Tables 3** and **4**.

85

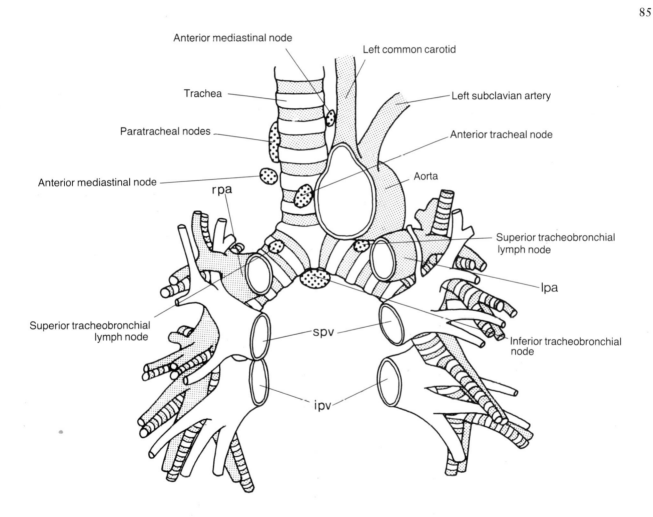

85   Diagram of the mediastinal structures showing relationship of the main lymph nodes, vessels and major proximal airways. The arrangement of the pulmonary arteries (shaded), pulmonary veins (unshaded) and bronchi (striped) represents the most common relationship; there is individual variation. Note that on the right the arrangement of the structures from front to back runs: vein, artery, bronchus. On the left the sequence is vein, bronchus, artery. The pulmonary artery and the bronchi run close to each other in the same connective tissue sheath, whereas the pulmonary vein is almost everywhere separate in its course through the lung. (lpa = left pulmonary artery, rpa = right pulmonary artery, spv = superior pulmonary veins, ipv = inferior pulmonary veins.)

Table 3. Unilateral hilar lymphadenopathy.

Causes	Confirmation
Bronchial carcinoma	Bronchoscopic biopsy Sputum cytology Mediastinoscopy
Tuberculosis	Strongly positive tuberculin test Pulmonary lesion (Ghon focus) Sputum culture
Sarcoidosis Histoplasmosis Coccidioidomycosis	As for bilateral hilar lymphadenopathy

Table 4. Bilateral hilar lymphadenopathy.

Causes	Confirmation
Sarcoidosis	Erythema nodosum/uveitis/ Bronchial/lung biopsy Mediastinoscopy Kveim test Serum angiotensin-converting enzyme
Tuberculosis	Migrant communities Tuberculin skin test conversion Search for mycobacteria
Lymphoma	Ill, febrile, losing weight Mediastinoscopy Lymph node biopsy
Metastases	Lymph node biopsy
Histoplasmosis	Endemic zones Erythema nodosum/uveitis
Coccidioidomycosis	Skin test Serum antibodies
Beryllium disease	History of exposure Accompanying pulmonary lesions Skin test Normal angiotensin-converting enzyme

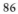

86

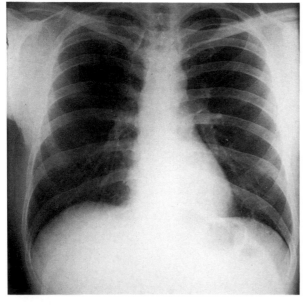

87

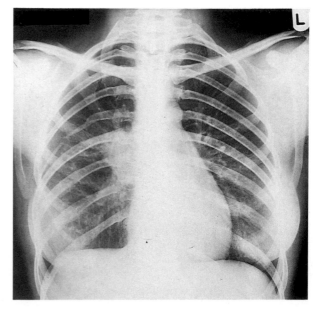

86 Normal hilar shadows. These are usually of equal density and size, the left hilum being 1–1.5 cm higher than the right.

87 Unilateral right hilar gland enlargement. The enlarged right paratracheal gland in this 25-year-old was caused by tuberculosis. Carcinoma of the bronchus gives a similar appearance.

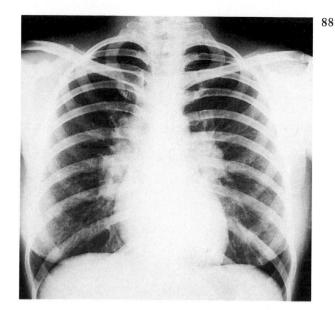

88 Bilateral hilar gland enlargement in sarcoidosis. The hilar and right paratracheal nodes are most commonly involved in sarcoidosis and also in lymphoma. A clear uninvolved zone is visible between the right hilar node and the mediastinum.

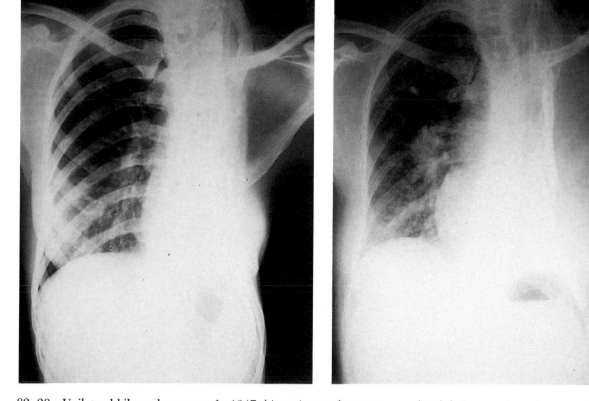

89, 90 Unilateral hilar enlargement. In 1947 this patient underwent a complete left thoracoplasty for extensive left lung cavitating pulmonary tuberculosis. Recovery was satisfactory and good health was maintained for many years. In 1960 the posteroanterior chest x-ray showed a normal right hilum and cardiac silhouette (**89**). Breathlessness secondary to hypoxic pulmonary hypertension developed and by 1989 the posteroanterior chest x-ray showed cardiomegaly due to right ventricular hypertrophy and massive enlargement of the pulmonary artery (**90**).

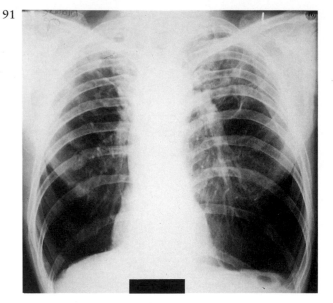

91 Elevated hilar shadows. These may occur as a consequence of upper lobe shrinkage caused by pulmonary tuberculosis, extensive allergic alveolitis or allergic bronchopulmonary aspergillosis.

6 Mediastinal masses

The mediastinum comprises those structures situated between the lungs at the centre of the thorax. It is bounded superiorly by the thoracic inlet, inferiorly by the diaphragm, on each side by the parietal pleura, posteriorly by the thoracic spine and anteriorly by the sternum. For descriptive purposes, it is divided into four compartments: superior from a line drawn above the fourth intervertebral disc, and below this lies the inferior mediastinum divided into anterior, middle and posterior compartments.

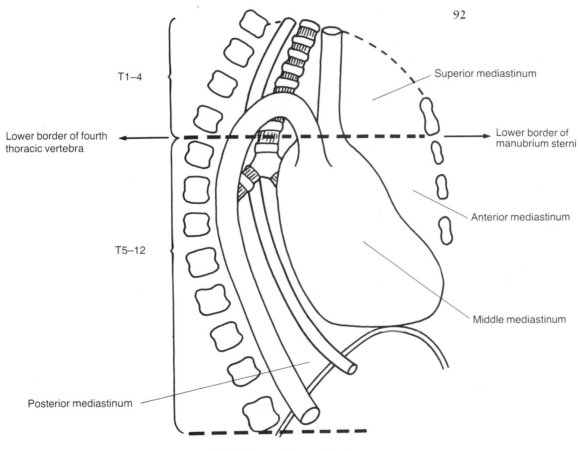

92   Subdivisions of the mediastinum.

Hilar and mediastinal nodes
Sarcoidosis
- Symmetrical, bilateral, asymptomatic

Tuberculosis
- Usually asymmetrical, mediastinal
- Primary infection in children often symptomatic
- Common in Asians (also those who are immigrants to Western countries)

Lymphoma
- Asymmetrical, often symptomatic

Hodgkin's disease
- Nodes can be huge
- Anterior mediastinum may be involved

Metastatic carcinoma
- Almost always bronchial primary
- Occasionally primary in breast or colon

Bronchogenic cyst
Arise from tracheobronchial tree
Usually close to carina

Enterogenous cyst
Arise from oesophagus but are rare

Retrosternal goitre
Thyroid tissue
- Identified with iodine-131 scan

Thymic mass
Commonly hyperplasia in infants
Benign or malignant thymoma
- 40% associated with myasthenia gravis
- Sometimes associated with pure red cell aplasia, systemic lupus erythematosus, thyrotoxicosis, polymyositis, haemolytic anaemia, Cushing's syndrome

Aortic aneurysms
Usually descending
Occasionally ascending and syphilitic

Neurogenic tumours
Most common mediastinal tumour
May splay or erode ribs
Neurilemmoma
- Benign, from Schwann cell

Neurofibroma
- From intercostal nerve (von Recklinghausen's disease)
- Thoracic scoliosis

Ganglioneuroma
- Arising in peripheral autonomic nervous system
- Usually benign

Neuroblastoma
- Arising in sympathetic nervous system
- Usually malignant
- Usually found in children under 12 years of age

Paravertebral abscess
Usually tuberculous
Loss of disc space an early sign

Teratodermoid
Germ cell tumour
- High serum β-human chorionic gonadotrophin
- High serum α-fetoprotein
- Malignant

Dermoid
- May contain teeth, bones, calcium
- May become malignant
- Cystic tumours, rarely malignant

Pericardial cyst
Well-defined
Ovoid or round
Usually on right side
'Spring water cysts'
Harmless

Hiatus hernia
Often visible fluid level
Confirm with barium swallow

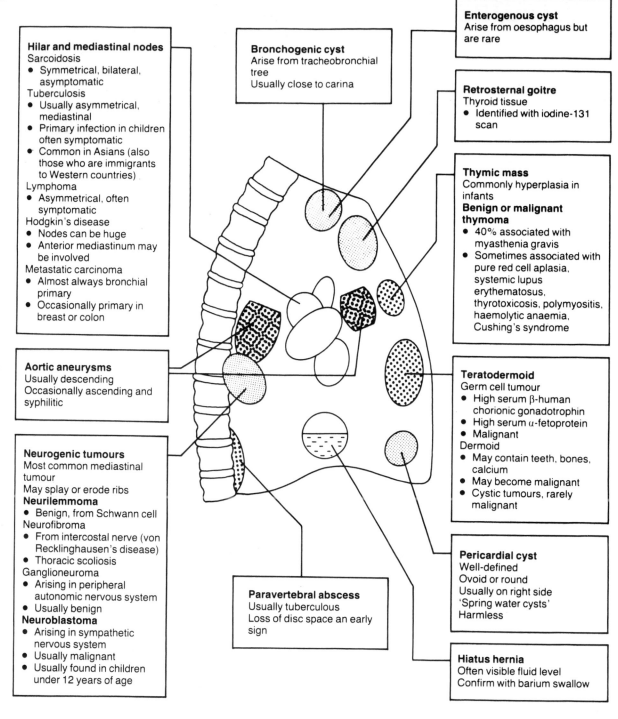

93 Schematic representation of the mediastinum, showing some causes of abnormal chest radiograph appearances. CT scanning is a good technique for identifying mediastinal anatomy, particularly in difficult cases. MRI scans may provide additional information. (With kind permission of Dr S.G. Spiro, adapted from *Medicine International* 1986; **36**: 1475, by courtesy of The Medicine Group Journals Ltd.)

Idiopathic mediastinal fibrosis

This rare disorder is of uncertain aetiology and causes progressive fibrosis of the mediastinum with compression of the vena cava, oesophagus, trachea and proximal airways.

The onset is usually in middle age. The clinical features are determined largely by the amount of fibrous tissue present but the most common presentation is with dyspnoea, dysphagia or superior vena cava obstruction.

In most instances no cause is found, but the condition may be associated with *Histoplasma capsulatum* or *Mycobacterium tuberculosis*.

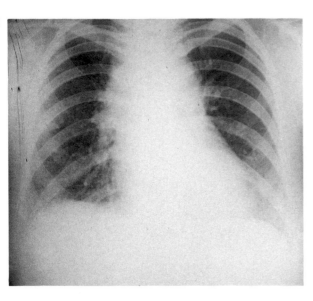

94 Idiopathic mediastinal fibrosis causing superior vena cava obstruction. Note the swollen arms and the tortuous venous collaterals over the anterior chest, which remained unchanged for five years.

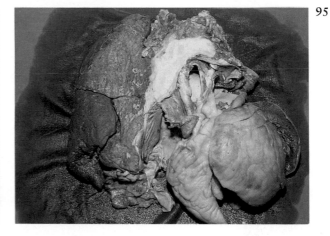

95 Idiopathic mediastinal fibrosis. Necropsy specimen. A firm mass of pale tissue surrounds and compresses the mediastinal structures. The dense fibrous tissue has strangled the superior vena cava, the right pulmonary artery and hilum. The superior vena cava is stenotic and only admitted a 1mm probe. The right pulmonary artery is narrowed by extrinsic compression.

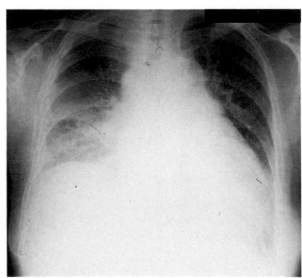

96 Idiopathic mediastinal fibrosis. Chest radiograph showing mediastinal widening in a middle-aged woman who presented with breathlessness and superior vena cava obstruction.

97 Idiopathic mediastinal fibrosis. Mediastinal widening. The same patient as shown in **96**, 15 years later. The right lung has contracted and the mediastinum widened. The clinical appearance is shown in **94**.

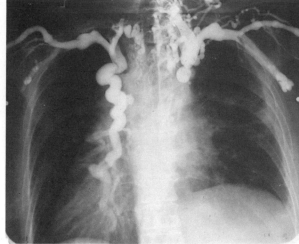

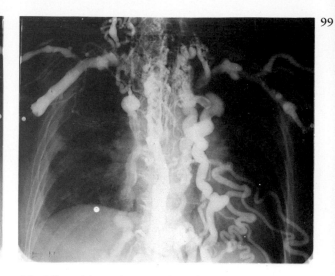

98 Idiopathic mediastinal fibrosis. Superior vena cavogram. The early film shows no dye in the superior vena cava and gross dilatation of vessels to the left of the mediastinum.

99 Idiopathic mediastinal fibrosis. Superior vena cavogram. The late film shows that some dye has reached the inferior vena cava. Flow in the superior vena cava is reduced to a trickle.

7 Pulmonary nodules and masses

These may be single or multiple, may vary considerably in size and sometimes may cavitate or contain calcium.

Solitary pulmonary nodules

The solitary circumscribed pulmonary nodule presents a common diagnostic dilemma. Benign lesions seldom warrant surgery, whereas early excision of a localised carcinoma may be curative. Calcification is common in benign hamartomas or healed granulomas. Stable uncalcified lesions and calcified nodules in patients under 35 years of age seldom require surgery and may be observed. In the older patient a solitary nodule is more likely to be malignant, so tissue diagnosis is essential. The solitary nodule is spherical or oval, relatively well defined, less than 5 cm in diameter, and lies within the lung. The causes and diagnostic measures are listed in **Table 5**.

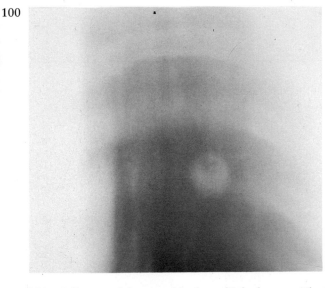

100 **Solitary nodule caused by bronchial adenoma.** The sharply circumscribed margin occurs in about 25% of bronchial carcinomas and in some tuberculomas (tomographic view).

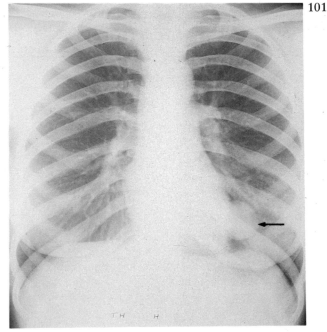

101 **Solitary nodule caused by hamartoma.** Hamartoma, the most common benign pulmonary tumour, is composed of different tissues that are normally present in the lung, but are abnormally organised to form a tumour. It is usually peripheral in position and found by chance on a routine x-ray. Calcification is common (40%).

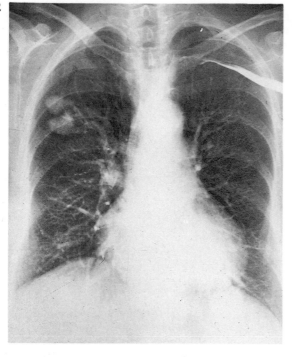

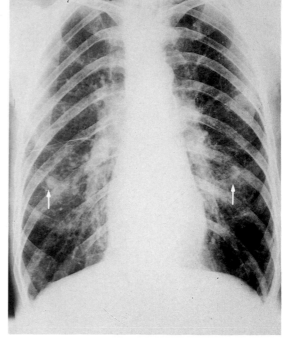

102 Arteriovenous fistula shown by pulmonary angiography. Often well circumscribed and never calcifies. This vascular abnormality, often multiple, is caused by the persistence of foetal capillary anastomosis between the arterial and venous pulmonary circulation.

103 Soft tissue shadows may simulate an intrapulmonary nodule. Nipple shadows are often seen on standard chest radiographs (arrowed).

Pulmonary masses

A large intrathoracic opacity that is more than 5 cm in diameter is usually malignant and is caused by a bronchial carcinoma, metastases, lymphoma, plasmacytoma or a mesothelioma. Benign tumours include hamartoma, fibroma, leiomyoma, lipoma, neurofibroma and chondroma. Granulomas rarely cause such large lesions, but cryptococcoma (torulosis) may occur in the lower lobes, and an aspergilloma (fungus ball or mycetoma) may occupy a chronic lung cavity. Intrapulmonary sequestration may appear as a fluid-filled cyst in the posterobasal segment of the right lower lobe. Large solitary masses may also be caused by hydatid cyst, encysted interlobar pleural effusion and pulmonary infarcts (**Table 6**).

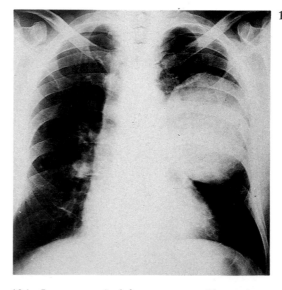

104 Large mass in left upper zone. The patient was asymptomatic and declined any investigations. Postmortem examination revealed a large fibroma.

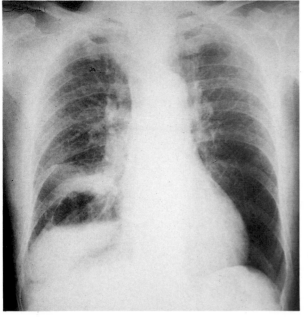

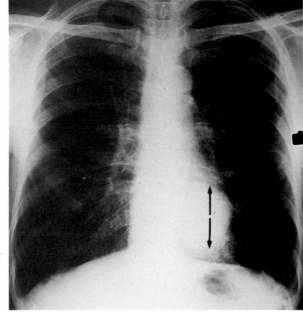

105 **Bleeding into a basal cyst** simulated a large tumour in the right lower lobe. Aspiration biopsy revealed blood and this repeat film demonstrates a fluid level.

106 **Neurolemmoma (neurofibroma).** This penetrated posteroanterior film shows a dense circular retrocardiac opacity. These benign tumours are for the most part clinically silent. Adjacent ribs may be splayed or eroded as the tumour increases in size.

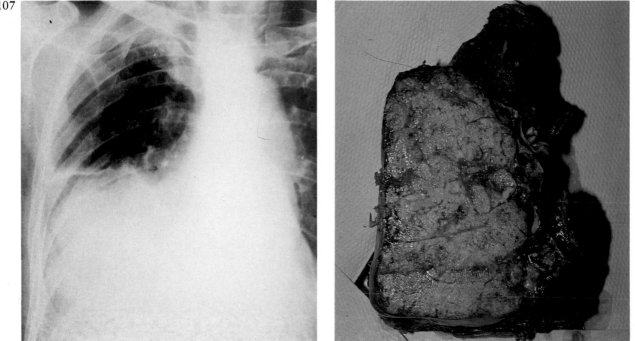

107, 108 **Squamous cell carcinoma infiltrating the right lower lobe.** The necropsy specimen of a whole adult lung shows a tumour invading the whole lower lobe. A mass of this size is unlikely to be benign, but lipomas or neurogenic tumours may attain a massive size.

Table 5. Some causes of solitary pulmonary nodules.

Causes	Confirmation
Bronchial carcinoma	Fibreoptic bronchoscopy
Alveolar cell carcinoma	Transbronchial lung biopsy Aspiration needle biopsy Sputum cytology
Metastasis	Transbronchial lung biopsy Aspiration needle biopsy Search for primary neoplasm
Bronchial adenoma (carcinoid)	Bronchoscopy Aspiration needle biopsy
Granuloma caused by tuberculosis, histoplasmosis or coccidioidomycosis	Endemic zones Calcification in tuberculosis and histoplasmosis but uncommon in coccidioidomycosis Skin tests Serum antibodies
Hydatid cyst (echinococcal)	Endemic zones Lobulated; lower lobe distribution Casoni skin test Complement fixation test Eosinophilia Liver scan for hepatic cysts
Arteriovenous aneurysm	Telangiectasia of lips and nasal mucosa Angiography
Hamartoma	Calcification frequent Aspiration biopsy
Rarities	Parasite, fungus ball, amyloid, gumma, mastocytosis

Table 6. Some causes of multiple pulmonary nodules.

Metastatic malignancy
Lymphoma
Granuloma
– tuberculosis
– sarcoidosis
– Wegener's granulomatosis
– coccidioidomycosis
– histoplasmosis

Rheumatoid nodule
Pneumoconiosis
Hydatid cysts
Pulmonary infarcts
Haematogenous pneumonia
Fluid-filled cysts/bullae

Multiple pulmonary nodules

One or both lungs may contain two or more spherical lesions. The nodules may differ in size, duration, presence of calcium and may have well-circumscribed or ill-defined margins.

109 Secondary deposits from a carcinoma of the colon. Well-demarcated 'cannon ball' shadows are present throughout both lung fields. Metastatic carcinoma is the most common cause. They may also reflect tuberculosis, lymphoma, rheumatoid lung, sarcoidosis, histoplasmosis, coccidioidomycosis, hydatid cysts, Wegener's granulomatosis and septicaemic pneumonia. At least two of the nodules should exceed 1 cm in diameter. Smaller sized multiple nodules are classified as diffuse disseminated miliary or reticulonodular infiltration.

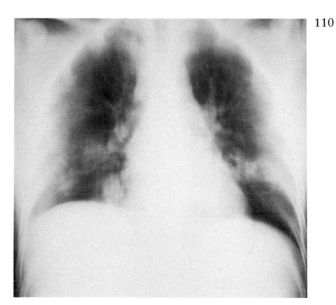

110 Multiple pulmonary nodules with cavitation in Hodgkin's disease.

8 Diffuse interstitial or miliary patterns

Table 7. Some causes of diffuse interstitial shadows.

1 *Infections*

Virus	**Parasite**	**Bacterial**
Influenza	Pneumocystis	Gram-negative bacilli
Varicella	Schistosoma	Staphylococcus
Smallpox	Microfilaria	Legionella
Measles		Psittacosis
Q fever	**Fungal**	
Cytomegalovirus	Histoplasma	**Mycobacteria**
	Coccidioides	– tuberculosis
	Blastomyces (South American)	– atypical
	Candida	
	Cryptococcus	
	Aspergillus	

2 *Pneumoconiosis*

Silicosis	Beryllium	Aluminium (bauxite)
Coal miners'	Talc	Silo fillers'
Asbestosis	Graphite	

3 *Allergic alveolitis*

Farmers' lung	Suberosis	Pituitary snuff
Bagassosis	Detergent	Cheese washer
Air conditioning	Maple bark	Malt worker
Bird fanciers' lung	Sequoia tree	Mushroom worker

4 *Malignancy*

Alveolar cell carcinoma	Leukaemia	
Metastases – haematogenous	Hodgkin's disease	
– lymphatic		

5 *Cardiovascular disease*

Mitral stenosis	Goodpasture's syndrome	Talc emboli
Haemosiderosis		

6 *Fibrosing alveolitis*

Desquamative alveolitis	Neurofibromatosis	**Drugs**
Rheumatoid arthritis	Dermatomyositis	Gold
Systemic lupus	Polymyositis	Nitrofurantoin
Systemic sclerosis		Busulphan
(Scleroderma)		Methotrexate
		Bleomycin

7 *Autoimmune disease*

Sjogren's syndrome	Fibrosing alveolitis	

8 *Miscellaneous*

Sarcoidosis	Thesaurosis	
Histiocytosis X	Alveolar proteinosis	
(eosinophilic granuloma)	Macroglobulinaemia	

Diffuse shadowing may be caused by widespread inflammatory or infiltrative involvement of the alveolar walls, blood vessels, lymphatics, bronchioles and the connective tissue framework.

Bilateral interstitial patterns are often termed reticular, fishnet or honeycomb, or, alternatively, as diffuse miliary or micronodular shadows. The radiographic appearance is composed of a huge number of minute overlapping nodules, each up to 5 mm in diameter. The patterns may vary.

A classification of mixed diffuse miliary or interstitial patterns of disease indicates that widely differing disorders produce confusingly similar radiographic patterns (**Table 7**). This chapter on the radiographic patterns of disease should be read with Chapter 22, where interstitial lung diseases are described in more detail.

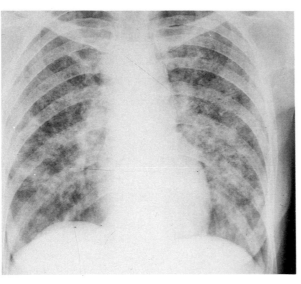

111 Widely disseminated micronodular shadows in miliary tuberculosis. This appearance with well-defined and widely distributed nodular shadows that are 2–5 mm in diameter is typical, but not exclusive, in miliary tuberculosis.

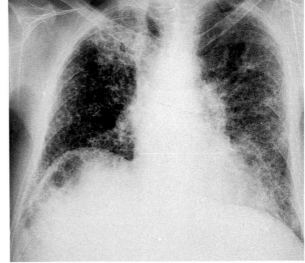

112 Scleroderma lung or honeycomb-like cystic spaces and nodular shadows.

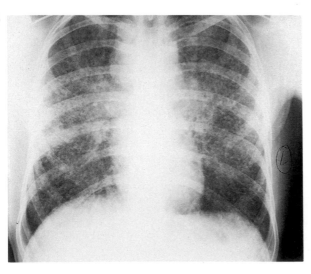

113 Miliary mottling with hilar and right paratracheal lymphadenopathy. The radiological diagnosis was of tuberculosis or sarcoidosis. It was established to be the latter.

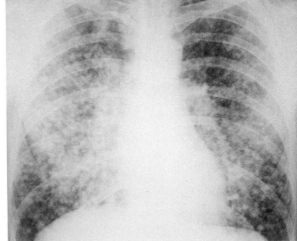

114 Miliary nodular shadows from metastatic adenocarcinoma of the pancreas in a symptom-free man aged 52 years.

Extrapulmonary radiographic shadowing

Confusing radiographic shadows may be produced by soft tissues, clothing or artefacts. There are several possible causes.

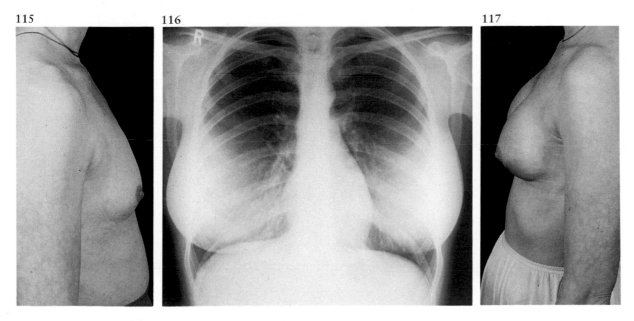

115–117 Breast shadows after cosmetic mammary augmentation. Bilateral opaque silicone-filled prosthetic implants are seen on the x-ray (**116**). **115** and **117** show the presurgical and postsurgical states. The radiographic opacities from such prostheses seldom cause diagnostic confusion, but may obscure lesions in the underlying lung.

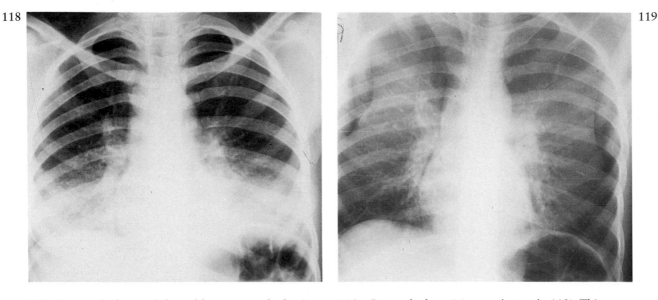

118 Breast shadows – bilateral lower zone shadowing. In adolescent girls the breasts are often relatively radio-opaque, in spite of their small size. The soft tissue radiographic shadow may simulate consolidation or bilateral basal lung fibrosis.

119 Breast shadows (same patient as in 118). This x-ray was taken after the patient had elevated the breasts. The normal lung bases are clearly seen. A lateral radiograph would also localise the breast shadows.

9 Consolidation

Consolidation of the lung occurs when alveolar air has been replaced by fluid, exudate or cells. Airlessness without shrinkage occurs in all types of pneumonia, in pulmonary oedema, when bleeding occurs into the alveoli, or when the alveoli are filled by neoplastic cells. The radiograph shows dense homogeneous opacification occupying the normal position of a lobe or segment. When consolidation occurs in association with atelectasis, the possibility of malignant bronchial obstruction should be considered. The anatomical localisation of consolidation could be established by CT scanning, but in conventional clinical practice a posteroanterior and lateral chest x-ray suffice. Two signs on the latter assist localisation and should be looked for:

1 The silhouette sign. This is based upon the premise that an intrathoracic opacity in anatomical continuity with the border of the heart, aorta or diaphragm will obscure that border.
2 The air bronchogram. Intrapulmonary bronchi are not visible on the normal chest x-ray because they contain air, and their walls are too thin to cast a significant radiographic shadow. Consolidation may allow visualisation of the patent bronchi, which appear as dark branching structures lying within adjacent opaque alveolar air spaces. The presence of an air bronchogram can help localise the abnormality to the lung rather than the pleura. This chapter is illustrated by examples of consolidation in which associated collapse is minimal.

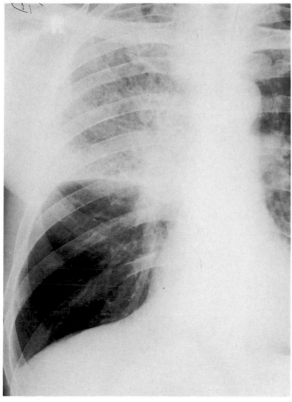

120

120 **Right upper lobe consolidation caused by pneumococcal pneumonia.** Consolidation of the whole right upper lobe is commonly seen in children. The homogeneous shadow extends from the apex downwards, to end in a well-defined inferior margin at the horizontal fissure, which in this example is normally placed.

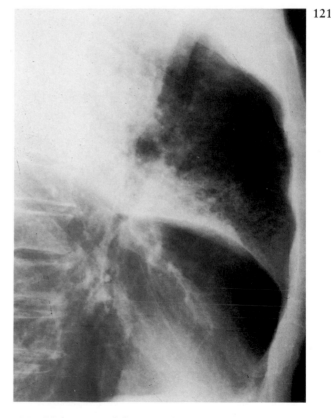

121

121 **Right upper lobe consolidation.** The lateral film shows a well-defined posterior and inferior border corresponding to the oblique and horizontal fissures. Consolidation involves the posterior and anterior segments.

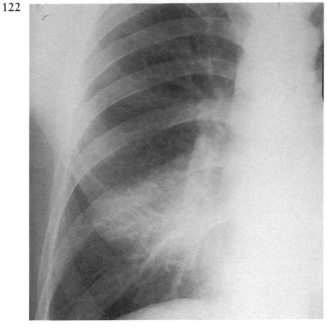

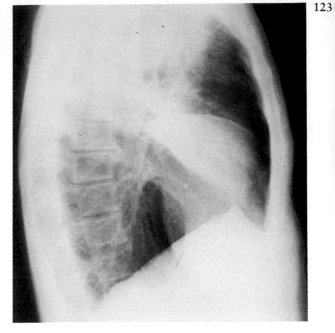

122 **Consolidation in right middle lobe.** The right heart border is indistinct because of the overlying consolidation causing the 'silhouette sign'.

123 **Consolidation in right middle lobe.** The lateral film shows the wedge-shaped area of consolidation overlying the heart, bounded by the horizontal and oblique fissures.

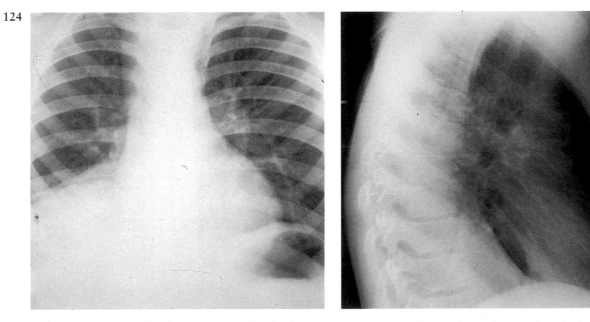

124 **Consolidation of right lower lobe.** The diaphragm and right cardiac border are partially obscured.

125 **Consolidation of right lower lobe.** The lateral film localises the consolidation. There is slight loss of volume.

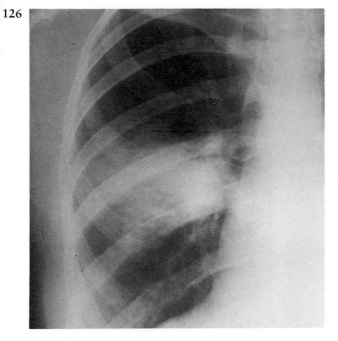

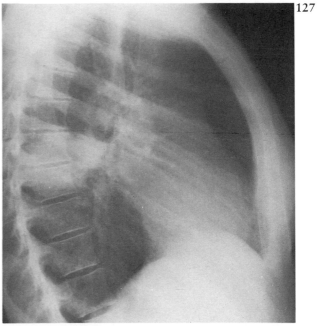

126 Consolidation in apical segment of right lower lobe. The posteroanterior film shows a circumscribed homogeneous area in the right mid-zone which could be caused by involvement of the lateral segment of the right middle lobe or of the apical segment of the right lower lobe.

127 Consolidation in apical segment of right lower lobe. The lateral film localises the consolidation to the apical segment of the right lower lobe.

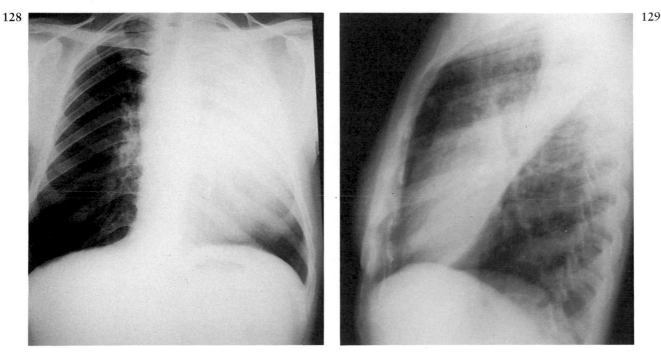

128 Consolidation of left upper lobe, with involvement of the lingula. The posteroanterior film shows a dense homogeneous opacity continuous with the mediastinum and left heart border.

129 Consolidation of the left upper lobe. The lateral film shows a well-defined fissure, with consolidation in the posterior segment of the left upper lobe and lingula.

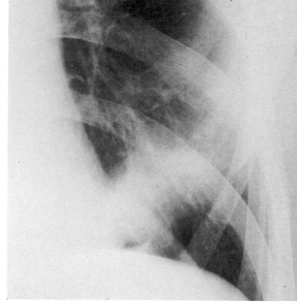

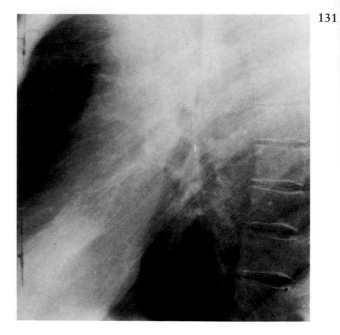

130 Consolidation in lingula. The shadowing lies against the left heart border.

131 Consolidation in lingula. The lateral film localises the consolidation.

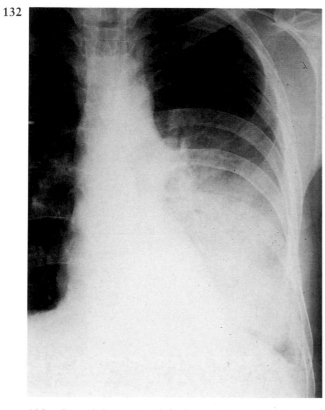

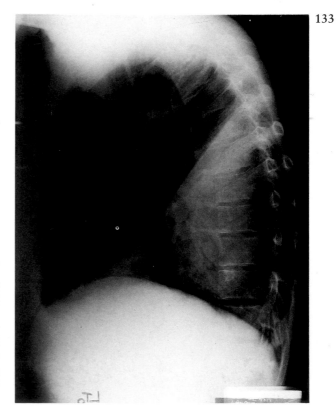

132 Consolidation in left lower lobe. Neither the diaphragm nor the left heart border is obscured by the consolidation (a negative silhouette sign).

133 Consolidation in left lower lobe. This lobar consolidation was due to pneumococcal pneumonia.

10 Collapse or atelectasis

The term 'collapse' is used to indicate loss of volume of the lung, lobe or segment, accompanied by reduced aeration (atelectasis). Collapse may result from fibrosis (contraction collapse), as in tuberculosis or silicosis, and from extrinsic pressure (compression collapse) following a tension pneumothorax. It is most commonly due to intrinsic obstruction caused by tumours or foreign bodies blocking a proximal bronchus, or by extrinsic compression from pathologically enlarged encircling lymph glands.

The collapsed portion of lung may be readily seen on a chest x-ray, but if it is not visible, several secondary radiographic features may indicate loss of lung volume. These include:

1 Shift of the mediastinum
2 Crowding of rib spaces
3 Unilateral diaphragmatic elevation
4 Displacement of the major fissures
5 Displacement of the hilar shadow
6 Crowding of the bronchial markings
7 Displacement of the vascular pattern

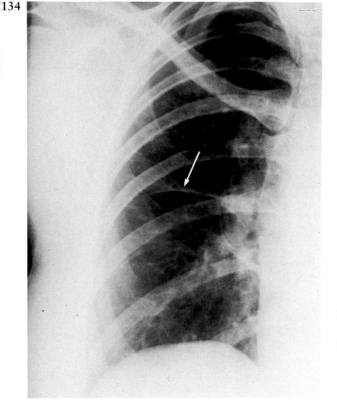

134 Atelectasis of anterior segment of the right upper lobe.

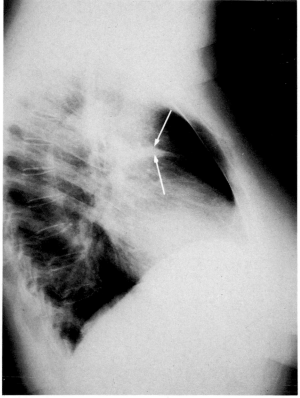

135 Atelectasis of anterior segment of the right upper lobe. Lateral view.

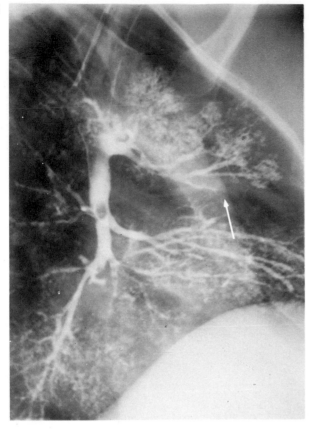

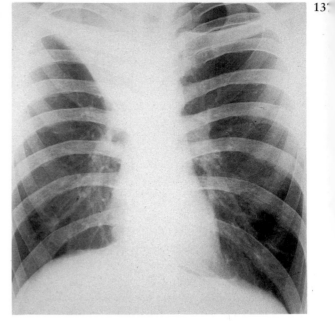

137 Partial collapse of the right upper lobe. The lung re-expanded when a mucus plug was aspirated from the bronchus of this asthmatic patient.

136 Atelectasis of anterior segment of the right upper lobe. The bronchogram shows narrowing of the segmental bronchus caused by fibrosis after pneumonia.

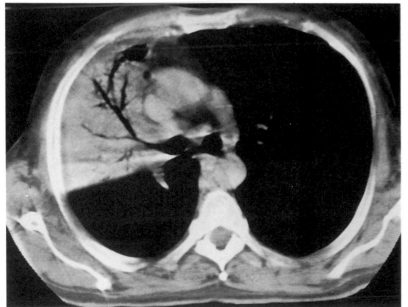

138 Air bronchogram within partial collapse of the right upper lobe. The scan, at carina level, shows narrowing of the right upper lobe bronchus due to a carcinoma. The partially collapsed lobe is sharply demarcated by the oblique fissure posteriorly. The mediastinum has shifted towards the collapsed lobe. Intrapulmonary bronchi are not visible on the normal chest radiograph because they contain air, are surrounded by alveolar air and their thin walls do not cast a significant shadow. Parenchymal consolidation may result in the visualisation of the bronchi which stand out against the opaque lung as dark bands.

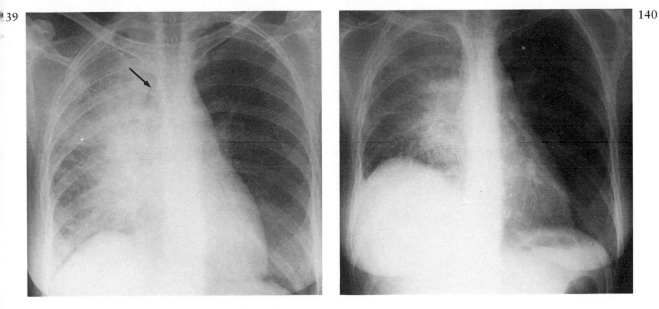

139, 140 Collapse of right upper lobe caused by a proximal small cell carcinoma. Diffuse shadowing and elevation of the right diaphragm are visible, and herniated left lung (arrowed) occupies the clear space anterior to the arch of the aorta (**139**). Five weeks later (**140**) the diaphragm is more elevated and the shadowing less apparent. There is a small right pleural effusion. Both **139** and **140** show right hilar adenopathy.

141 Collapse of right upper lobe. The lateral view shows displacement of the oblique fissure upwards and forwards to cross the thoracic spine at the level of the first thoracic vertebra. A gastric air bubble is present below the left diaphragm (arrowed).

142 Partial collapse of right middle lobe. The horizontal fissure is pulled down.

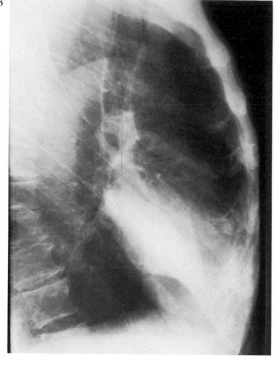

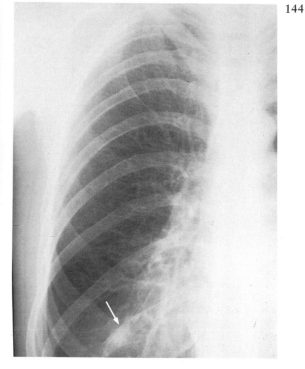

143 Partial collapse of right middle lobe. The lateral view shows a narrow homogeneous shadow lying over the heart shadow.

144 Complete collapse of right middle lobe. The right heart border is blurred. Note the well-defined nipple shadow (arrow).

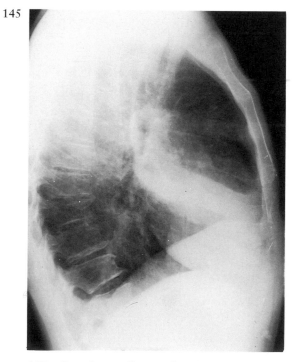

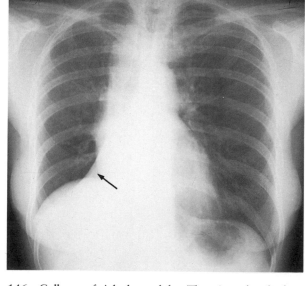

145 Complete collapse of right middle lobe. Lateral view.

146 Collapse of right lower lobe. The triangular shadow at the right cardiophrenic angle continues towards the costophrenic angle. A negative silhouette sign with clear right heart border localises the collapsed lobe.

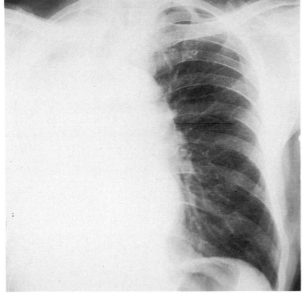 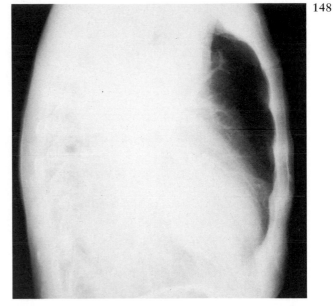

147 Collapse of right lung caused by an obstruction of the main bronchus by an oat-cell carcinoma. The trachea and heart are deviated to the right towards the side of the collapse.

148 Collapse of right lung. Lateral view of **147**. The anterior mediastinal translucency is caused by the over-inflated left lung.

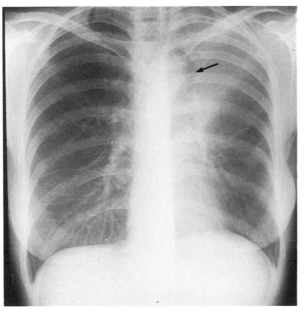 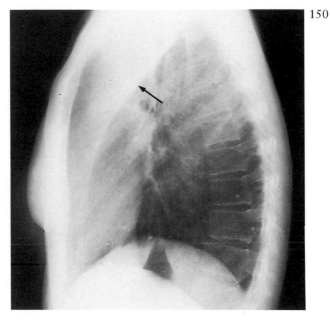

149 Collapse of left upper lobe. Bronchostenosis of the left upper lobe often includes the lingula. This postero-anterior view shows a hazy homogeneous opacity in the left upper zone obliterating the left heart border. The right lung is herniated across the midline (arrowed).

150 Collapse of left upper lobe. This lateral film shows upwards and forwards displacement of the interlobar fissure (arrowed).

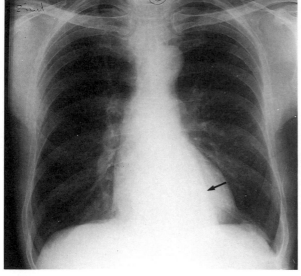

151 Collapse of left lower lobe seen as a dense shadow behind the heart, with a well-defined left margin sloping downwards and outwards. The left hilum is displaced downwards.

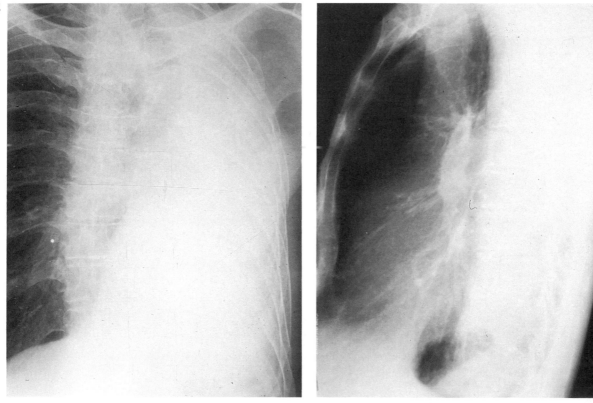

152 Complete collapse of left lung. The mediastinum and trachea are markedly deviated to the left, and the diaphragm is obscured.

153 Complete collapse of left lung. The lateral view shows a large radiolucent area anterior to the heart, as a result of compensatory expansion to the left of the aerated right lung. The left diaphragm is elevated and the collapsed lung lies posteriorly.

11 Hypertransradiancy

The normal radiographic appearance of the lung is a composite shadow picture comprising pulmonary vessels and soft tissue shadows of the body wall muscle and ribs. Bilateral hypertransradiancy (hypertranslucency) is difficult to see, but a local loss of lung density may be detected by comparison with other areas of normal lung. Comparisons can also be made between equivalent matching areas in both lungs.

Table 8. Some causes of radiographic hypertransradiancy.

Hypertransradiancy	Possible causes
Extrathoracic (usually unilateral)	Absent female breast Absent pectoral muscle Severe scoliosis Increased density of other side Rotation of body
Intrathoracic Extrapulmonary	Pneumothorax Diaphragmatic hernia
Intrathoracic Intrapulmonary (unilateral)	Obstructive emphysema (foreign body, neoplasm) MacLeod's syndrome (see page 70) Bronchogenic cyst or bulla Post lobectomy
Intrathoracic Intrapulmonary (bilateral)	Simple emphysema Cystic bronchiectasis

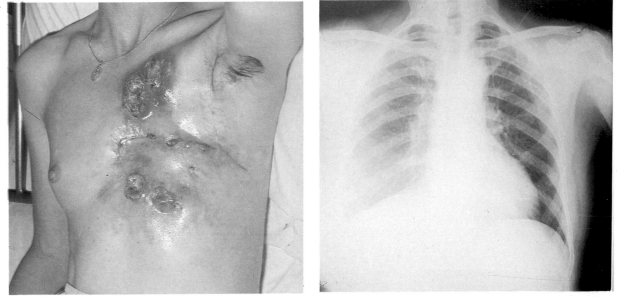

154, 155 Mastectomy with recurrent local tumour (154). An example of a chest wall abnormality causing radiographic hypertransradiancy of the lung field. The x-ray (155) taken 3 years previously shows the difference in radiodensity produced by the loss of soft tissue between the right and left lower lung fields.

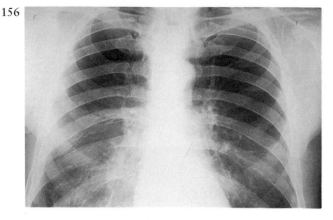

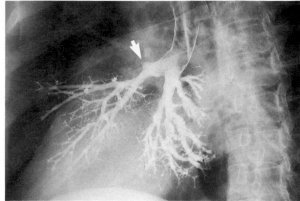

156 Early obstructive emphysema of the left upper lobe. A comparison of both upper zones shows fewer vessels on the left.

157 Bronchogram of 156 – lateral oblique view. Filling of the left lower lobe and lingula is normal, but a carcinoma is causing obstruction at the origin of the left upper lobe bronchus. A ball valve mechanism allows air to enter on inspiration, but it is retained during expiration. Collapse of the lobe usually follows.

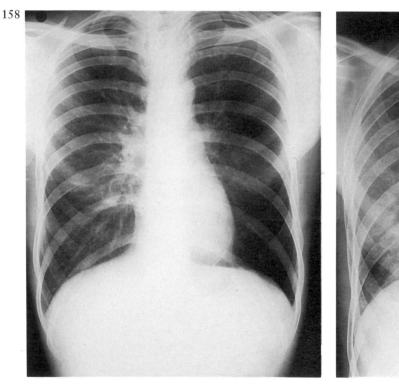

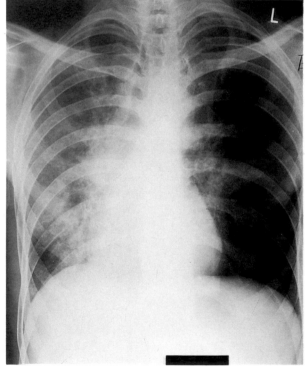

158 Macleod's syndrome – inspiratory film. The left lung is hypertransradiant because the pulmonary artery and peripheral vessels are hypoplastic. The underlying abnormality is due to bronchiolitis in infancy, resulting in airway obstruction and poor function in the affected lung.

The bronchi are normal to the respiratory bronchioles, but there is a diminished number of alveoli, suggesting alveolar injury before 8 years of age; the total adult number of alveoli develop at about this age.

159 Macleod's syndrome – expiratory film. The mediastinal structures are deviated to the right as a consequence of air trapping in the left lung.

Lung damage probably occurs during childhood respiratory infections, especially in measles or whooping cough. The hypoplastic lung is most damaged, but necropsy may show patchy fibrosis in the radiographically normal lung.

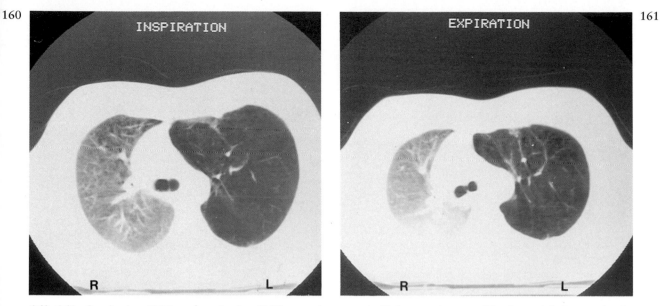

160, 161 Inspiration (160) and expiration (161) scans in congenital lobar emphysema. The degree of air trapping in the affected left upper lobe is clearly demonstrated in the expiration film, in contrast to the increased density and decreased size of the normal right upper lobe.

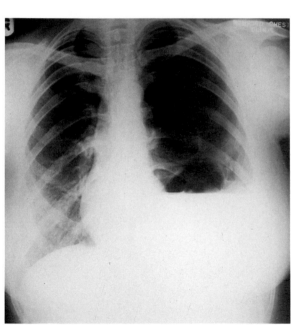

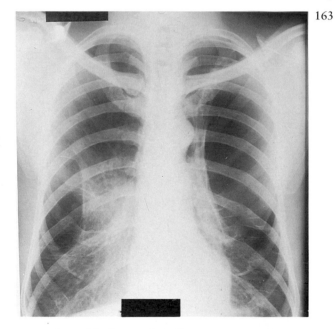

162 Fluid level in huge bulla which was mistaken for a tension hydro-pneumothorax because of the mediastinal shift to the right.

163 Bilateral bullae. Both bullae were removed giving significant improvement in lung function. Note the considerable hyperinflation, with a low, flat diaphragm.

Radiographic features of widespread emphysema

The radiograph correlates poorly with functional changes in moderate emphysema and even severe structural changes may not produce significant radiographic abnormalities.

The following features are typical of severe panlobular (panacinar) emphysema.

Hyperinflation
- Low diaphragms. The right diaphragm lies below the anterior end of the sixth rib.
- Flat diaphragm (see **165**).
- Visible phrenocostal muscle attachments.
- Deep posteroanterior diameter on lateral chest x-ray.
- Increased retrosternal transradiancy on lateral chest x-ray.
- Bullae or hypertransradiant bullous areas.

Cardiovascular changes
- Peripheral lung vessels diminished in size and number.
- Prominent hilar vessels.
- Narrow vertical heart.

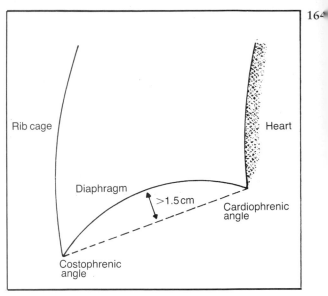

164 Measuring the diaphragm curve. The costophrenic and cardiophrenic angles are joined by a line drawn between them. A vertical line drawn from this to the highest point on the curve of the diaphragm is normally in excess of 1.5 cm.

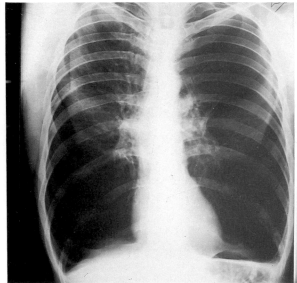

165 Hypertransradiant lung caused by severe emphysema. The diaphragm is low and flat and the prominent right upper zone 'marker vessels' contrast with the few narrowed vessels elsewhere.

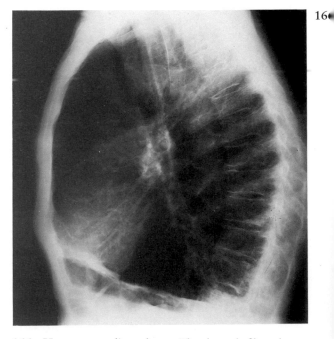

166 Hypertransradiant lung. The lateral film shows large anterior translucency with deep posteroanterior measurements (same patient as in **165**).

12 Calcification

Dense radiographic opacities are commonly caused by calcification. The size, shape, position and relationship to adjacent structures may point to the cause of the calcium deposits.

Identification of calcium in a solitary pulmonary nodule is of great importance in management and diagnosis (see page 49). Central calcification is a fairly reliable sign that the lesion is benign; usually arising from healed fungal or tuberculous infections. Calcification at the periphery usually indicates a benign lesion, but rarely may represent a pre-existing healed granuloma engulfed by a neoplasm arising in a lung scar.

Peripheral 'egg shell' calcification of lymph nodes is a feature of sarcoidosis, silicosis and treated lymphoma.

Calcification in multiple pulmonary nodules is also commonly caused by healed fungal or tuberculous infections. Rarely, multiple pulmonary metastases from osteosarcoma, thyroid, ovary, testis or breast may calcify.

Unilateral pleural calcification occurs as linear or oval plaques predominantly on the diaphragmatic or lateral chest wall visceral pleura. Haemothorax, empyema or tuberculosis are common causes.

Bilateral pleural calcified plaques on the parietal pleura, especially involving the diaphragm, may signify asbestosis or other pneumoconioses (talc, bakelite, mica). Damaged heart valves and athero-sclerotic blood vessels may calcify, as may hilar lymph nodes and the lung parenchyma.

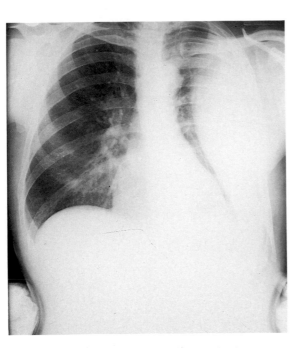

167 Pleural calcification. Old calcified artificial pneumothorax. A dense homogeneous shadow occupies most of the left lung field. This rare occurrence sometimes followed intrathoracic bleeding induced by repeated artificial pneumothoraces.

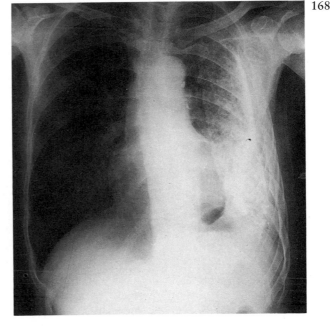

168 Pleural calcification caused by an old tuberculous pleural effusion. The left lung is shrunken and encased by thickened calcified pleura.

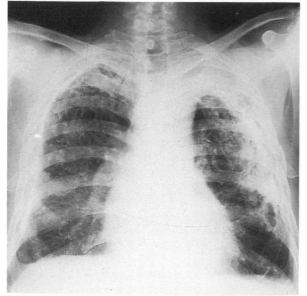

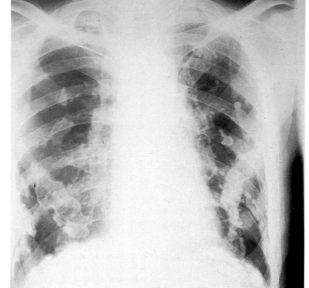

169 Bilateral pleural calcification after tuberculosis.
There was no history of occupational exposure to asbestos.
Note that the calcium is deposited near the inner surface
of the greatly thickened pleura. This results in a clear
linear radiolucent space between the calcification and the
bony thorax on tangential projection.

170 Extensive parietal pleural calcification from asbestos
exposure in a shipbuilding worker. Bilateral diaphragmatic
calcification is extensive and characteristic. It may herald
a subsequent mesothelioma.

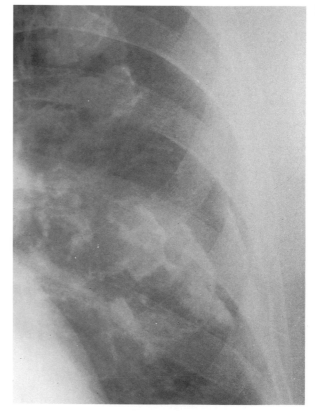

171 Calcification of the diaphragmatic pleura, caused
by asbestos exposure.

172 Irregular pleural shadowing provides a 'holly leaf'
appearance that is typical of asbestos exposure. The calcification occurs on the parietal pleura.

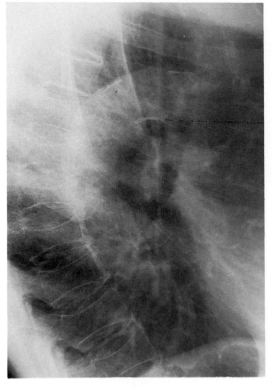

173 **Calcified aortic arch** is commonplace with ageing.

174 Calcified aortic arch.

175 **Bilateral hilar calcification** due to sarcoidosis. This patient suffered from chronic sarcoidosis with persistent hypercalciuria. Calcified hilar lymph nodes are frequently caused by tuberculosis, but may also occur in silicosis and chronic sarcoidosis.

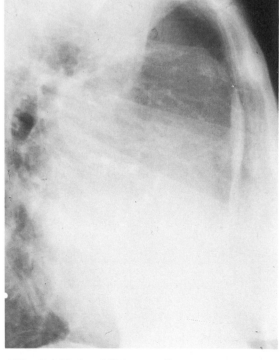

176 Calcified syphilitic ascending aorta.

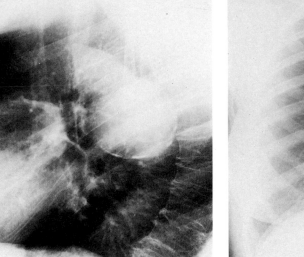

177 Calcification in a traumatic aortic aneurysm which resulted from a road traffic accident.

178 Healed tuberculosis 'primary complex' (Ghon focus). There is a dense localised area of calcification in the left mid-zone and in the draining left hilar lymph node.

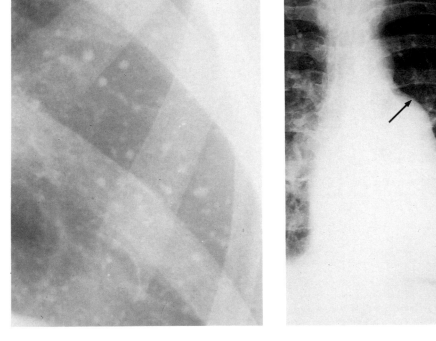

179 Discrete dense shadows about 2 mm in size may follow haemorrhagic chickenpox pneumonia, particularly in the adult. The dense calcification usually appears within 2 years of acute severe adult infection. Similar (1–2 mm) circular calcified shadows may follow histoplasmosis.

180 Dense uniform opacities caused by ectopic bone formation may occur in mitral stenosis or, rarely, after acute rheumatic fever without valve disease. Note the characteristic appearance of the cardiac silhouette which accompanies severe mitral stenosis. The left atrium and left atrial appendage (arrowed) are enlarged.

13 Tube, band and line shadows

These common radiographic shadows are all essentially linear, varying in width from barely discernible lines of 1–2 mm to well-defined bands of 1–2 cm.

Tubular shadows are evident when a couple of line shadows are closely parallel. The diagnostic challenge constantly facing the physician is whether these shadows reflect diseases or normal structures and artefacts.

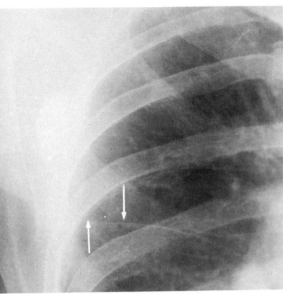

181 The horizontal fissure may appear as a line shadow on a posteroanterior x-ray.

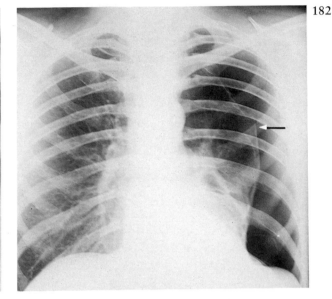

182 A fine linear shadow of visceral pleura marks the lung edge of a pneumothorax.

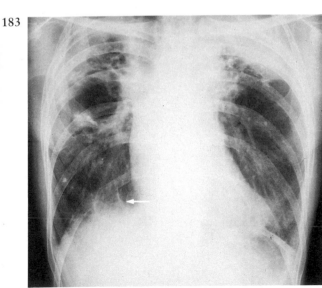

183 A vertical line shadow extending upwards from the diaphragm is due to indrawn visceral pleura.

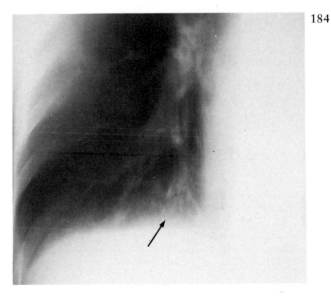

184 Tubular 'tram line' shadows caused by localised lower lobe bronchiectasis. The bronchial walls are thickened and dilated.

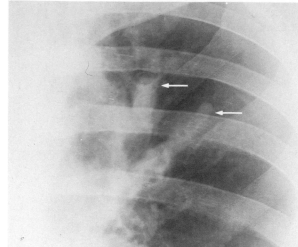

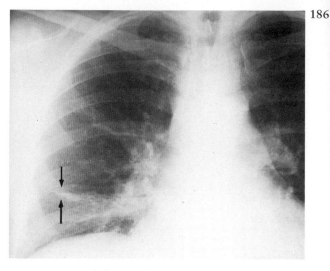

185 Band-like and tubular shadows. Two dilated upper lobe bronchi are filled with secretions, producing a V-shaped band shadow. Tubular or ring shadows of air-filled, dilated, thick-walled bronchi are seen adjacent to the hilum. The diagnosis was allergic bronchopulmonary aspergillosis.

186 Horizontal linear shadows (discoid atelectasis). These shadows represent atelectasis caused by obstruction of the medium-sized bronchi, developing when diaphragmatic movement is limited by postoperative pain, pleurisy, rib fracture and pulmonary embolism.

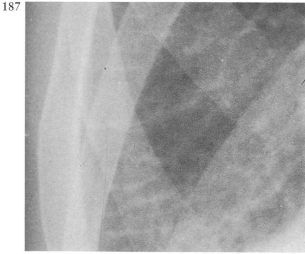

187 Kerley 'B' septal line shadows at the right lung base in a patient with left ventricular failure. The fine transverse lines represent oedema and thickening in the interlobular septa and appear as horizontal lines 1–3 cm in length and 1–2 mm in width, located perpendicular to a pleural surface. These transient lines are caused by raised pulmonary venous pressure. They may persist if the lymphatic channels are obstructed by tumour, choked by dust particles in pneumoconiosis, or thickened by fibrosing alveolitis.

188 Kerley 'A' lines reflect thickened intercommunicating lymphatics and appear as thin, non-branching lines extending out from the hilum. These persistent 'A' lines were caused by lymphangitis carcinomatosa. Transient 'A' lines may be seen when left ventricular failure develops rapidly or in pulmonary oedema caused by drug hypersensitivity.

14 Apical lesions

It is often difficult to disentangle the apex because of the overlying first and second ribs and clavicle, so tomography, lordotic views and CT scanning are invaluable in identifying normal structures, artefacts and disease. MRI provides better contrast resolution and is superior to CT scans in detecting tumour involvement of the brachial plexus or displaying the soft tissues of the chest wall.

Apical lesions lie within the circle of the first rib; subapical lesions lie between the circle of the first and second ribs.

Table 9. Some causes of radiographic apical shadowing.

Normal structure and artefacts	Apical and subapical lesions
Azygos lobe (right)	Pleural cap fibrosis
Cervical rib	Pancoast superior sulcus tumour
Sternomastoid muscle	Tuberculosis
Lock of hair	Mycoses
Clothing	Aspergillosis
Retrosternal thyroid	Mycetoma
Subclavian artery	Neurofibroma
	Ankylosing spondylitis
	Irradiation fibrosis
	Alveolar cell carcinoma
	Metastases
	Cysts, blebs, bullae

189

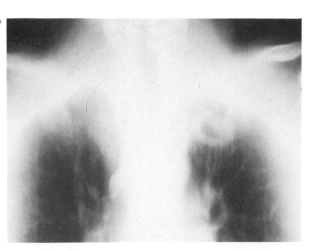

189 Tomogram of lungs, revealing an apical cavity caused by tuberculosis.

190

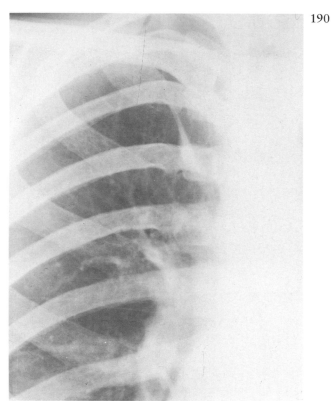

190 **Accessory lobe of azygos vein.** The hairline shadow extends from the apical pleura to a comma-like expansion near the hilum. The line shadow represents a double layer of visceral parietal pleura, which encloses the abnormally placed azygos vein.

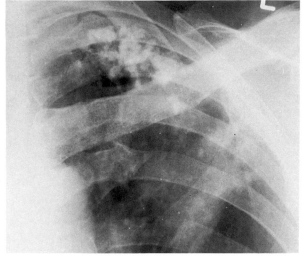

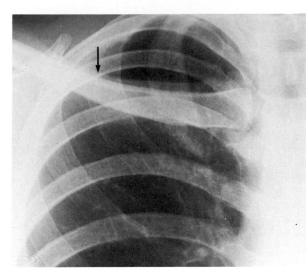

191 Bilateral apical and subapical calcification from healed pulmonary tuberculosis.

192 Companion shadows above the clavicle. A 2–3 mm wide companion shadow is often seen running parallel to the upper border of the clavicle. This shadow is lost if the supraclavicular lymph nodes are enlarged. It is caused by the fold of skin and subcutaneous tissue lying horizontally above the bone, which represents a considerable thickness of tissue to the x-ray beam.

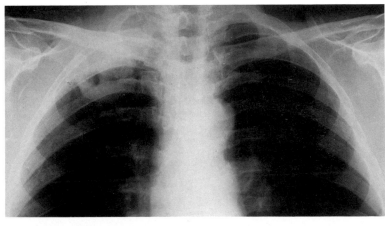

193 Pancoast tumour. Cavitating apical lesion with lysis of part of the first and second ribs due to a peripheral squamous cell carcinoma.

194 Left apical cavity with aspergilloma. A translucent halo surrounds a dense circular opacity.

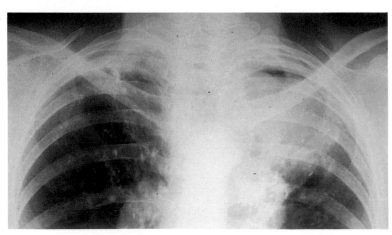

15 Pneumonia, lung abscess and empyema

After cardiovascular disease and malignant neoplasms, respiratory infection is the next most common cause of death. Mortality at the extremes of age is particularly high.

In temperate climates pneumonia is more common in the winter months, whereas in the tropics the peak is at the end of the dry season. Acute respiratory tract infections account for 57 deaths per 100,000 population in well-developed countries, compared with 76 per 100,000 population in less well-developed areas.

Pneumonia may be defined as inflammation in the lung parenchyma. Consolidation results in the alveolar air being replaced by a watery inflammatory exudate. Pneumonia may be classified as:

1 *Lobar pneumonia.* Areas of uniform consolidation present in lobules and lobes.
2 *Bronchopneumonia.* Inflammation of the terminal and respiratory bronchioles leads to airway damage, followed by spread of the inflammation into the surrounding alveoli.

The traditional classification of pneumonia into lobar, lobular and bronchopneumonia is of little help to the clinician in determining aetiology, guiding therapy or assessing prognosis. A clinical classification based upon the history, physical examination, chest radiograph, total and differential white blood cell count, immediate Gram stain of sputum and simple biochemistry usually suffices (**Table 10**). The seasonal variation in the frequency of some infections should also be considered (**196**). Blood cultures should be taken in all but the mildest cases, and arterial blood gas analysis should be per-

Table 10. Clinical classification of pneumonia.

Community acquired pneumonia
Hospital acquired (nosocomial) pneumonia
Aspiration and anaerobic pneumonia
Pneumonia in the immunocompromised
AIDS related pneumonia
Recurrent pneumonia

formed. Clinical and laboratory features associated with severe pneumonia and a poor prognosis are summarised in **Table 11**. A classification of pneumonia is given in **195** and **Table 12**.

In most cases, the initial therapeutic decision will be correct and the patient will show signs of substantial recovery in 48–72 hours. Further measures may be necessary in those patients who have not improved. Sputum cultures often yield upper airway flora, rather than the causative organism. Purer cultures may be sought by performing direct lung or transtracheal puncture or by obtaining lung washings through a sterile catheter during fibreoptic bronchoscopy.

Other possible infective agents disregarded at presentation should be looked for at this stage (**Table 12**). Acute serological studies for viral, mycoplasma, rickettsial or legionella infections may be useful. In the immunocompromised patient, coliforms, *Pneumocystis, Pseudomonas aeruginosa, M. tuberculosis* or pathogenic fungi may be present.

Finally, structural factors which may delay resolution, such as bronchial blockage by carcinoma or non-infective causes, should be considered.

Table 11. Features associated with severe pneumonia.

Clinical features	*Laboratory features*
Age more than 60 years	Hypoxaemia $pO_2 \leqslant 8\,kPa$ (60 mmHg)
Underlying disease	Leucopenia WBC $\leqslant 4000 \times 10^9/l$
Confusion	Leucocytosis WBC $\geqslant 20,000 \times 10^9/l$
Respiratory rate $\geqslant 30$/minute	Raised serum urea $\geqslant 7\,mmol/l$
Diastolic blood pressure $\leqslant 60\,mgHg$	Hypoalbuminaemia
Atrial fibrillation	Bacteraemia
Multilobar involvement	

Table 12. Respiratory infections.

Family	Pathogenic organism / Member	Isolation from	Blood test	Treatment	Remarks
Gram-positive cocci	Streptococcus – pneumoniae	Sputum Blood	Leucocytosis Specific poly-saccharide in blood and body fluids	Benzylpenicillin G or amoxycillin or a cephalosporin or erythromycin	Consider polyvalent pneumococcal vaccine for the immunosuppressed, the elderly and bronchitics
	– pyogenes	Sputum Blood		Benzylpenicillin G or amoxycillin or a cephalosporin or erythromycin	Usually found complicating influenza and other virus infections
	Staphylococcus aureus	Sputum Blood	Leucocytosis	Benzylpenicillin G or flucloxacillin or a cephalosporin or erythromycin	Complicating virus infections, cystic fibrosis, immunodeficient infants
Gram-negative bacilli	Klebsiella pneumoniae (Friedlander)	Sputum Blood		Cefoxitin Clarithromycin	Necrotising upper lobe pneumonia with redcurrent jelly sputum, pleurisy and abscesses particularly in the immunodeficient and alcoholic
	Haemophilus – influenzae	Sputum Blood Cerebrospinal fluid Pleural fluid	Anti-type B antibodies	Amoxycillin ± chloramphenicol	Epiglottitis necessitates tracheostomy
	Bordetella pertussis	Pernasal swab Cough plate	Leucocytosis Lymphocytosis	Erythromycin or chloramphenicol	Consider hyperimmune human gamma globulin in the unimmunised
	Pasteurella – tularensis	Sputum Blood Body fluids	Serum agglutinins	Streptomycin ± tetracycline	X-ray shows oval lesions with hilar adenopathy and pleurisy
	Bacteroides fragilis and fusobacteria	Sputum Pleural fluid Transtracheal aspiration Bronchoscopy Blood		Metronidazole or cefoxitin Ciprofloxacin	Pulmonary necrosis, foul-smelling sputum associated empyema. May be aspirated from peritonsillar abscess
Mycobacteria	– tuberculosis	Sputum		Rifampicin Isoniazid Ethambutol Streptomycin Pyrazinamide	Particularly in the immunodeficient elderly and certain ethnic groups
	– atypical	Sputum		Rifampicin Isoniazid Ethambutol Streptomycin Pyrazinamide	Usually white males over 45 years old with pre-existing chronic pulmonary disease or AIDS
Miscellaneous	Mycoplasma pneumoniae	Sputum Throat washings	Normal leucocyte count Cold agglutinins Mycoplasma CFT	Tetracycline or erythromycin	Usually accompanies myringitis with bulla on tympanic membrane
	Legionella pneumophila	Lung, sputum Pleural exudate Sputum Transtracheal aspirate	Normal leucocyte count Serum fluorescent antibodies	Rifampicin or erythromycin Ciprofloxacin	More frequent in male town-dwellers
	Chlamydia psittaci	Sputum Blood	Psittacosis CFT Normal leucocyte count	Tetracycline Ciprofloxacin	Contracted from birds. A penicillin-resistant pneumonia
	Pneumocystis carinii	Sputum Transbronchial or open lung biopsy	± leucocytosis ± eosinophilia Oxygen desaturation	Co-trimoxazole	Particularly in AIDS and immunosuppressed patients recipients of transplants
	Coxiella burneti	Special laboratories only	Complement-fixing and agglutinating antibodies	Tetracycline or chloramphenicol	Penicillin-resistant pneumonia. Contracted from sheep and cattle

Table 12. Respiratory infections continued.

Pathogenic organism					
Family	*Member*	*Isolation from*	*Blood test*	*Treatment*	*Remarks*
Actinomycetes	A-Israeli	Pus, sinus or empyema track		Benzylpenicillin G	Pneumonia with empyema and sinus
	Nocardia	Sputum, pus, bronchoscopy, sinus		Sulphonamide + streptomycin	Particularly in the immunodeficient, including alveolar proteinosis
Virus	Influenza	Sputum Throat washings	Serum antibodies	Oxygen therapy Antibiotics to control secondary bacterial pneumonia	Complicated by secondary bacterial bronchopneumonia

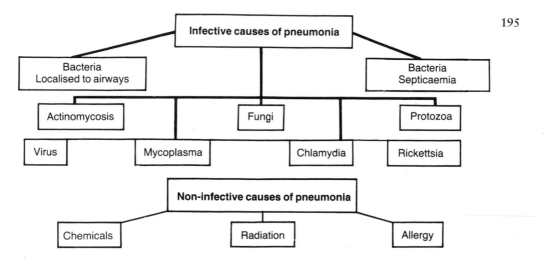

195

195   Aetiology of pneumonia.

Community acquired pneumonia

Primary pneumonia acquired in the community may occur at random or secondary to either a predisposing factor in the host, e.g. pre-existing chronic lung disease (COPD) or diabetes, or to environmental factors, e.g. an influenza epidemic. In the United Kingdom the incidence of respiratory infections and pneumonia rises dramatically during the first three months of the year (**196**).

Pneumococcal infection is by far the most common cause of community acquired pneumonia. Other bacterial pathogens include *Haemophilus influenzae* *Legionella*, *Staphylococcus aureus* and atypical infections, particularly with *Mycoplasma pneumoniae*. Viral chest infections are implicated in 10–20% of cases and are usually complicated by secondary bacterial infections.

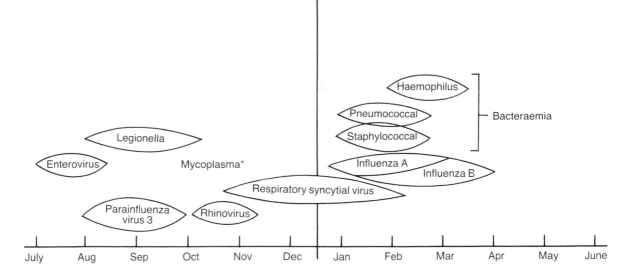

196 Seasonal patterns of various respiratory pathogens. *Mycoplasma epidemics also occur every 3–4 years. (Adapted from Macfarlane JT, *BJDC*, with permission.)

Pneumococcal pneumonia

The pneumococcus was first recognised by Pasteur in 1880 when he recovered it from sputum. The polysaccharide capsule is the main determinant of pathogenicity. At least 84 serotypes of pneumococci are recognised, based on the specific antigenic com-position of the pneumococcal polysaccharide capsule. Pneumococcal vaccine has been available for several years and in 1983 was changed to a 23 valent type covering the most common pneumococcal serotypes that cause disease.

Clinical features of pneumococcal pneumonia
S. pneumoniae is a common cause of lobar con-solidation, especially in previously healthy adult males. The onset of illness is abrupt over a few hours with rigors, high fever, malaise, tachycardia and tachypnoea, and a cough that is dry or pro-ductive of sticky pink sputum. Focal signs are heard in the chest, crackles being much more common than bronchial breathing. Herpetic cold sores are seen in over one-third of cases.

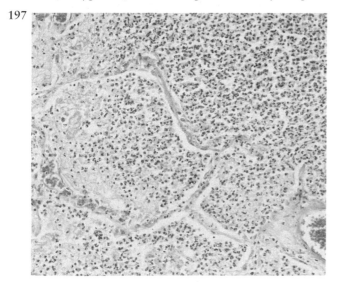

197 Pneumococcal pneumonia. The alveoli are con-solidated by polymorphonuclear leucocytes, fibrin and red cells. The capillaries are dilated at this early stage of inflammation (red hepatisation). (H & E × 140.)

Table 13. Physical respiratory signs of pneumonia.

Early physical signs
    Diminished expansion
    Impaired percussion note
    Diminished normal breath sounds
    Crackles

Physical signs after 24–36 hours
    Diminished expansion
    Dull percussion note
    High pitched bronchial breathing
    Increased tactile vocal fremitus and whispering
       pectoriliquy
    Widespread crackles
    A pleural rub may be present

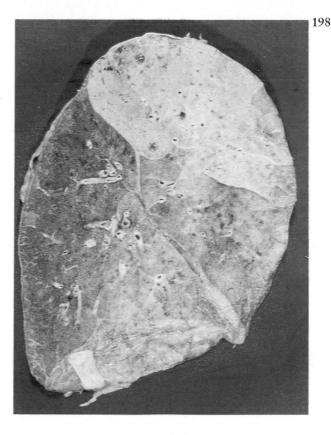

198

198 Pneumococcal pneumonia. Macroscopic section of whole lung showing uniform pale consolidation of the upper lobe. At this stage of grey hepatisation, the lobe is firm, the alveolar capillaries are inconspicuous and the pulmonary arterioles may become thrombosed. The alveoli are filled with fibrin and polymorphonuclear leucocytes.

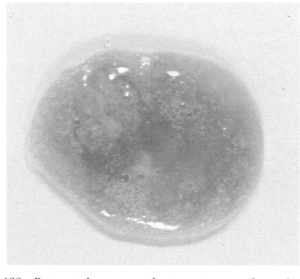

199

199 Rusty red mucopurulent sputum specimen in pneumococcal pneumonia. Sputum may be initially scanty or absent, later becoming purulent.

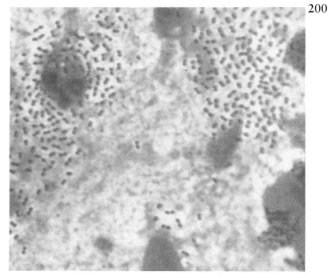

200

200 Gram-positive, lancet-shaped diplococci in association with polymorphonuclear leucocytes in sputum specimen. (Gram stain×1000.)

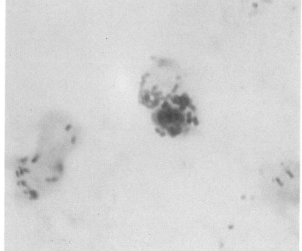

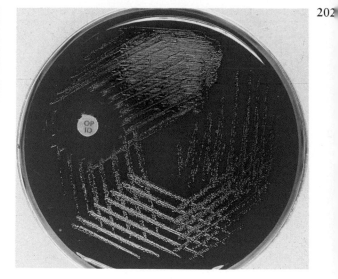

201 Cerebrospinal fluid containing *S. pneumoniae* and pus cells in purulent pneumococcal meningitis. Bacteraemia is evident in about one-quarter of patients with bacterial pneumonia. Ideally, blood cultures should be part of the investigative routine. (Gram stain×1000.)

202 Culture of pneumococci on blood agar medium. Typical colonies are flat with raised margins, sometimes likened to 'draughtsmen'. The colonies are surrounded by a zone of green discoloration or alpha haemolysis caused by destruction of the red blood cells in the culture medium. The growth of *S. pneumoniae* is inhibited by optochin (ethyl hydriecuprein hydrochloride) which assists bacteriological confirmation (optochin disc = OP10).

203

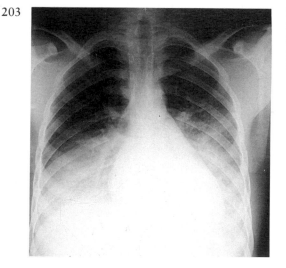

203 Bilateral lower lobe consolidation in an auto-splenectomised sickle-cell disease patient. Lobar consolidation frequently develops in pneumococcal pneumonia, although this extensive consolidation is unusual.

Treatment of pneumococcal pneumonia

The vast majority of pneumococci are exquisitely sensitive to penicillin, with minimum inhibitory concentrations (MICs) of 0.02 mg/ml or less. The response of patients with pneumococcal lobar pneumonia to benzylpenicillin is often dramatic, with a fall in temperature to normal within 24 hours. There have been occasional isolates of pneumococci from Australia, New Guinea, England and North America that have reduced sensitivity to penicillin with MICs of 0.1–2 mg/ml, and isolates of multiple resistant strains from South Africa. Cephalosporins and erythromycin are effective alternatives in penicillin-sensitive patients. All pneumococci are resistant to aminoglyclosides and a proportion are resistant to tetracyclines.

Staphylococcal pneumonia

Staphylococci cause less than 5% of all bacterial pneumonias, but the disease is especially important because of its high mortality rate. The onset can be dramatic. The chest x-ray shows patchy infiltrates and cavitation. Pneumothorax and empyema are common complications. Staphylococcal pneumonia may follow viral respiratory infections, especially influenza, or occur in the debilitated or immuno-suppressed.

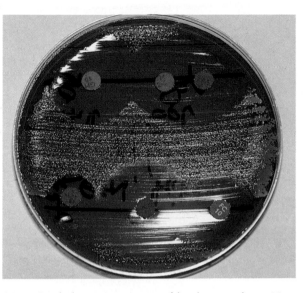

204 *Staphylococcus aureus* on blood agar culture. Note the inhibition of bacterial growth adjacent to the antibiotic impregnated discs.

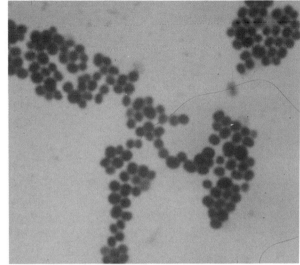

205 *Staphylococcus aureus.* Gram-positive organisms present on blood culture.

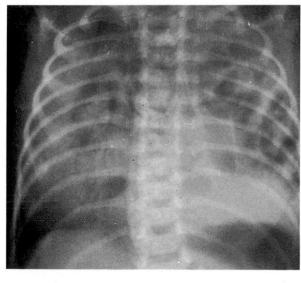

206 **Primary staphylococcal pneumonia** is more often seen in infants. Multiple pneumatoceles present on the chest radiograph. Pneumothorax or pyopneumothorax results from rupture of a pneumatocele.

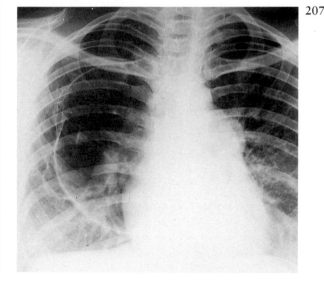

207 **Large right lung pneumatocele** after staphylococcal pneumonia. The large heart and pulmonary arteries are due to pulmonary hypertension which developed after repeated chest infections. A primary neutrophil disorder predisposed to infection. Pneumatoceles appear on the radiograph as air-filled, thin-walled cysts that change in size and appearance from day to day. Healing leads to radiographic resolution within a couple of weeks although, rarely, a stationary bulla-like shadow may remain.

Haemophilus influenzae

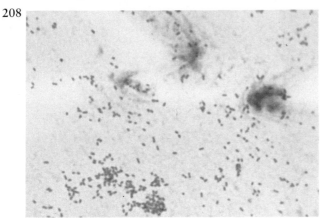

An occasional cause of pneumonia in adults. Infection occurs by aspiration of organisms from the upper respiratory tract or by inhalation of infected droplets from a carrier. A confident diagnosis requires isolation of the organisms from blood, pleural fluid or tracheal aspirates. Sputum culture can be misleading since the organisms are often present in the pharynx.

208 *Haemophilus influenzae.* Small Gram-negative bacilli present in sputum.

Atypical pneumonia

The term 'atypical pneumonia' is used to describe community acquired pneumonias that do respond to erythromycin and tetracycline but not to penicillin. It includes infection by *Mycoplasma pneumoniae*, *Coxiella burneti* (Q fever), *Chlamydia psittaci* (psittacosis), and a newly recognised *C. pneumoniae*, responsible for pneumonia, bronchitis, pharyngitis, sinusitis and otitis media. It is referred to as the TWAR (Taiwan acute respiratory) species because it was first isolated in Taiwan.

Mycoplasma pneumoniae

Mycoplasma pneumoniae infections are endemic worldwide and responsible for localised outbreaks of pneumonia, tracheobronchitis, pharyngitis or myringitis. *M. pneumoniae* produces illnesses ranging from mild upper respiratory infections to severe pneumonia which occasionally can be fatal.

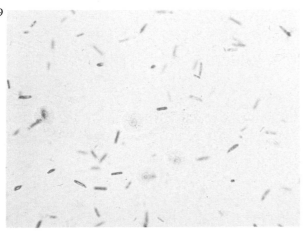

209 *M. pneumoniae* **culture on agar.** Mycoplasma may be isolated from sputum that does not appear purulent as in bacterial pneumonia. The organism grows on blood agar. It is the smallest free-living organism and does not have a rigid cell wall, relying on a three-layered membrane. It is indifferent to antibiotics that affect cell wall synthesis but generally sensitive to tetracycline and erythromycin, antibiotics that inhibit protein synthesis.

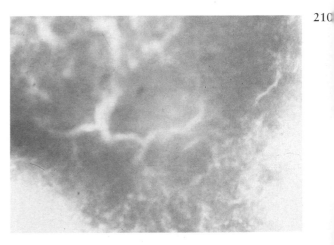

210 *M. pneumoniae* **colony** shown on a glass cover-slip imprint of blood agar culture. The single amorphous 'cotton wool' colony stains pink with Gram's stain.

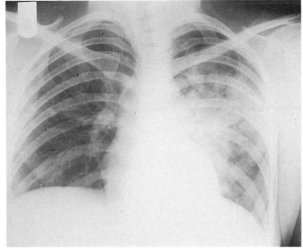

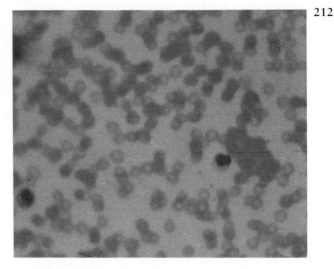

211 *Mycoplasma pneumoniae* pneumonia–consolidation and nodular opacities. There may be surprisingly few abnormal physical signs compared with widespread chest x-ray changes. The two dominant radiographic patterns are confluent areas of consolidation and nodular opacities. This radiograph was taken on the fifth day of illness. The incubation period lasts about 3 weeks, after which clinical illness comes on gradually over 2–4 days with malaise, headache, myalgia and pyrexia. The cough may be dry at first, after a few days becoming productive of small amounts of mucoid or mucopurulent sputum that is sometimes flecked with blood.

212 Cold agglutinins. Autoantibodies, which agglutinate human red blood cells at 4°C, will develop in the sera of 50% of patients with *M. pneumoniae* infection during the second week of illness. The diagnosis is confirmed by isolation of the organism and the raised mycoplasma complement fixation test. Cold agglutins are IgM antibodies that bind to the erythrocyte I antigen. *M. pneumoniae* has a selective affinity for the respiratory epithelial cells and produces H_2O_2 responsible for the epithelial respiratory tract damage and red cell haemolysis.

Table 14. Extrapulmonary manifestations of *Mycoplasma pneumoniae* pneumonia.

Cardiac	Pericarditis, myocarditis, conduction defects
Neurological (usually in first 2 weeks)	Headache encephalitis, aseptic meningitis, transverse myelitis, Guillain–Barré syndrome, cranial and peripheral neuropathy, cerebellar ataxia, psychosis
Gastrointestinal	Anorexia, nausea, vomiting, diarrhoea, hepatitis, pancreatitis
Haematological (second to third week)	Cold agglutinin production (50% of cases), haemolytic anaemia (5% of cases), disseminated intravascular coagulation
Dermatological (up to 25% cases)	Various rashes including erythema multiforme, Stevens–Johnson syndrome
Musculoskeletal (in first 2 weeks)	Migratory polyarthritis of large joints, Raynaud's phenomenon
Miscellaneous	Upper respiratory tract symptoms Myringitis Immune complex related interstitial or glomerulonephritis Splenomegaly Generalised lymphadenopathy

Viral pneumonia

Respiratory viral illnesses are caused by a large number of serologically distinct members of seven major virus families. They are spread by small particle aerosols, large droplets requiring close contact or by hand-to-hand transfer. Only a very small inoculum is needed to infect the ciliated columnar epithelial cells of the respiratory tract, which are progressively destroyed at the time of virus shedding.

The most frequent pneumonia in epidemic form is caused by the influenza virus. Other true virus pneumonias are caused by parainfluenza, measles, varicella, respiratory syncytial virus, cytomegalovirus and adenovirus. In clinical practice the differential diagnosis is from Q fever, psittacosis, *Mycoplasma pneumoniae* pneumonia and Legionnaires' disease. These diseases cannot be distinguished on clinical or radiographic evidence, and precise diagnosis entails isolation of the organisms and/or a fourfold rise in serum antibodies.

Various new antiviral drugs act at different points in the absorption and penetration of the virus into a cell, its intracellular synthesis, assembly and release.

213

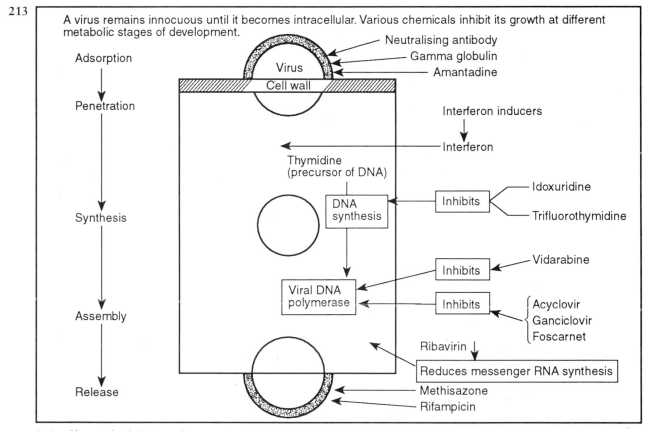

213 Chemical inhibition of viruses. A virus remains innocuous until it becomes intracellular. Viruses are obligate intracellular parasites that utilise biochemical pathways of the infected host cell, so that it is difficult to achieve clinically useful antiviral activity without adversely affecting host cell metabolism. Various antiviral agents inhibit viral growth at different metabolic stages of replication.

Primary influenza pneumonia

Epidemiology

The influenza virus, particularly type A, has a remarkable ability to undergo spontaneous antigenic changes in the haemagglutinin (HA) and neuraminidase (N) surface glycoproteins, resulting in minor antigenic drifts and major antigenic shifts. The minor changes cause sporadic infections but major antigenic drifts cause pandemic disease. Type B and type C influenza are much more stable antigenically.

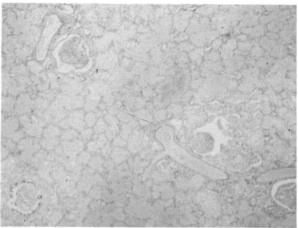

214 Fatal primary influenza virus pneumonia. Massive haemorrhagic oedema fills the alveoli and the respiratory epithelium is oedematous. The virus is spread in respiratory secretions which are infectious for 1–2 days after the onset of the illness. Virus from infected droplets penetrates columnar epithelial cells, resulting in necrosis and denudation of ciliated epithelium of the tracheobronchial tree. There is associated hyperaemia and haemorrhage. If the infection reaches as far as the alveoli, there is alveolar oedema and leucocyte exudation with capillary thrombosis.

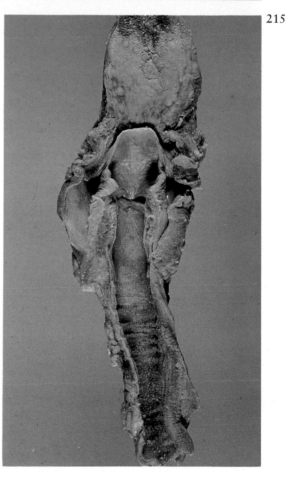

215 Influenza tracheobronchitis. Influenza virus infection damages the ciliated respiratory epithelium, which degenerates and desquamates, leaving a thin layer of basal replacement cells. Mucociliary clearance is markedly reduced and bacterial adherence to mucosal cells is increased. In addition to these defects in physical defence mechanisms, abnormalities of humoral and cellular immunity occur with impaired chemotaxis, reduced monocyte and macrophage phagocytic function, and a decrease in circulating T lymphocytes.

216 Combined influenza virus and bacterial pneumonia. Whole lung section. Widespread consolidation and focal abscesses are caused by staphylococcal pneumonia complicating influenza. Secondary bacterial pneumonia may be caused by *S. pneumoniae*, *S. aureus*, *H. influenzae*, *S. pyogenes* and *P. aeruginosa*.

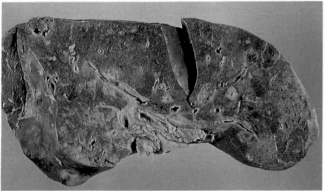

Herpes virus infections

These include varicella–zoster, herpes simplex, Epstein–Barr virus and cytomegalovirus.

Varicella–zoster infection

This is a highly contagious infection, primarily of children. Most cases of varicella pneumonia occur in adults, with three-quarters of cases occurring in 20–30-year-olds. The incubation period lasts up to 21 days and symptomatic pneumonia usually develops early in the course of the illness, particularly in those with severe skin involvement.

Cough, dyspnoea and chest pains develop, and the chest x-ray shows progressive fluffy infiltrates. Pneumonia is a serious complication of chickenpox in adults, with a reported mortality of up to 20% prior to the recent availability of specific antiviral therapies such as acyclovir and vidarabine.

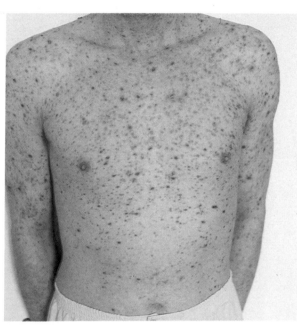

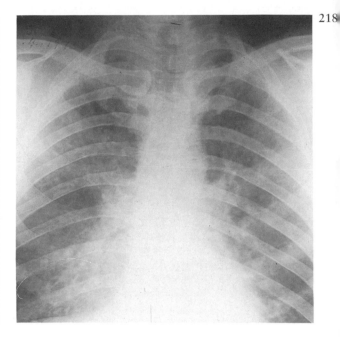

217 Varicella skin eruption. Centripetal crops of umbilicated vesicles at different stages of development, with macules, papules and scabs.

218 Varicella pneumonia. Severe adult chickenpox. Diffuse bilateral nodular infiltration, which may heal with miliary calcification, is shown.

Giant cell pneumonia

Almost all giant cell pneumonias result from infection with measles virus, although many patients do not have a classic attack of measles. Conditions in which measles giant cell pneumonia may occur include acute lymphoblastic leukaemia, neuroblastoma, lymphomas, hypogammaglobulinaemia and cytotoxic therapy.

Three to four weeks after exposure to measles, the patient presents with a cough, high fever and tachypnoea. Fine crackles may be heard over the lung bases. As the disease progresses, these become more widespread.

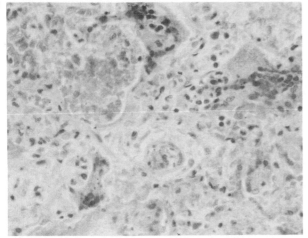

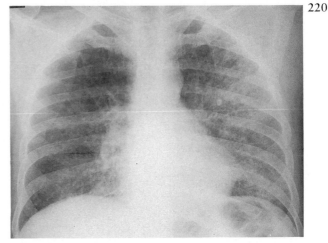

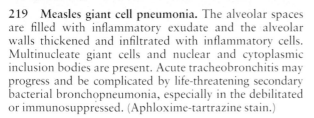

219 **Measles giant cell pneumonia.** The alveolar spaces are filled with inflammatory exudate and the alveolar walls thickened and infiltrated with inflammatory cells. Multinucleate giant cells and nuclear and cytoplasmic inclusion bodies are present. Acute tracheobronchitis may progress and be complicated by life-threatening secondary bacterial bronchopneumonia, especially in the debilitated or immunosuppressed. (Aphloxime-tartrazine stain.)

220 **Measles giant cell pneumonia.** Chest x-ray with widespread coarse nodular pulmonary infiltrates. The diagnosis is usually suspected in those who develop bronchopneumonia of this type and who have depressed cellular immunity, particularly if they are known to have been exposed to measles.

Legionella infections

Legionnaires' disease is a form of severe pneumonia caused by an aerobic Gram-negative flagellated bacillus, *Legionella pneumophila*, which has been shown to be a significant cause of both community and hospital acquired infection. Outbreaks may be epidemic, endemic or, most commonly, sporadic.

Legionella organisms are ubiquitous, widely disseminated and isolated from natural and domestic water systems. Multiplication is enhanced in stagnant water systems with a temperature ideally between 20 and 45°C. Transmission of infection is by inhalation of airborne organisms disseminated from infected cooling systems, defective air conditioning systems, showers, respiratory therapy equipment and spray caps.

The incubation period is up to 14 days. The illness starts abruptly with high fever of more than 39°C, rigors, malaise and myalgia. Respiratory symptoms are initially overshadowed by severe headache, confusion and delirium in more than half the patients. Cough may be absent or slight, with scanty mucoid sputum. Asymptomatic infections occur. Investigations may show moderate leucocytosis with lymphopenia, hyponatraemia, abnormal liver function and haematuria. Histology shows a confluent bronchopneumonia.

The diagnosis can be made on detecting a fourfold rise in titre or an initial positive titre of greater than 1:256 of specific antibodies by the indirect fluorescent antibody test, by direct fluorescent antibody staining of the organisms in lower respiratory secretions, in lung tissue and by culture. Death occurs in up to 20% of cases, mortality being highest in the elderly and immunosuppressed.

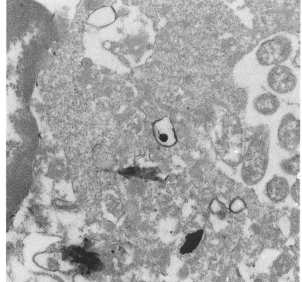

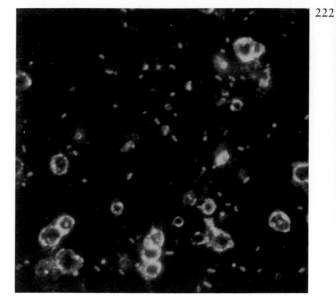

221 *Legionella pneumophila* organisms in lung tissue. The organisms are frequently intracellular and stain poorly, if at all, with Gram's stain. Complicated staining techniques are required if the organisms are to be reliably identified. Direct immunofluorescence is preferable; the test becomes positive during the second week of infection and IgM antibodies may persist for 18 months. (EM× 10,000.)

222 *Legionella pneumophila.* Smear of formalin-fixed lung tissue from a fatal case of Legionnaires' disease (stained with FTIC – conjugated rabbit serum raised against *L. pneumophila* serogroup 1 stain). The organisms are shown by fluorescence.

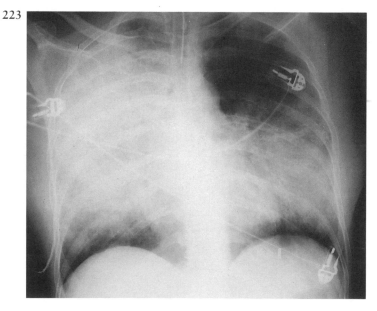

223 *Legionella pneumophila.* Extensive bilateral **pneumonic shadowing** with sparing of the lung bases and left upper zone. Legionnaires' disease should be considered in any patient with severe pneumonia that fails to respond to conventional antibiotic therapy.

Nosocomial (hospital acquired) pneumonia

Lower respiratory tract infection acquired during a hospital admission, especially in the debilitated, or after anaesthesia, is most commonly due to Gram-negative organisms. Staphylococci and anaerobes are occasionally found.

Klebsiella pneumonia

Klebsiella pneumoniae is a capsulated, non-motile bacillus which is a cause of acute pneumonia with a predilection for the right upper lobe. It produces an extensive haemorrhagic necrotising consolidation of the lung, which may be fatal. It most often afflicts middle-aged men, alcoholics, diabetics, the malnourished and those with chronic lung disease.

The sputum can be thick, blood-stained and tenacious, and is sometimes described as 'redcurrant jelly'. Leucocytosis is common and blood cultures are positive in one-quarter of cases. *K. pneumoniae* is sensitive to cephalosporins, aminoglycosides and chloramphenicol, although the choice of antibiotic depends on the local prevalence of resistant strains.

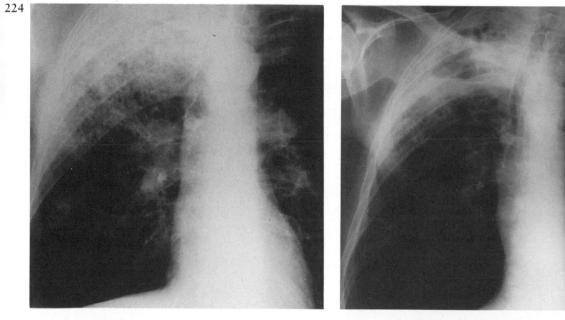

224, 225 Klebsiella pneumonia. Severe constitutional symptoms and right upper lobe cavitating pneumonia (**224**) in a 66-year-old alcoholic with severe chronic obstructive lung disease. After 10 days the upper lobe abscess cavity is clearly seen (**225**).

226 Klebsiella pneumonia colonies on agar culture plate. Large mucoid coalescing colonies are present. The infected sputum is thick, gelatinous, and like redcurrant jelly. (MacConkey agar B.)

Aspiration and anaerobic pneumonia

The conditions most frequently associated with aspiration pneumonia are: dysphagia due to neurological or mechanical lesions of the upper gastrointestinal tract; and impaired consciousness, when the cough reflex is depressed or lost, such as in alcoholic stupor, hypnotic drug overdose, epilepsy, general anaesthesia and neurological disease. Most commonly affected are the right upper lobe and the apical segments of the lower lobe, which are susceptible to aspiration by virtue of their dependent position in subjects who are lying supine. The severity of the pneumonia depends upon the pathogenicity of the organisms inhaled, the efficacy of the local defences by bronchopulmonary macrophages and the general resistance of the patients.

Aspiration anaerobic pneumonia is most common in the elderly and may be unrecognised because it presents with features similar to any bacterial pneumonia. It is often a necrotising pneumonia in which multiple small abscesses develop, usually in more than one lobe, and is associated with foul and purulent sputum. Empyema may develop by contiguous spread or by rupture of an abscess and development of a bronchopleural fistula.

Pneumonia after inhalation

Pneumonia after inhalation from the upper gastrointestinal tract is a far more serious event. If the aspirated fluid is acidic (the stomach has a pH of less than 2.4), alveolar oedema and destructive chemical pneumonitis will develop rapidly, resulting in hypoxia and respiratory failure. Inhalation of lesser amounts may lead to haemoptysis, haemorrhagic pneumonia and pulmonary oedema (acute adult respiratory distress syndrome).

227

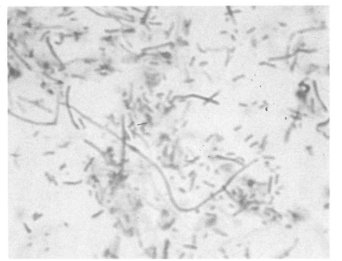

227 Anaerobic organisms in sputum. Aspiration contaminates the lower respiratory tract with a complex aerobic and anaerobic bacterial flora. The important aerobic bacteria include Gram-negative Enterobacteriaceae and *Pseudomonas aeruginosa*, both of which are related to nasopharyngeal colonisation. The important anaerobes include Gram-positive anaerobic cocci, peptostreptococcus and Gram-negative bacilli of the *Fusobacterium* and *Bacteroides* species. (Gram stain.)

228

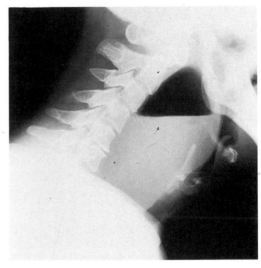

228 Secondary pneumonia was caused by aspiration from this huge retropharyngeal abscess.

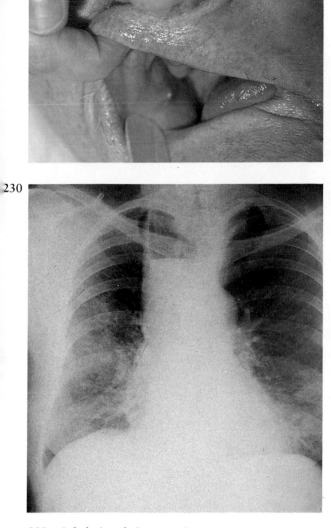

229

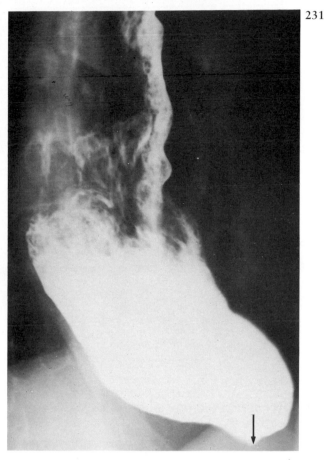

231

229 Bacterial parotitis. Elderly cachectic lady with terminal aspiration bronchopneumonia from bacterial parotitis. Pus can be seen exuding from the parotid duct.

230 Achalasia of the oesophagus. Note the widened mediastinum, the fluid level in the upper oesophagus and the bilateral lower lobe shadowing caused by chronic overspill infection.

231 Achalasia of the oesophagus. The barium contrast study demonstrates terminal narrowing of the oesophagus (arrowed).

Lipoid pneumonia

This is an uncommon form of aspiration pneumonia, whereby inhaled lipid incites lung inflammation and pneumonitis. Liquid paraffin has been responsible for most cases as a consequence of its relatively common usage for aperient purposes over long periods of time. Other causes include the use of mineral oil based nasal drops, aspiration of milk feeds or cod liver oil in children with feeding difficulties, inhalation of diesel oil by shipwrecked sailors, smoking of black fat tobacco that contains mineral oil, and exposure to fine mists of mineral oil used in industry for coolant or lubricating purposes.

Inhaled mineral and vegetable oils are emulsified in the lungs, engulfed by alveolar macrophages and slowly cleared into the lymphatics. A chronic low-grade inflammatory response can develop, complicated by secondary infection and fibrosis. In contrast, animal fats are broken down by lung lipases to release more toxic fatty acids that produce a brisk inflammatory pneumonitis.

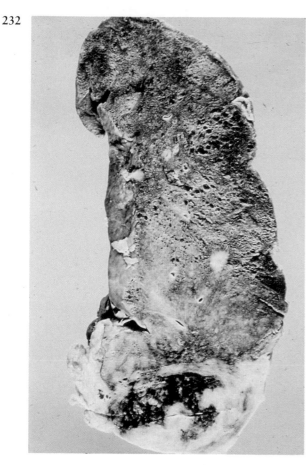

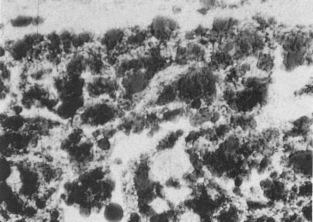

232 Lipoid 'paraffin' granuloma in the lower lobe developed as a result of the patient's long-standing ingestion of liquid paraffin in the mistaken hope of improving oesophageal achalasia. Similar lesions may follow aspiration of milk in infants, inhalation of oily nose drops, smoking of black fat tobacco or, usually, after intrabronchial injection of oil-based contrast medium for bronchography.

233 Pulmonary 'paraffin' granuloma. Microscopy shows diagnostic lipoid material stained red in this biopsy specimen of 'paraffin' granuloma. (Sudan IV×100.)

Recurrent pneumonia

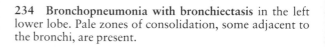

Pneumonia recurring in one part of the lung suggests a localised bronchopulmonary abnormality, perhaps due to an endobronchial malignancy or bronchi-ectatic segment. More generalised pneumonia may also be due to bronchiectasis, as well as aspiration, mucociliary or immune deficiency, or chronic obstructive lung disease. The latter is often caused by *S. pneumoniae* and *H. influenzae* infections. Other causes include recurrent pulmonary emboli and eosinophilic pneumonia.

234 Bronchopneumonia with bronchiectasis in the left lower lobe. Pale zones of consolidation, some adjacent to the bronchi, are present.

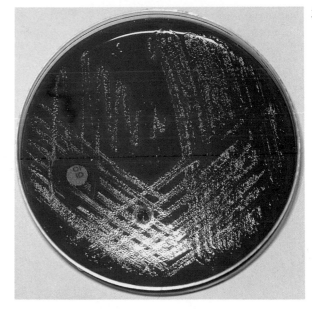

235 Sputum culture. Mixed growth of *S. pneumoniae* and *H. influenzae* in a bronchitic patient. The smaller *H. influenzae* colonies are inconspicuous against the larger *S. pneumoniae* colonies which are surrounded by their halo of gamma haemolysis. (Blood agar – reflected light.)

Lung abscess

A lung abscess is a cavitated infected necrotic lesion of the lung parenchyma, which results when infection causes intense tissue necrosis with inflammatory vasculitis. The more compromised the blood supply, the more severe, suppurative, cavitatory or gangrenous is the pneumonic process ending in abscess formation. Empyema occurs if the abscess discharges into the pleural space. According to this strict definition, infected bullae and bronchogenic cysts are not true lung abscesses because necrosis is absent, but their presentation and clinical management will in most instances be exactly the same as that of a true lung abscess.

Table 15. Causes of lung abscess.

Aspiration from the oropharynx
Bronchial obstruction
Immunocompromised state
Pneumonia
Septicaemia
Infected pulmonary infarcts
Trauma
Transdiaphragmatic spread
Vasculitis

Bacteriology
Pathogens include bacteria, mycobacteria, fungi and parasites. The microbiology reflects the mechanism by which the lung abscess has arisen. Most common are mixed anaerobic infections from aspiration of oropharyngeal contents (**Table 16**).

Table 16. Microbiological classification of lung abscess.

Bacteria	Mycobacteria	Fungi	Parasites
Staphylococcus aureus	*M. tuberculosis*	Histoplasma	*Entamoeba histolytica*
Streptococci	*M. kansasii*	Coccidiodes	Paragonimiasis
Klebsiella	*M. intracellulare*	Sporothrix	Echinococcus
Proteus		Aspergillus	
Anaerobes		Cryptococcus	
H. influenzae		Phycomycetes	
Legionella		Nocardia	
Pseudomonas aeruginosa			
Pseudomonas pseudomallei			
Actinomyces			

Pathology

Lung abscesses begin in an area or areas of pneumonia, within which small areas of necrosis or micro-abscesses develop, consolidating the lung. Some of these areas coalesce to form a single area, or sometimes multiple areas, of suppuration. Abscesses arising as a result of aspiration usually occur close to the visceral pleural surface and favour dependent parts of the lung. Lung abscesses that occur as a result of predominantly aerobic infection, with no clear episode of aspiration, may arise in any part of the lungs.

Table 17. Principal differential diagnoses of lung abscess.

Cavitating pulmonary tumour
Infected bulla or bronchial cyst
Localised saccular bronchiectasis
Aspergilloma
Wegener's granulomatosis
Hydatid cyst
Cavitated pneumoconiotic lesion
Cavitating rheumatoid nodule
Gas fluid level in the oesophagus, stomach or bowel

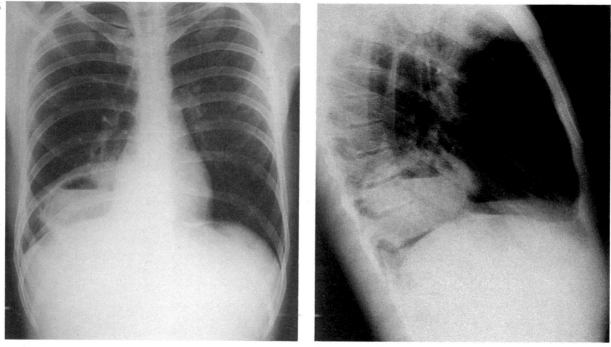

236, 237 Lung abscess. Intrapulmonary cavitating mass with fluid level lying posteriorly in the right lower lobe.

Empyema thoracis

This is defined as the presence of pus within the pleural cavity. Infection of the pleural space is most commonly a complication of bacterial pneumonia. It is convenient to consider the pleural response to infection as:

- Dry pleurisy, with pain and a pleural rub.
- Serous exudate (parapneumonic effusion).
- Empyema.

The transition from parapneumonic effusion to empyema involves the appearance of organisms in the fluid, an increase in polymorphs and a drop in pH and glucose.

Clinical

In a patient with pneumonia, the development of empyema is suspected if the clinical state is slow to improve, if there is persistent or recurrent fever, and if there is a persistently raised white cell count. There may be marked weight loss, chest pains in the region of the infection and rapid development of finger clubbing. A more insidious illness may occur in patients who have received inadequate antibiotic therapy for a preceding pneumonia, which may have been misdiagnosed as 'influenza' or 'bronchitis'.

The diagnosis is supported by radiological evidence of an effusion and confirmed by aspiration of characteristic fluid.

Management of empyema

The two basic principles for successful management of thoracic empyema are:

- Control of infection with appropriate antibiotics.
- Adequate drainage of pus by either closed or open procedures. Closed drainage may be by repeated aspiration (thoracocentesis) or may be continuous by placing an intercostal tube connected to an underwater seal drainage. If the empyema does not respond to aspiration, it is likely to become loculated; aspiration then becomes more difficult, and even the insertion of a chest drain may not provide complete drainage. The pleura becomes thickened and the lung trapped. In these circumstances thoracotomy and decortication may be required. Early surgical intervention and effective drainage reduces the frequency of complications.

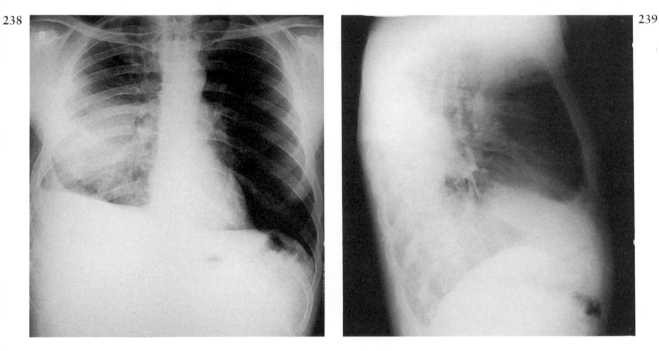

238, 239 Encysted postpneumonic pleural effusion. Ill-defined mid-zone shadowing and right basal pleural reaction. The lateral projection film (**239**) shows a posterior pleurally based mass shadow. Aspiration obtained 250 ml of foul smelling pus. The patient had been treated with antibiotics for a chest infection some 3 months previously.

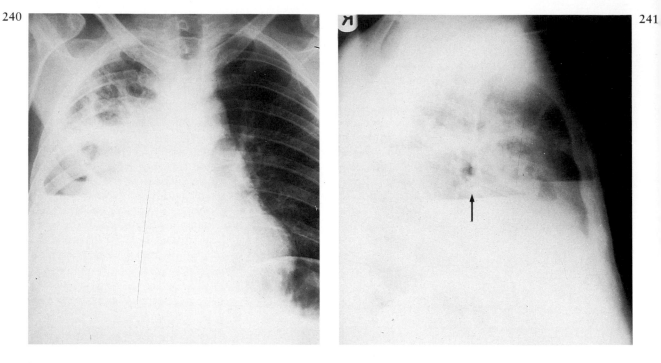

240, 241 **Empyema and pyopneumothorax.** Right lower lobe abscess cavity rupturing into the pleural space, following neoplastic right bronchus intermedius obstruction complicated by volume loss and secondary pneumonia. The lateral projection film (**241**) shows a fluid level (arrowed) in the pleural space.

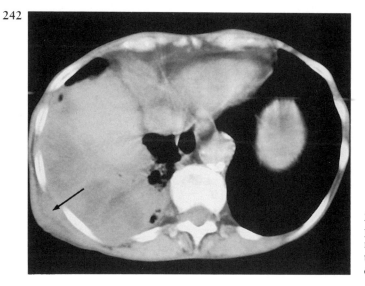

242 **Chronic empyema.** CT scan showing loculated postpneumonic effusion. Note the soft tissue involvement as the empyema tracks through the chest wall to produce a fluctuant mass (arrow) on the posterior chest wall (empyema necessitans).

16 Tuberculosis

Tuberculosis has a worldwide distribution. It is a common cause of morbidity or death in many developing countries, and in some communities 1% of the population have tubercle bacilli in their sputum.

In developed countries, higher standards of nutrition and accommodation, together with chemotherapeutic and other control measures practised during the past 40 years, have helped to reduce both the mortality and overall prevalence of the disease. It remains high in certain groups of patients – the diabetic, alcoholic, malnourished, those receiving corticosteroids or immunosuppressive drugs and in patients who have undergone gastrectomy. In spite of the decline of tuberculosis in certain countries, the pandemic of HIV infection and AIDS has had a major impact with a rising incidence of active tuberculosis in Central Africa and some cities in the USA, in association with an increase in HIV seropositivity. It still has numerous masquerades (**Table 18**), particularly in immigrants and in the ageing population.

Compared with an incidence of 7 per 100,000 in Britain's native white population, the incidence is 200 per 100,000 in Britain's Asian population, rising to 500 per 100,000 in Asian males over 55 years of age. In addition to this increased incidence, bacilli found in members of the Asian community also carry an increased resistance to streptomycin and isoniazid.

Mycobacterium tuberculosis and *M. bovis* are responsible for the majority of human infections.

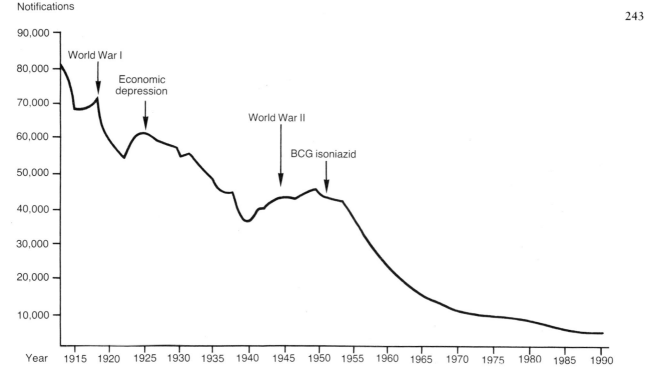

243 Tuberculosis notifications – England and Wales 1912 to 1990.

Table 18. Masquerades of tuberculosis

Myocardial disease
Crohn's regional ileitis
Sarcoidosis
Opportunist mycobacterial disease
Lymphocytic meningitis
Peritonitis
Breast cancer
Liver granulomas
Lymphadenopathy

Transmission of tubercle bacilli

Patients with active cavitating pulmonary tuberculosis frequently expel an aerosol of tubercle bacilli. The bacteria are suspended in droplets that are produced when speaking, sneezing or coughing, or in dust from dried sputum droplets disseminated by clothes or handkerchiefs.

Droplets of about 1 μm in diameter may penetrate directly to the alveoli and produce local infection, whereas large aggregates containing many bacteria impact in large airways and are cleared by mucociliary transport mechanisms.

Transmission by direct inoculation through the skin, cornea or buccal mucosa is rare. *Mycobacterium bovis* infection occurs through the alimentary canal via infected milk. Infection of cattle has been almost eliminated in developed countries by pasteurisation of milk, and by tuberculin testing and slaughter of infected animals.

Diagnostic tests

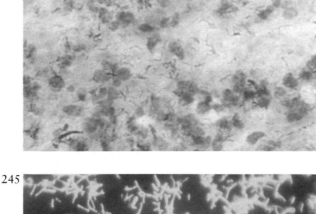

244 *Mycobacterium tuberculosis* **direct sputum smear stain by Ziehl–Nielsen method** (hot carbol fuchsin). The organisms are rod-shaped, usually about 5 μm in length, and 0.2–0.6 μm in width. They do not stain readily, but once stained, resist decolorisation by alcohol or strong mineral acid solution. This quality of 'acid and alcohol fastness' is a feature of the intact cell's waxy lipid-rich wall. If the direct smear is negative, the centrifuged sputum sediment may be stained and examined. The number of organisms must exceed 5,000 per ml before the direct smear is reliably positive, and such numbers are rarely present, except in cavitating pulmonary disease. (×1,000.)

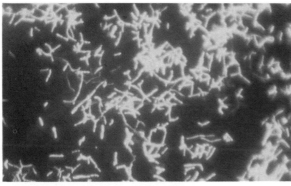

245 *Mycobacterium tuberculosis* **fluorescent staining with auramine.** Acid-fast bacilli appear as glowing fluorescent spots at low magnification. A large number of specimens may be rapidly examined using this technique. Culture is essential for diagnosis, as saprophytic non-pathogenic acid-fast bacilli will also be stained by auramine and Ziehl–Nielsen methods. (×1000.)

246 *Mycobacterium tuberculosis* **culture on Löwenstein–Jensen medium slopes** (egg and oleic acid–albumin agar medium). In culture, tubercle bacilli grow slowly, taking 2–6 weeks to form colonies. *M. tuberculosis* is an obligate aerobe which grows best at 37°C and pH 6.5–6.8, in an atmosphere of 5–10% carbon dioxide. Culture is likely to be positive when the number of organisms in the inoculum exceeds 100 per ml.

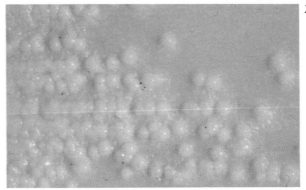

247 *Mycobacterium tuberculosis* **culture.** The slow-growing colonies are visible within 3–4 weeks. They are cream coloured and dry and wrinkled with irregular edges. *M. tuberculosis* does not develop orange or yellow pigment in the presence of light and is positively identified by its ability to produce niacin. Isolated tubercle bacilli should be tested for drug sensitivity.

Opportunist mycobacterial infections

There are many mycobacteria which may be confused with *M. tuberculosis*. They are ubiquitous and exposure is unavoidable. Some are free-living saprophytes, some are associated with animals and some produce unequivocal disease closely resembling tuberculosis. The opportunist mycobacteria are low-grade pathogens and as such do not constitute a threat to most people. They are divided into groups according to pigmentation and growth rate (**Table 19**).

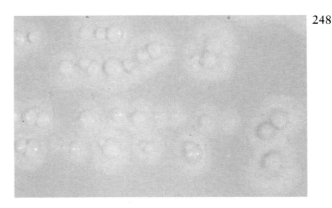

248 *Mycobacterium kansasii*, 'the yellow bacillus', is non-pigmented when grown in the dark, but forms rough yellow colonies in the light (photochromogen). Up to 60% of atypical mycobacteria infections are caused by *M. kansasii*. The organism shows a predilection for older males, pneumoconiotic coal miners in France and Wales, and silicotic sandblasters in New Orleans.

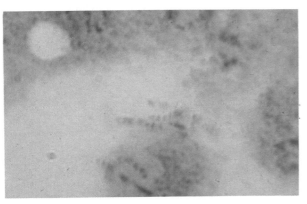

249 *Mycobacterium kansasii.* The direct smear shows acid-fast rods that are identical to those of *M. tuberculosis*.

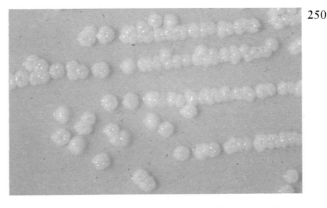

250 *Mycobacterium fortuitum.* White, glistening colonies rapidly develop at 37°C (non-chromogen). This rapidly growing mycobacterium may contaminate wounds or postinfection abscesses, but is only rarely associated with lymphadenopathy or pulmonary disease.

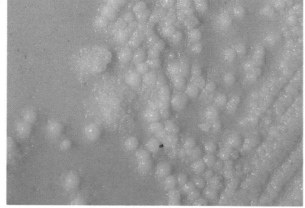

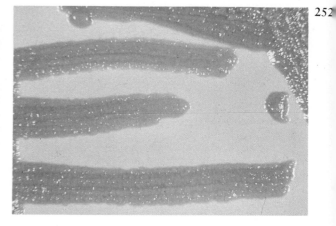

251 *Mycobacterium avium – intracellulare.* Micro-aerophilic, non-photochromogenic slow-growing myco-bacteria. DNA probes discriminate between *M. avium* and *M. intracellulare*. Mycobacteria of these species are responsible for most non-tuberculous infections.

252 *Mycobacterium scrofulaceum.* The organisms are microaerophilic. Slow-growing yellow/orange pigmented colonies develop at 37°C (scotochromogen).

Table 19. The opportunist mycobacteria causing human disease.

Group	Mycobacterium species	Habitat and constitution	Human infection
Runyon I Photochromogen	M. kansasii	Water but not soil. Rarely isolated from animals. South to Central America, Europe	Pulmonary disease in middle-aged males with chronic underlying lung disease and poor defensive bronchopulmonary macrophages
Runyon II Scotochromogen	M. scrofulaceum	Soil and water worldwide	Lymphadenopathy Rarely lung disease
Runyon III Non-chromogen	M. xenopi (weak chromogen)	Water: river estuaries and coastal areas	Pulmonary disease and lymphadenopathy *M. avium–intracellulare* generalised systemic infection in AIDS
	M. intracellulare (non-chromogenic)	Soil W. Australia and southeast USA	
	M. avium (non-chromogenic)	Soil	
Runyon IV	M. malmoense (non-chromogenic)	UK and Sweden	
	M. fortuitum (non-chromogenic)	Soil Common contaminant	Skin abscess Wound infections
Skin pathogens only	M. marinum (1) M. balnei M. ulcerans (III) (weak chromogens)	Water Swimming pools Fish tanks	Skin granulomata

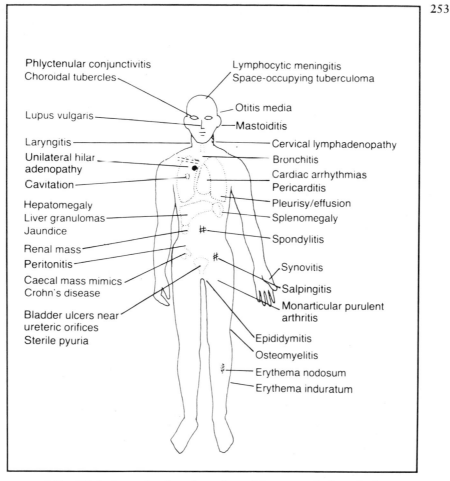

Phlyctenular conjunctivitis
Choroidal tubercles

Lymphocytic meningitis
Space-occupying tuberculoma

Lupus vulgaris

Otitis media
Mastoiditis

Laryngitis

Cervical lymphadenopathy

Unilateral hilar adenopathy

Bronchitis

Cavitation

Cardiac arrhythmias
Pericarditis

Hepatomegaly
Liver granulomas
Jaundice

Pleurisy/effusion
Splenomegaly

Renal mass
Peritonitis

Spondylitis

Caecal mass mimics
Crohn's disease

Synovitis
Salpingitis

Bladder ulcers near ureteric orifices
Sterile pyuria

Monarticular purulent arthritis

Epididymitis
Osteomyelitis
Erythema nodosum
Erythema induratum

253   Clinical examination of a patient with suspected tuberculosis.

Primary pulmonary tuberculosis

The first phase, the primary infection, occurs in those without specific immunity. The primary intrathoracic complex or Ghon focus consists of a subpleural lesion, most commonly in the lower two-thirds of the lungs in which ventilation is greatest and, hence, the deposition of airborne infection most likely. At an early stage, bacilli are transported through the lymphatics to the regional lymph nodes, where there is a marked reaction, often with caseation. Organisms tend to escape into the bloodstream, with widespread dissemination.

Uncomplicated primary tuberculosis seldom causes significant illness and may pass unnoticed unless routine x-rays of the chest or tuberculin test demonstrate a conversion from negative to positive carried out at the appropriate time.

Erythema nodosum or phlyctenular conjunctivitis may follow tuberculin conversion. Most primary infections heal with or without calcification of the primary complex. Occasionally, the infection progresses either locally in the lung or systemically with dissemination through the bloodstream. In young children, tuberculous bronchopneumonia or life-threatening haematogenous miliary spread may occur. In adolescents and adults, local extension with apical cavitation and fibrosis is more common.

Table 20. Complications of primary tuberculosis.

Progressive disease at site of the lung lesion
Tuberculoma formation
Atelectasis from bronchial compression
Tuberculous bronchopneumonia following lymph node rupture
Tuberculous pleural effusion
Tuberculous pericardial effusion
Miliary tuberculosis

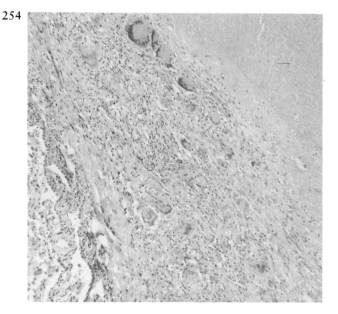

254 Tuberculous granuloma with caseation and giant cells. Deposition of tubercle bacilli in the alveoli is followed by vasodilation and by influx of neutrophils and macrophages. After several weeks the neutrophils, which characterise the initial inflammatory response, are replaced by macrophages that eventually fuse into Langhans' multinucleate giant cells. Granulation tissue supervenes and central caseous necrosis (top right of picture) may subsequently heal with fibrosis and calcification. (×100.)

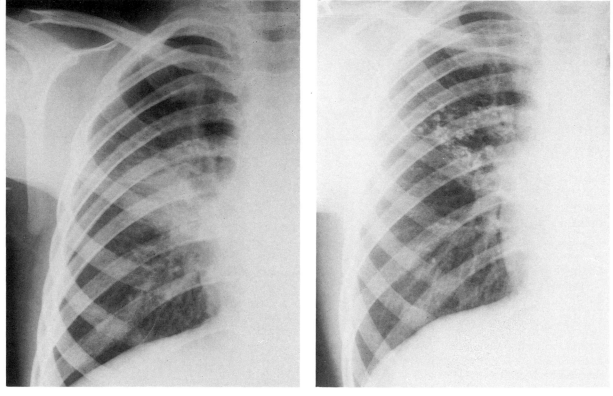

255, 256 **Primary infection in right upper lobe.** Healing left extensive calcification in the lung parenchyma.

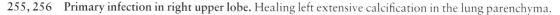

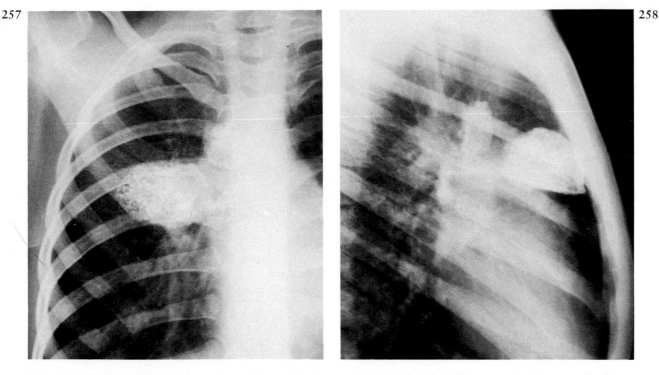

257, 258 The healed primary complex, with calcification in the lung and draining lymph node. This example shows an unusual amount of calcification in the healed tuberculoma and associated lymph node.

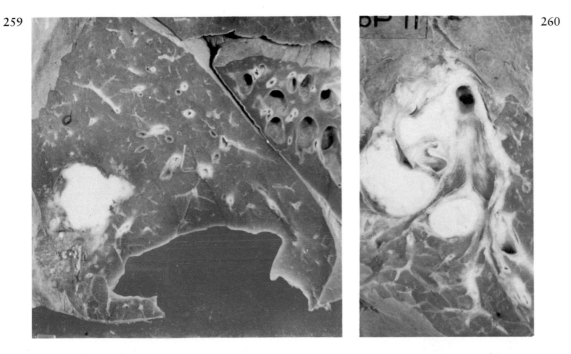

259 Peripheral Ghon focus in healed primary tuberculosis. The focus appears as a white scar near to the lung periphery.

260 Tuberculous lymph nodes encircling and narrowing the right middle lobe bronchus. Caseous material discharged from the nodes into the bronchial lumen resulted in widespread tuberculous pneumonia.

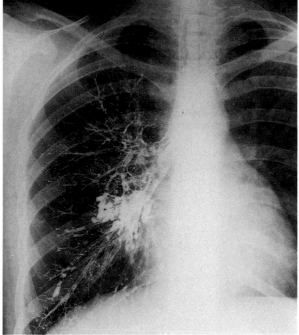

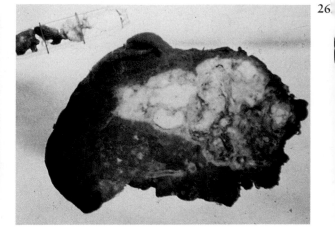

26

261, 262 'Middle lobe syndrome'. The bronchogram (**261**) demonstrates bronchiectasis in the middle lobe. This is also shown in the resected right middle lobe surgical specimen. The enlarged tuberculous lymph nodes, present in the glass specimen tube (**262**), compressed the right middle lobe bronchus, causing distal collapse and infection. This commonly affects the middle lobe bronchus because it is encircled by lymphatic tissue.

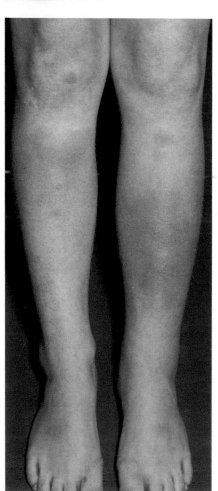

263 **Erythema nodosum** is a manifestation of the presence of circulating immune complexes. It may infrequently accompany primary tuberculosis, being most common in adolescent girls. Erythema nodosum is a non-specific hypersensitivity phenomenon. It is particularly common in women of childbearing age. There are numerous causes for the physical sign (**Table 21**).

Table 21. Conditions associated with erythema nodosum.

Associated disease	Age	Clinical features	X-ray	Skin test	Laboratory confirmation
Sarcoidosis	20 to 40 Rare below 20 or over 50	Female preponderance Lymphadenopathy, uveitis or conjunctivitis	Bilateral hilar adenopathy ±pulmonary infiltration	Kveim–Siltzbach test positive Tuberculin test negative	Histology of inflamed scar tissue Hypercalcaemia Serum angiotensin converting enzyme
Streptococcal infection	Any	Preceding upper respiratory tract infection	—	—	β-haemolytic strepto-coccus in throat Raised anti-strepto-lysin titre
Tuberculosis	Under 20	Asian migrant close contact with tuberculosis Primary complex	Unilateral hilar adenopathy Ghon focus	Tuberculin conver-sion to high degree of positivity	Isolation of *Mycobacterium tuberculosis*
Drugs	Any	Transfer factor Sulphonamides Oral contraceptives Sulphones Penicillin Levamisole	—	—	Recurs when rechallenged with drug
Histoplasmosis	Any	From Ohio Respiratory symptoms Lymphadenopathy	Miliary mottling	Histoplasmin	Complement-fixation test Fungal hyphae in sputum or lung biopsy
Coccidioido-mycosis	Any	From California Respiratory symptoms Flu-like illness	Miliary mottling Hilar glands or cavitation	Coccidioidin	Complement-fixation test Fungus in sputum or lung biopsy
Leprosy (lepromatous)	Any	From 'tropics' Symmetrical nodular rash Iridocyclitis Patchy sensory loss	Normal	Lepromin	Isolate *M. leprae*: skin or nerve biopsy
Ulcerative colitis	15 to 40	Diarrhoea	Barium enema	—	Rectal biopsy
Crohn's disease	15 to 40	Abdominal pain, fever, fistulae	Barium follow-through Barium enema	Depression of delayed-type hypersensitivity	Intestinal biopsy
Yersinia infection	Any	Particularly France and Scandinavia Abdominal pain, diarrhoea	Normal chest x-ray and barium studies	—	Stool culture: *Y. enterocolitica* Raised agglutinin titres
Pregnancy	15 to 40	First trimester	—	—	Recurs with next pregnancy
Circulating immune complex	Any	Polyarthralgia Uveitis Meningism	—	—	High ESR Positive tests by various techniques Raji, Ciq, etc.

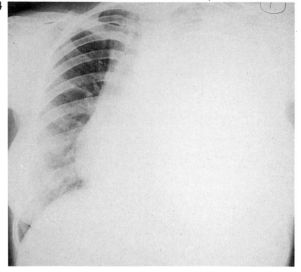

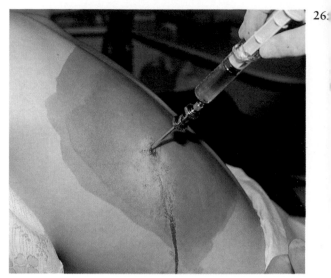

264 **Tuberculous pleural effusion** presenting with pleural pain and fever 3–6 months after a primary infection. The massive effusion has displaced the mediastinum.

265 **Therapeutic aspiration of a tuberculous effusion.** Pleural biopsy is performed at the same time. It may be diagnostic in tuberculosis. Note the characteristic straw-coloured fluid in the syringe. The protein content was 4.3 g/l and lymphocytes were present in large numbers, but the smear for acid-fast bacilli was negative. Culture for acid-fast bacilli proved to be positive.

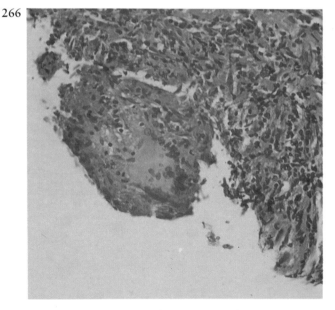

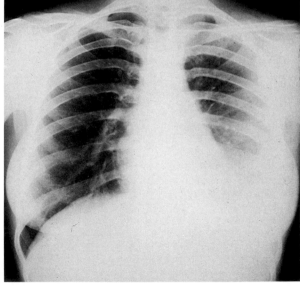

266 **Pleural biopsy specimen**. Caseating granulomas in pleural biopsy tissue confirmed the diagnosis of tuberculosis. Tuberculous pleural effusion is associated with very extensive pleural seeding by tubercles, and a small biopsy specimen frequently provides diagnostic histology.

267 **Tuberculous pleural effusion** after aspiration of 5 litres of fluid. Note the central position of the mediastinum. (Same patient as in **264**.)

268 Tuberculous pericardial effusion. The cardiac silhouette is widened and has a globular shape. Culture of the aspirated fluid grew tubercle bacilli. One clue to the diagnosis was the enlarged right paratracheal lymph gland (arrowed).

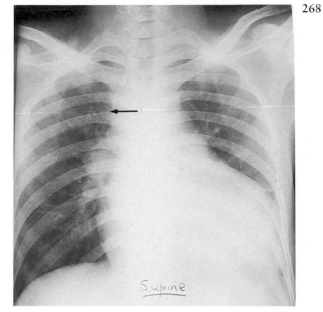

269 M-mode echo scan of the heart, showing a large posterior pericardial effusion. LA = left atrium, AO = aorta, S = septum, AMV = anterior leaflet of mitral valve, LV = left ventricular cavity, PW = posterior cardiac wall, EFF = pericardial effusion.

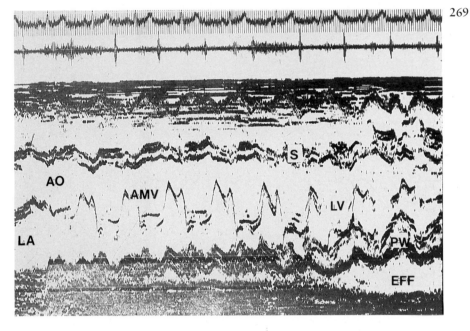

Table 22. Treatment regimens for pulmonary tuberculosis

Drugs for pulmonary tuberculosis	Regimens		
	1 HRE/HR	2 HRZE/HR	3 HRZ/HR
Isoniazid (H)	← 9/12 →	← 6/12 →	← 6/12 →
Rifampicin (R)			
Ethambutol (E)	← 2/12 →	← 2/12 →	
Pyrazinamide (Z)		← 2/12 →	← 2/12 →

Primary tuberculosis – acute miliary

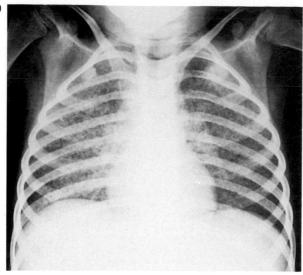

Miliary tuberculosis results from the rupture of a caseating primary focus or from a caseating lesion in the intima of a blood vessel that discharges bacilli throughout the bloodstream. This is most likely to occur in young children at the time of the primary infection.

270 Acute and fatal miliary tuberculosis in a 6-year-old child. The right paratracheal lymph node gland is enlarged and miliary shadows are present in both lung fields. Miliary tuberculosis implies blood-borne dissemination. The lung is uniformly seeded with tubercles which are usually relatively small (about 2–3 mm in diameter).

271

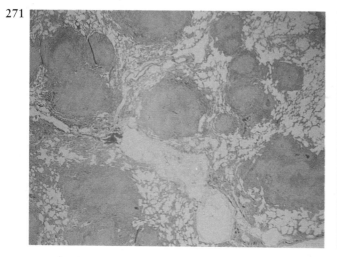

271 Miliary tuberculosis. Numerous caseating pulmonary granulomas.

27

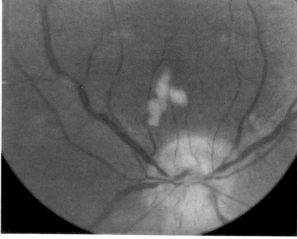

272 Choroidal tubercles in acute miliary tuberculosis. Their presence is pathognomonic. In adult chronic miliary tuberculosis, choroidal tubercles are rarely present.

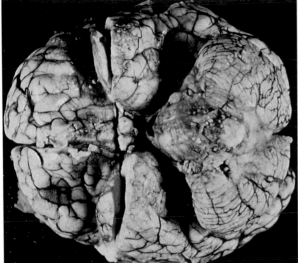

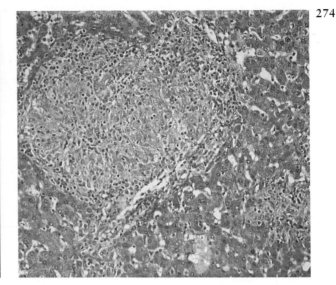

273 Tuberculous meningitis. The meninges are studded with small tubercles and the base of the brain covered by a fibrinous exudate. Miliary spread to the brain is most common in childhood and occurs within the first year of infection. This classic case presented with fever, hepatosplenomegaly and choroidal tubercles.

274 Miliary tuberculosis. Hepatic involvement with caseating granulomas. In difficult cases, liver biopsy may be diagnostic.

Bone and joint tuberculosis

Orthopaedic tuberculosis is common in developing countries. The spine is involved in about half the cases (other less common sites being the knee, ankle and hip), but any bone can be involved and multiple sites are frequent. A remarkably low bacterial population is a feature of bone tuberculosis, and positive cultures are found in only one-third of aspirates.

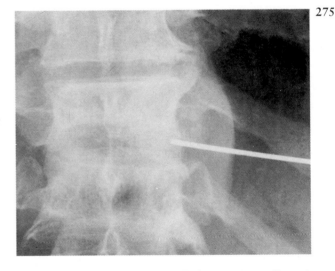

275 Tuberculous paravertebral abscess (Pott's disease) involving the lumbar vertebrae in an adult. The needle lies in the abscess cavity. Narrowing of the disc space is soon followed by destruction of adjacent vertebral bodies. This patient experienced troublesome back pain for two years before the correct diagnosis was made.

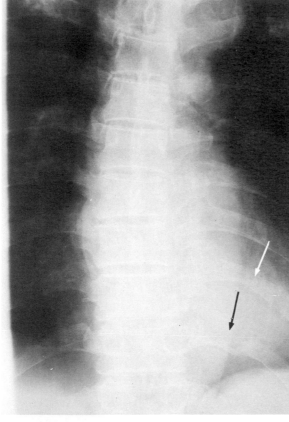

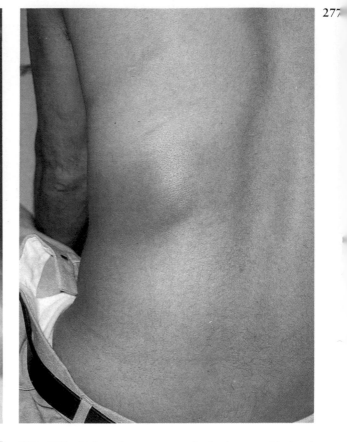

276, 277 Tuberculous paravertebral abscess with local lysis and sclerosis of the ninth and tenth ribs (arrowed) associated with an inflammatory swelling over the posterior chest wall.

Think of tuberculosis when an 'at risk' patient presents with fluctuant or inflammatory chest wall swellings.

278

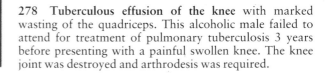

278 Tuberculous effusion of the knee with marked wasting of the quadriceps. This alcoholic male failed to attend for treatment of pulmonary tuberculosis 3 years before presenting with a painful swollen knee. The knee joint was destroyed and arthrodesis was required.

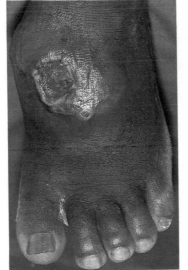

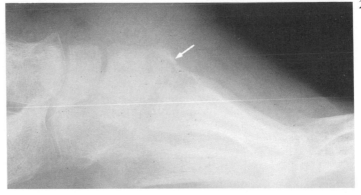

279, 280   Tuberculous osteomyelitis presenting with a deep ulcer in the foot. Bone involvement, as in this case, usually occurs within 3 years of the primary infection. The x-ray shows bone destruction (arrowed).

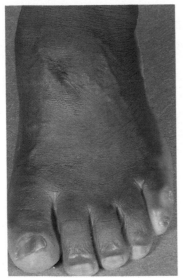

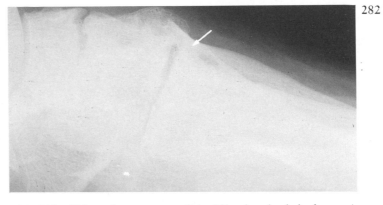

281, 282   Tuberculous osteomyelitis. The ulcer healed after antituberculous chemotherapy, with pathological arthrodesis of the underlying joint (arrowed).

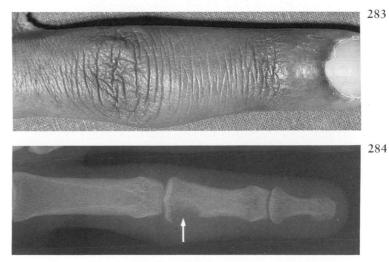

283, 284   Tuberculous dactylitis commonly involves the metaphysis (arrow).

Post primary tuberculosis

Although the primary infection heals, the organisms that produced the infection persist in the tissues in a dormant form. The organisms causing post primary disease are usually those disseminated by the circulation at the time of the primary infection. Post primary disease is most common in tissues with high oxygen tension. The lungs are most frequently involved; this is important because smear-positive infected sputum is the main source of infection responsible for the persistence of the disease in the community. Other common sites include bone and lymph nodes, but any tissue may be involved.

In the lungs, the earliest lesions are aggregations of tubercles, with collapse and consolidation of alveoli. In those with normal immunity the lesions may remain localised and confined by fibrosis, presenting a compromise between destruction and repair. Many tuberculous patients remain asymptomatic, their disease only being detected by routine chest x-ray. Caseation may occur and cavities form if the caseous pus is discharged into a bronchus. Cavitation may be accompanied by weight loss, productive cough, purulent sputum, haemoptysis and fever. Haemoptysis may be slight if due to inflamed bronchial walls, or brisk from cavitated lesions traversed by incompletely obliterated bronchovascular bundles.

Post primary tuberculosis may arise from:

- Progression of a primary lesion. In Europe and North America the primary infection often occurs in adolescence or adult life.
- Reactivation of a quiescent primary or post primary lesion. The poor cellular immunity which occurs with immunosuppressant drugs, certain diseases and old age may lead on to reactivation of dormant infection.
- Haematogenous spread to the lungs.
- Exogenous re-infection. Most patients with a healed primary complex mount a successful immune response when re-exposed to tuberculosis. Superinfection may overwhelm these defences.

285

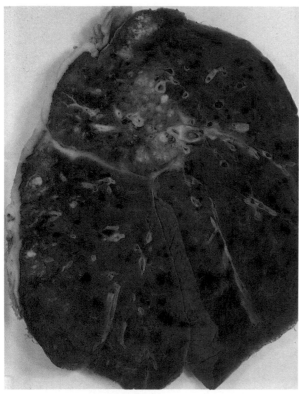

285 Post primary tuberculosis with chronic cavities and fibrosis in the upper lobe.

286

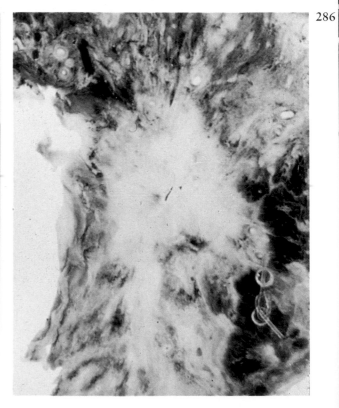

286 Post primary tuberculosis. The cavity has healed and dense fibrous tissue has formed.

Radiology

There are no absolute diagnostic radiographic appearances. The following findings support the diagnosis:

- Nodular patchy shadows in the upper lobes, particularly in the posterior and apical segments.
- Bilateral upper zone shadows.
- Cavitation in the upper lobes.
- Pulmonary/pleural calcification.

- Linear shadows indicating fibrosis in the upper lobes associated with soft shadows suggesting active process.
- Mediastinal lymph node enlargement.

287

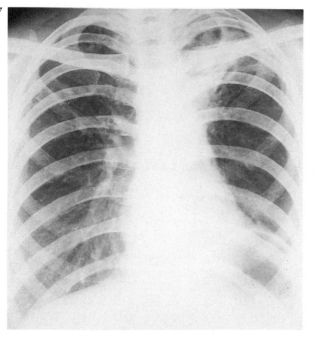

288

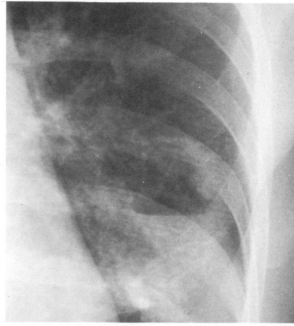

289

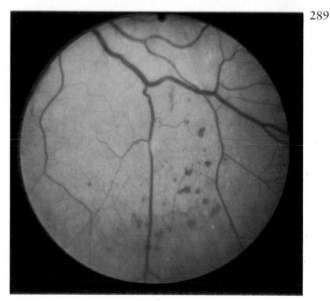

287 Pulmonary tuberculosis. Upper lobe consolidation and an apical cavity. Sputum was heavily infected with acid-fast bacilli.

288 Cavitating tuberculosis. A fluid-filled cavity lies in the left lower lobe; the sputum was positive. In cavitating tuberculosis, large numbers of organisms are expectorated. Diagnosis should be made readily on examining the sputum.

289 Diabetic retinopathy. Microaneurysms and exudates in the retina. There is an increased incidence of tuberculosis among diabetic patients. The possibility of diabetes should be considered in all patients with tuberculosis.

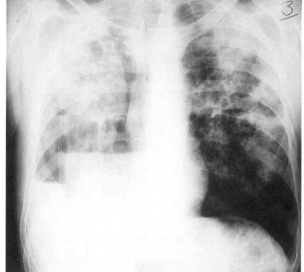

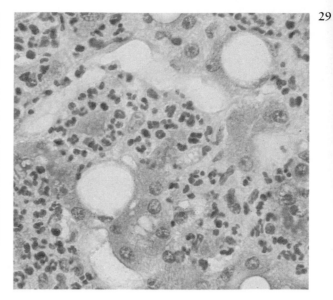

290 Tuberculous empyema and widespread bilateral bronchopneumonic shadowing. Rupture of a cavity or caseous pleural lesion produces a loculated empyema with pyopneumothorax and bronchopleural fistula. The healed rib fractures are a common finding in alcoholics. The effusion was haemorrhagic. The alcoholic cirrhotic malnourished vagrant is prone to reactivation of tuberculosis and to discontinuing therapy abruptly before a cure is effected. The serum total bilirubin concentration was elevated.

291 Micronodular cirrhosis. Many of the hepatocytes are necrotic and there is marked fatty infiltration. The biopsy was taken from a patient with alcoholic cirrhosis and tuberculosis. Hepatotoxic antituberculous drugs should be given under close supervision with serial measurements of liver function. Most cirrhotic patients tolerate antituberculous drugs well; their liver function improves with abstinence from alcohol and provision of adequate diet.

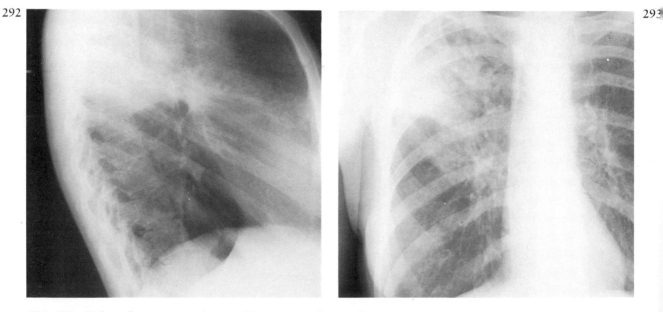

292, 293 Tuberculous pneumonia resembling an acute bacterial pneumonia is seen when the alveoli are flooded with bacilli from an area of liquid necrosis. The patient presented with rigors, fever, pleuritic chest pain and a productive cough. The radiographic clue to a diagnosis of tuberculosis is the involvement of the posterior and apical segments of the upper lobe.

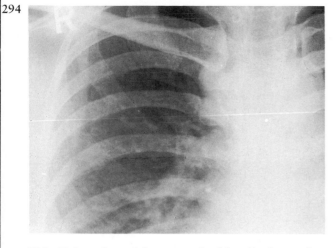

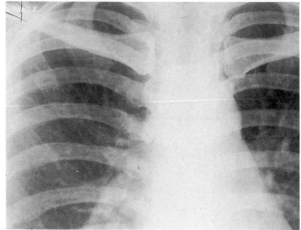

294 Tuberculous right paratracheal lymphadenopathy. This patient presented with night sweats, malaise, weight loss and a strongly positive tuberculin test. Routine 'first line' antituberculous treatment was begun.

295 Tuberculous right paratracheal lymphadenopathy. The clinical response to 8 weeks of drug treatment was satisfactory. The x-ray shows shrinkage of the previously enlarged nodes. (Same patient as in **294**.)

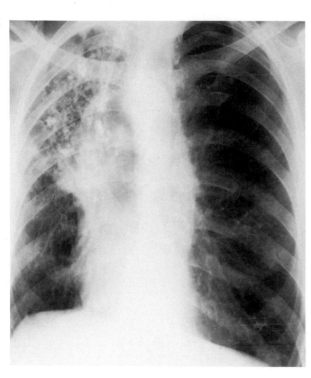

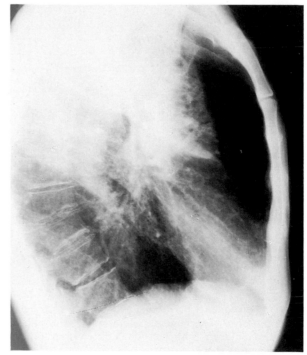

296 Extensive fibrosis of right upper lobe with calcification as a sign of old pulmonary tuberculosis. The mediastinum is deviated to the right.

297 Extensive fibrosis of right upper lobe. The lateral film shows a large anterior window caused by the left lung herniating across to the right. (Same patient as in **296**.)

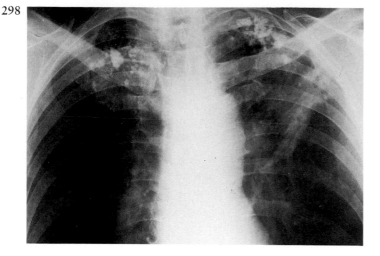

298 Extensive bilateral apical calcification from healed tuber-culosis. Modern antituberculous chemotherapy, combined with public health measures, should reduce the numbers of patients whose lungs are extensively damaged by tuberculosis.

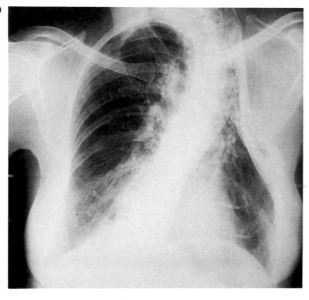

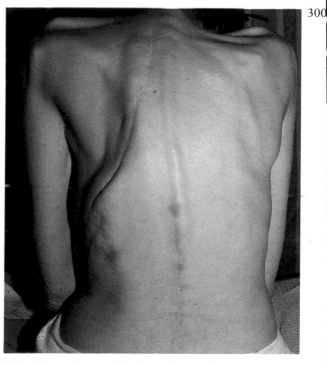

299 Thoracoplasty performed to collapse the left upper lobe cavity; 25 years later the lateral spine curvature has increased and there is calcification in the collapsed portion of the lung, but the patient is otherwise well. Since the advent of modern chemotherapy, extensive collapse surgical treatment of this type is only of historical interest.

300 Deformity resulting from thoracoplasty.

Lymph node tuberculosis

Cervical adenitis in Asian, African and West Indian populations
is often associated with pulmonary or extrathoracic tuberculosis.

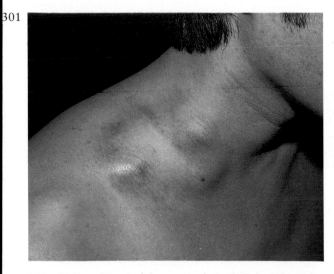

301 Tuberculous involvement of cervical lymph nodes
(scrofula). Glandular tuberculosis is now rare in Europeans,
but still relatively common in Asians. Usually of insidious
onset, lymph node swelling may progress to the formation
of abscesses and chronic discharging sinuses.

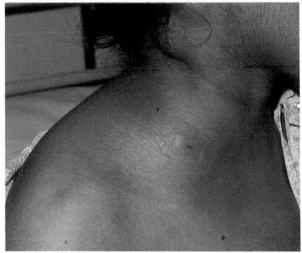

302 Tuberculous cervical and post auricular adenopathy.
This patient went on to develop tuberculous peritonitis
and osteomyelitis.

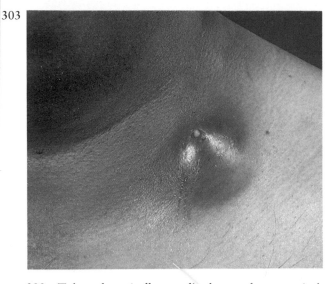

303 Tuberculous 'collar stud' abscess from cervical
lymph nodes pointing in the neck. Cervical node enlargement is a particularly common extrapulmonary manifestation in Asian immigrants, caused by secondary rather
then 'primary complex' tuberculosis. Evidence of tuberculosis elsewhere may not be found.

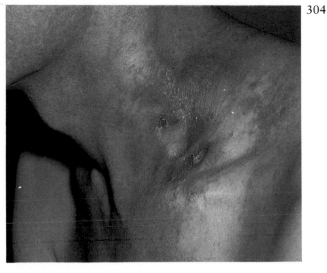

304 Tuberculous abscess. A ragged chronic discharging
sinus. Tuberculous glands often lie beneath the deep
fascia, and discharge caseous pus. Diagnosis is best established by gland biopsy; culture of the lymph node or pus
is less successful. Surgical drainage with curettage and
routine antituberculous therapy is curative.

Mediastinal lymph node tuberculosis

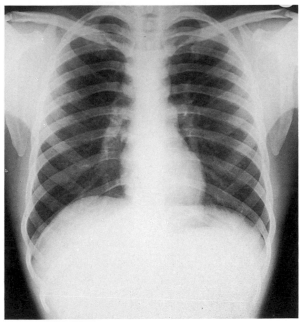

Mediastinal lymphadenopathy, although characteristic of primary tuberculosis, is not a common feature of adult post primary disease in Europeans. However, among Asian, African and West Indian populations, mediastinal lymph node enlargement is much more common and in the majority of cases there is no obvious accompanying radiological lung involvement. The same ethnic groups are much more likely to suffer cervical or extrapulmonary tuberculosis.

305 Tuberculous paratracheal gland enlargement. Strongly positive tuberculin test. Confirmation by lymph node biopsy obtained at mediastinoscopy may be required in some cases. The progress of the same patient on antituberculous chemotherapy is shown in 306, 307.

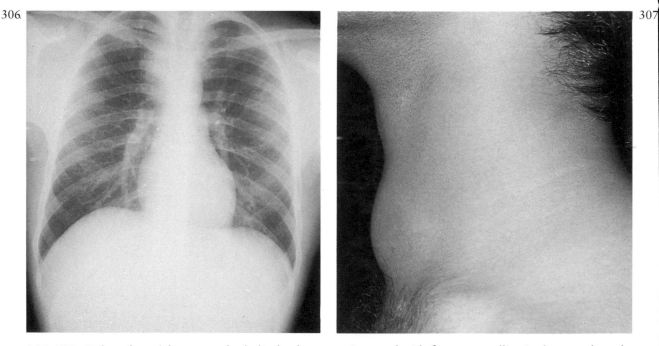

306, 307 Tuberculous right paratracheal gland enlargement increased with fluctuant swelling in the sternal notch, from which 60 ml of sterile caseous pus was aspirated after 140 days of antituberculous chemotherapy.

The behaviour of lymph nodes during treatment is notoriously unpredictable, with abscess formation and discharging sinuses or node enlargement in about a quarter of cases. The reasons for this are not fully understood, but may include hypersensitivity to tuberculoprotein released at intervals from disrupted macrophages. Prolonged chemotherapy and curettage were necessary to settle this patient's tuberculosis.

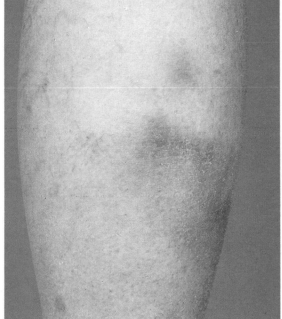

308 Erythema induratum (Bazin's disease). Symmetrical chilblain-like lesions develop on the calves of young women. The attack usually begins in cold weather. The lesions may ulcerate. Bazin gave the name 'erythema induratum' to this condition when histological examination revealed caseation and necrosis associated with tuberculosis.

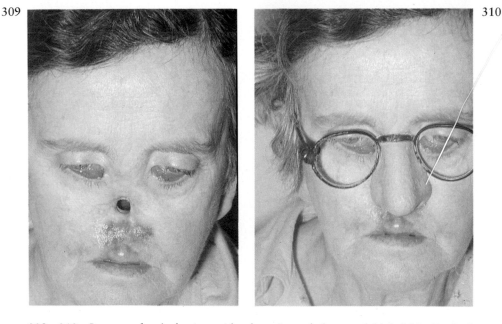

309, 310 Lupus vulgaris begins with ulceration of the nasolabial fold. Gradual extension of this tuberculous inflammation leads to complete destruction of the nose. This patient was fitted with an artificial nose (310) which proved to be a cosmetic success.

Skin tests for tuberculosis

Cell-mediated delayed hypersensitivity to tuberculoprotein develops 4–8 weeks after infection with tubercle bacilli and is demonstrated by intradermal injections of a purified protein derivative of tuberculin (PPD) or heat-concentrated tuberculin (HCSM). The potency of PPD is expressed in terms of international units (IU) per ml. Tests using tuberculin detect individuals with host immunity to tuberculosis. A positive reaction may mean previous infection with tubercle bacilli, current active tuberculosis or successful BCG vaccination.

Standard Mantoux test dilutions (UK)

Labelled dilution on container	Labelled potency on container	Potency of 0.1 ml dose injected
1/10,000	10IU per ml	1IU
1/1,000	100IU per ml	10IU
1/100	1,000IU per ml	100IU

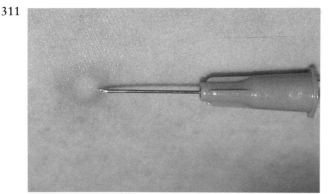

311 Mantoux skin test. 0.1 ml of a standard dilution of PPD prepared from *M. tuberculosis* is injected intradermally, using a tuberculin syringe with intradermal needle (25 gauge, 16 mm long, with short bevel). Routine testing in the UK is performed with PPD 10IU, whereas PPD 5IU (intermediate strength) is used for the standard test in the USA. A more dilute solution containing 1IU is available to test those who may be expected to show a strong reaction, especially children (first strength PPD). In doubtful cases the test may be repeated with 100IU (UK) or 250IU (USA, second strength). PPD prepared from atypical and avian mycobacteria is available.

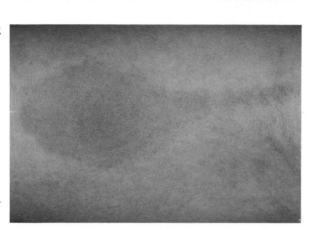

312 Mantoux 10IU positive reaction at 48 hours. 30 mm induration and central vesiculation in a strongly hypersensitive subject. The Mantoux skin test is read 48–72 hours after injection. The UK recommendations imply that the widest diameter of induration is measured; induration of 6 mm or greater indicates a positive reaction. In the USA it is recommended that the diameter of the induration is measured in millimetres transversely to the long axis of the forearm; 5–9 mm induration is regarded as a doubtful positive, and 10 mm induration or greater as positive. A doubtful positive is equated with the alternative possibility of non-specific atypical mycobacterial infection. A reaction of 15 mm to a standard 10IU Mantoux is equivalent to a Grade 3–4 Heaf reaction.

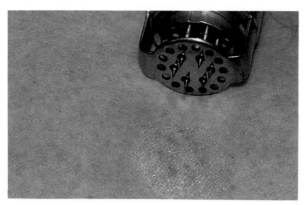

313 The Heaf multiple tuberculin test. This simple instrument has six spring-loaded needles which introduce undiluted tuberculin (PPD 100,000IU per ml) into the skin. The depth of penetration can be adjusted; 1 mm is recommended for infants and 2 mm for older children and adults. A drop of undiluted PPD (100,000IU per ml) is applied to the cleansed dry skin of the forearm. The instrument is applied at right angles to the skin and the end plate firmly pressed on the centre of the film of tuberculin. The release of the mechanism allows the needles to pierce the skin and carry with them some tuberculin. The test, which is at least as strong as a Mantoux 10IU test, is read after 48–96 hours. There are four well-defined grades of reaction (see **314**).

314 Results of multiple puncture tuberculin test (Heaf test), read 4–7 days after puncture.

Reactions are graded as follows:

0 No reaction or up to three discrete papules
1 Four or more discrete papules
2 Confluent papules to form a ring
3 A disc of induration
4 Induration greater than 10 mm or vesiculation

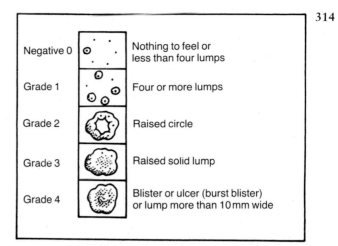

Negative 0		Nothing to feel or less than four lumps
Grade 1		Four or more lumps
Grade 2		Raised circle
Grade 3		Raised solid lump
Grade 4		Blister or ulcer (burst blister) or lump more than 10 mm wide

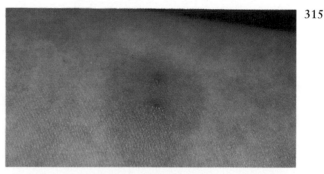

315

315   Heaf test – grade 1. Discrete palpable induration at four or more of the puncture points.

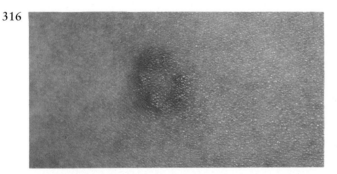

316

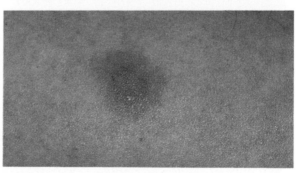

317

316   Heaf test – grade 2. The papules are larger and have coalesced to form a ring.

317   Heaf test – grade 3. More intense induration. The papules are larger still and have formed a solid central plaque.

318   Heaf test – grade 4. Extensive induration greater than 10 mm, or vesiculation and surrounding erythema. This is a severe reaction. The plaque is surmounted by vesicles which have fused, resulting in early central ulceration with lymphangitis and regional lymphadenitis.

When tuberculosis is suspected, Mantoux PPD 1IU should be used as a first test to prevent unnecessarily severe reactions.

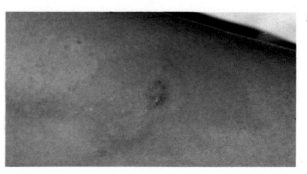

318

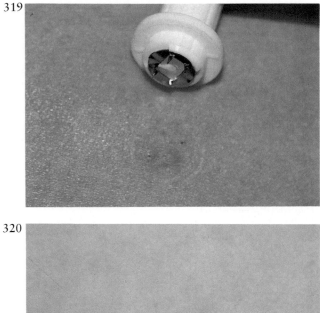

319

319 **The tuberculin tine test** is a disposable multi-puncture test comparable to a Mantoux 5IU PPD test. The four tines, coated with highly purified undiluted old tuberculin (OT), are firmly pressed on the skin of the forearm for 2 seconds. When the unit is lifted, there are four visible puncture sites. The reaction, ranging from grade 1 to grade 4, is similar to that obtained by the Heaf test and is measured after 48 hours.

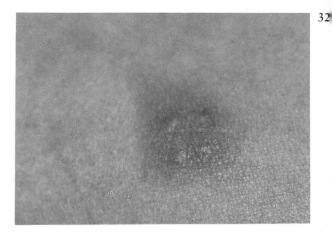

320 **Tine test – grade 1.** Palpable induration around at least two puncture sites.

321 **Tine test – grade 2.** The papules just touch. If there are four papules, they are found to form a four-leafed clover shape with a central depression.

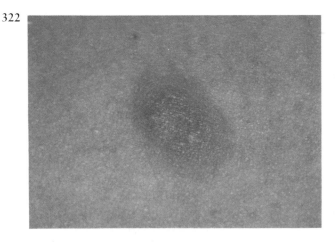

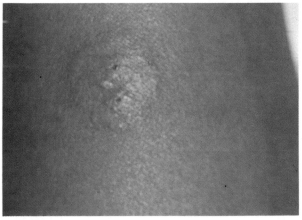

322 **Tine test – grade 3.** The papules are larger and have filled in the centre to form a solid plaque.

323 **Tine test – grade 4.** A plaque surmounted by vesicles at the original puncture points.

BCG vaccination

The organism used in this vaccine is derived from an attenuated strain of the bovine bacillus originally developed by Calmette and Guérin. The vaccine has been widely used throughout the world and the indications for its use vary considerably according to the epidemiology of tuberculosis. Tuberculin testing before vaccination is undertaken in the UK (except in the newborn). Individuals whose Heaf test grade is 0–1 or whose Mantoux test reaction to 10IU is less than 6mm in induration are eligible for BCG. Vaccination is contraindicated if there is hypogammaglobulinaemia, in atopic patients with eczema and in patients with AIDS, tuberculosis or positive tuberculin tests. The vaccine provides protection from the complications of primary tuberculosis.

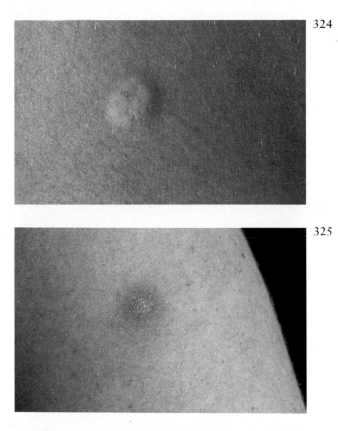
324

324 Intradermal immunisation using BCG vaccination. The vaccine must be injected strictly intradermally, avoiding subcutaneous injection as this may result in abscesses and ulceration. A separate 1ml syringe and short, bevelled 25 gauge needle are used for each patient and 0.1ml of vaccine is injected into the superficial layers of the dermis, raising a blanched skin weal of about 7mm in size. The preferred injection site is at the insertion of the deltoid muscle into the humerus.

A cutaneous primary complex forms at the vaccination site. After about a week a small swelling appears at the injection site, progressing to a papule or to a benign ulcer approximately 10mm in diameter after 3 weeks and healing in 6–12 weeks. A dry dressing should be used if the ulcer discharges, but the air should not be excluded.

It is estimated that BCG confers an 80% protection against tuberculosis and this lasts for about 15 years.

In developing countries BCG vaccination can provide a cheap and effective method of reducing the incidence of tuberculosis. Vaccinations against smallpox, polio or yellow fever within the previous 3 weeks constitute relative contraindications to BCG vaccination. The World Health Organisation recommends BCG vaccination at birth in all developing countries.

325

325 BCG fourth week. Indurated papule which becomes scaly and may ulcerate.

326

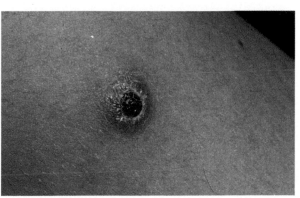

326 BCG sixth week. Crusting and a dry scab develop.

327

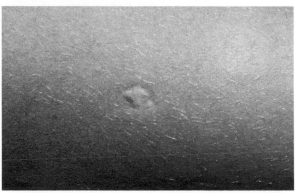

327 BCG scar. The ulcer heals leaving a depressed white scar.

Adverse reactions to BCG vaccination

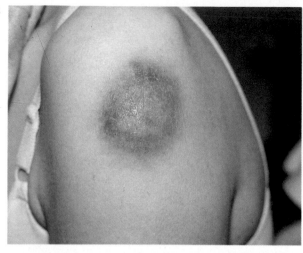

Large ulcers or abscesses can form following inadvertent subcutaneous injection of the vaccine. Local lymphadenitis is rare and more likely to occur in infants. Local secondary infection is the most common complication and can be controlled with courses of erythromycin. Keloid scarring tends to occur in dark-skinned individuals and where injection is administered on the shoulder tip. Disseminated BCG in immunologically deficient subjects and anaphylactic reactions are rare complications.

328 BCG abscess. This indolent abscess developed at the site of BCG injection 2 years after vaccination.

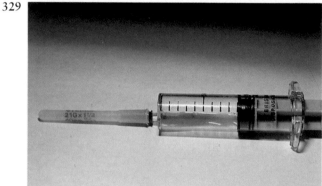

329 BCG pus aspirated from arm of patient shown in **328**.

Indications for BCG vaccination in the UK

- Hospital workers (doctors, nurses, laboratory staff).
- Travellers to areas of high prevalence.
- Immigrants from areas of high prevalence.
- Infants born of African or Asian parents.
- Schoolchildren aged 11–14 years (about 5% of UK children are tuberculin positive at this age.

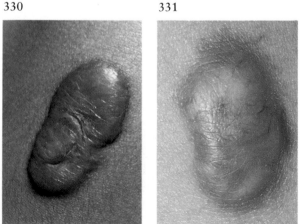

330, 331   Post BCG vaccination keloid scars.

17 Other infections

Coccidioidomycosis

Coccidioidomycosis is an infectious disease that is caused by *Coccidioides immitis,* a saprophytic fungus which normally dwells in alkaline soils of semi-arid regions of the Americas. It is endemic to parts of California, Arizona, New Mexico, Texas, Nevada and Utah (see **332**). Synonyms include San Joaquin fever, valley fever or desert rheumatism.

C. immitis is dimorphic, existing in living tissues as spherules, and as a mycelial form in soils and on routine culture, where it grows as a mould with septate hyphae. Certain hyphae form thick-walled, barrel-like, 2×5μm arthroconidia (spores) that are extremely resistant to drying and are gas-filled, rendering them so light that the merest breeze secures airborne dissemination. Inhaled arthroconidia that survive phagocytosis grow as spherules, reproductive structures 50–100μm in diameter that on maturation release as many as 10^5 endospores, each 2–3μm in diameter. Endospores that are not expectorated or destroyed by the host form new spherules.

In some patients the evidence for infection is the development of precipitating antibodies and positive skin tests, while others will develop an influenza-like illness with fever, malaise and arthralgia. Hypersensitivity reactions with erythema nodosum may develop in 5–10% of infected individuals. Although most infections are mild and self-limiting, *C. immitis* may cause persistent and chronic progressive pneumonia or fatal widely disseminated miliary disease, especially in the immunocompromised.

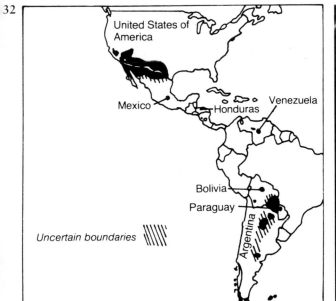

332   Distribution of coccidioidomycosis (shaded areas).

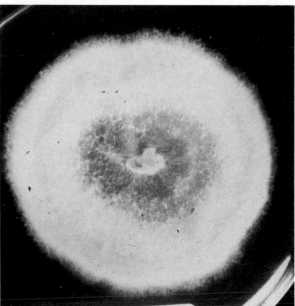

333   *Coccidioides immitis* grows on culture as white-to-tan fluffy mycelium composed of septate hyphae. The culture has no specific characteristics and therefore identification is made by demonstrating spherules in the tissues of an infected host.

334

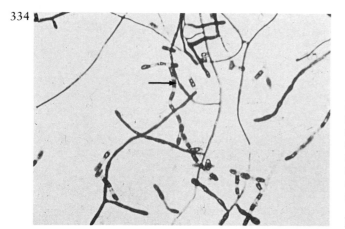

334 *Coccidioides immitis* **hyphae** form alternating arthro-spores and empty cells (arrowed). The arthrospores are light and, if inhaled, are highly infectious, developing into tissue spherules. They are produced on specialised lateral branches of the vegetative hyphae. The fertile part of these branches expands and septation occurs. Alternate cells grow larger and develop into arthrospores, while cells between the spores lose cytoplasm.

Arthrospores have the ability to change into spherules in host tissue and also in special culture conditions.

335

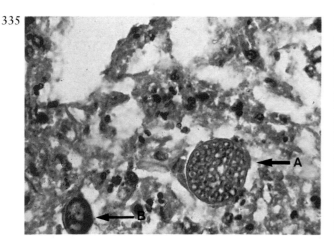

335 *Coccidioides immitis* **mature spherule with endo-spores (arrow A).** Tissue from a lung biopsy. Spherules vary from 20 to 100μm in diameter and develop only in animal hosts. When mature, up to 10 endospores may be released. An immature spherule is also shown (arrow B). It has a clear centre with peripheral cytoplasm and a prominent thick wall. (H & E × 100.)

33

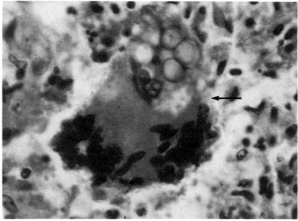

336 *Coccidioides immitis* granuloma with spherules. A lung biopsy from a patient with pulmonary coccidioido-mycosis. This spherule has ruptured (arrowed) and only a small portion of the wall remains. The spherules lie adjacent to a Langhans' giant cell. (H & E × 200.)

337

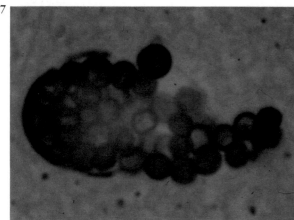

337 *Coccidioides immitis.* Percutaneous needle biopsy aspiration specimen showing the ruptured wall of the mature spherule and mass of endospores. (Grocott × 200.)

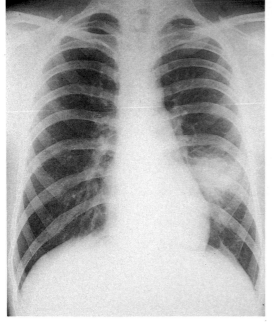

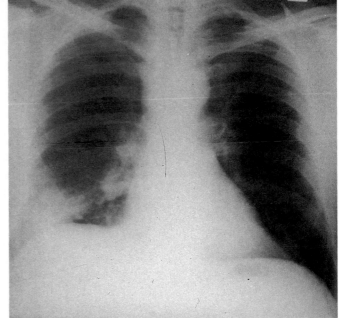

338 **Chronic coccidioidomycosis.** This coin lesion was a coccidioidoma. The diagnosis was made by aspiration needle biopsy.

339 **Acute coccidioidomycosis** with hilar and paratracheal lymphadenopathy and right basal pneumonia. Effusions may also occur.

Skin test
Delayed hypersensitivity to intradermal injection of coccidioidin (a filtrate of broth culture of *C. immitis*) or spherulin (a sterile filtrate from culture spherules) develops 3 days to 3 weeks after the onset of symptoms. Maximum induration is reached 24–48 hours after injection. IgM precipitins are detectable in 90% of patients within 4 weeks of infection and are followed by complement-fixing IgG antibodies. The persistence of precipitins or increasing titres of complement-fixing antibodies are associated with dissemination and a poor prognosis.

Histoplasmosis

Histoplasmosis occurs in many parts of the world and is endemic in central and eastern states of the USA, Canada, the Far East and Australia.

The causative organism is the dimorphic fungus *Histoplasma capsulatum*, which can be isolated from soil that has been contaminated by bird and bat droppings. In its mycelial phase the fungus produces spores of two sizes; microconidia (2–5μm in diameter) are infectious whereas the macroconidia (8–14μm in diameter) are not. If inhaled into the lungs, the microconidia germinate to a yeast form which attracts and is phagocytosed by macrophages. A granulomatous response is typical, sometimes with caseation and healing by fibrosis. The initial respiratory infection may be followed by widespread dissemination to the reticuloendothelial system.

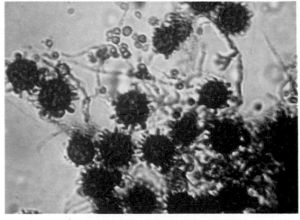

340 *Histoplasma capsulatum.* Mycelial phase with microconidia and macroconidia (Sabouraud's medium 25°C.)

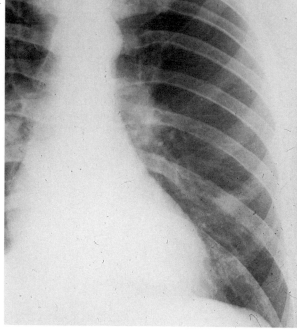

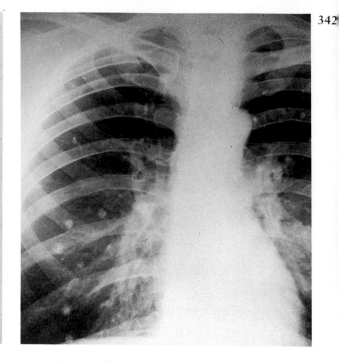

341 Primary pulmonary histoplasmosis. Primary contact with *H. capsulatum* may result in a transient influenza-like respiratory tract infection or, less commonly, pneumonia. Lassitude may be severe. This patient suffered an attack of suspected 'viral pneumonia' after exploring caves in Venezuela. One month later there was a small primary lesion in the left lower lobe and left hilar lymph node enlargement; a histoplasmin skin test became positive. The primary lesion and associated hilar lymphadenopathy are reminiscent of the primary complex of tuberculosis.

342 Primary pulmonary histoplasmosis. Severe infections lead to an acute bronchopneumonia which may follow a protracted course, healing with residual fibrosis and multiple calcified lesions ('buck shot' calcification). Chronic pulmonary histoplasmosis with cavitation and progressive fibrosis is common in patients with chronic airways disease, resembles pulmonary tuberculosis and may lead to respiratory failure. Disseminated histoplasmosis is uncommon, affects those with defective cell-mediated host immunity and is variable in severity.

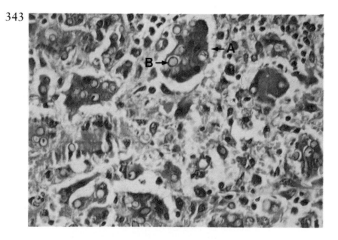

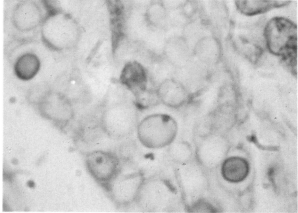

343 A chronic granuloma caused by *Histoplasma capsulatum.* The reticuloendothelial system is particularly involved by histoplasmosis, with fever, lymphadenopathy, splenomegaly and anaemia. Granulomata may develop in the tissues (arrowed A). *H. capsulatum* lies within numerous foreign body giant cells (arrowed B).

344 *Histoplasma capsulatum* in the lung. Spherical uninuclear yeast cells with irregularly distributed cytoplasm and thick double contoured walls. The cell wall stains poorly, giving the impression of a capsule. (H & E × 1000.)

Pulmonary aspergillosis

Aspergillus fumigatus, a ubiquitous mould of decaying vegetation, and, less commonly, other species of aspergillus (*A. clavatus, A. flavus, A. niger, A. terreus*) cause a variety of respiratory disorders. The fungi liberate an abundance of respirable spores which, if inhaled, may cause a hypersensitivity immediate type I (asthmatic) or type III reaction between the spores and circulating antibodies.

Aspergillosis, the disease caused by the fungus, may present in the following forms:

1 Allergic aspergillosis.
  - Bronchial asthma.
  - Allergic bronchopulmonary aspergillosis.
  - Allergic alveolitis.
2 Colonising aspergilloma.
3 Locally invasive aspergillosis.
4 Disseminated aspergillosis.

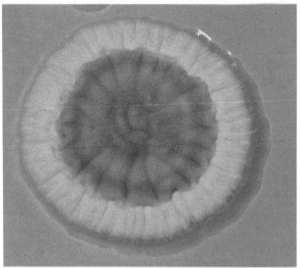

345 *Aspergillus fumigatus.* Grey-green colonies with a central dome of conidiophores (fruiting heads). Sabouraud's medium incubated at 37–40°C.

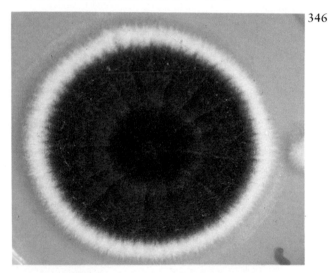

346 *Aspergillus niger.* Black colonies. Sabouraud's medium incubated at 37–40°C.

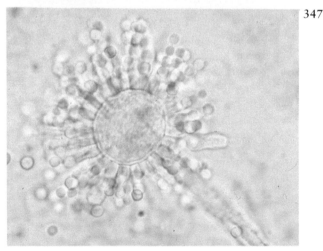

347 *Aspergillus fumigatus.* Conidiophore and chains of conidia (spores)×40.

Aspergillus spores are 2–3μm in diameter and readily respirable. Their size and the wide temperature range in which they can grow make the spores of *A. fumigatus* uniquely suited for colonisation of the human bronchial tree, where they germinate and form vegetative elements (hyphae).

Allergic bronchopulmonary aspergillosis (ABPA)

The diagnosis of ABPA should be suspected in any asthmatic patient who has an abnormal chest radiograph and a high peripheral blood eosinophil count. The diagnostic criteria include:

1 Asthma (in the majority of cases).
2 Peripheral blood eosinophilia of $>0.5 \times 10^9$/litre.
3 Presence or history of chest radiographic abnormalities.
4 Positive skin test to an extract of *A. fumigatus*.
5 Serum precipitating antibodies to *A. fumigatus*.
6 Elevated total serum IgE, significantly higher than in uncomplicated bronchial asthma.
7 Fungal hyphae of *A. fumigatus* on microscopic examination of sputum.

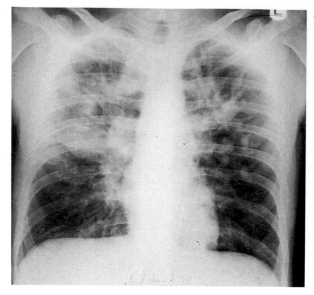

348 **Allergic bronchopulmonary aspergillosis.** Widespread non-segmental predominantly upper zone shadows caused by eosinophilic pneumonia in a long-standing case of allergic aspergillosis. Malaise and fever are usual, although this patient was symptom free.

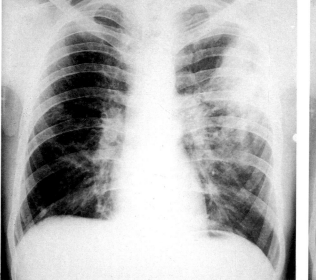

349 **Allergic bronchopulmonary aspergillosis.** Spontaneous clearing of most of the shadowing seen in 348 within a month. The fleeting nature of the shadowing is often emphasised, but fixed abnormal shadows may be found. Mucus impaction from masses of fungal mycelium blocks a segment of the left upper lobe.

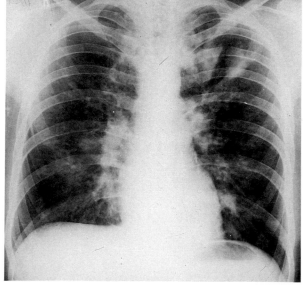

350 **Allergic bronchopulmonary aspergillosis.** Clearing of shadowing seen in 349 with corticosteroids. The mucus plug seen in the left upper zone was expectorated. Recurrent attacks leave a characteristic pattern of proximal bronchiectasis in their wake.

351 Bronchogram showing proximal bronchiectasis caused by allergic bronchopulmonary aspergillosis. Bronchial wall fibrosis may occur where mucus plugs have occluded the bronchi to provoke immune-based inflammation and produce tissue damage. Type III immune reactivity is evident from bronchial wall damage, pulmonary infiltrates, delayed type skin tests, precipitating antibodies and elevated serum aspergillus specific IgG. The presence of granulomas in the bronchi and lung indicates cell-mediated type IV reactivity.

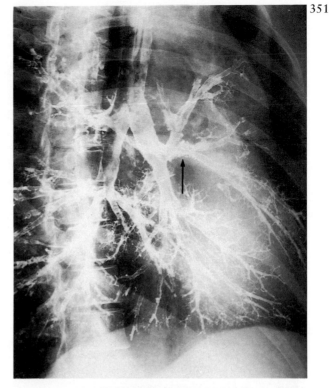

351

352 Allergic bronchopulmonary aspergillosis. The scan (at carina level) shows a marked degree of dilatation of the lobar and segmental bronchi from near their points of origin. This proximal dilatation of larger bronchi, especially in the upper lobes, is more common in ABPA than in any other condition. The bronchial tree is usually normal beyond the areas of dilatation and the lung parenchyma is not often involved in secondary changes.

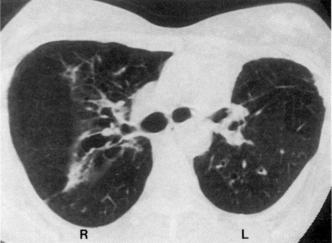

352

353 Skin prick sensitivity to aspergillus. Asthma is the most common disorder associated with *A. fumigatus*, and sensitisation is most frequent in atopic individuals with coincident sensitivity to pollen or dust. *A. fumigatus* colonises the bronchial tree, giving rise to a complex series of immunological reactions and presenting with asthma, eosinophilia and pulmonary infiltrates. Aspergillus is found in sputum and bronchial washings. The eosinophilia, asthma, elevated serum IgE levels, aspergillus specific IgE and positive immediate type skin test all reflect type I reactivity. (A, control: B, house dust mite; C, grass pollen; D, tree pollen; E, *Aspergillus fumigatus*.)

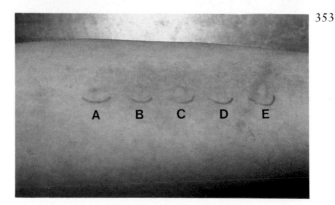

353

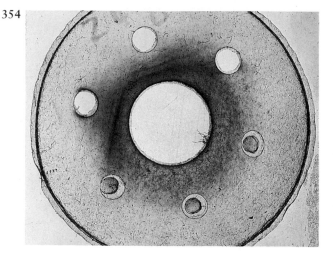

354 Allergic bronchopulmonary aspergillosis – precipitin arcs. Serum antibodies to *A. fumigatus*. Precipitating antibodies to *A. fumigatus* of IgG type are present in the serum of two-thirds of patients with allergic aspergillosis. The presence of precipitating antibodies is not diagnostic of aspergillosis since precipitins may be found in healthy individuals. The number of precipitin arcs varies from 1 to 3. Aspergillus antigen extracts are placed in the peripheral agar wells, and the patient's serum in the central well. As diffusion occurs through the agar disc, lines of precipitate form in the region where the serum antibodies and extract antigen are in optimal concentration. This stain preparation exhibits three 'weak' precipitin lines directed against two of the antigens. (Ouchterlony's method, amido schwartz stain, transmitted light.)

Colonising aspergillosis

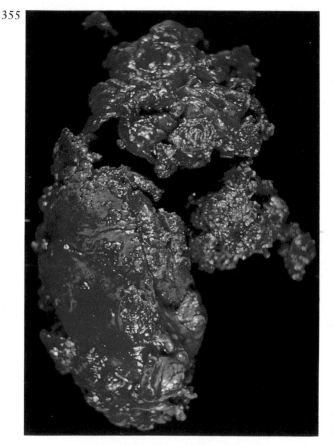

A. fumigatus is the most common organism to colonise abnormal cavities or spaces in the bronchi, lungs or pleural space, leading to the formation of a mass or ball of fungus (aspergilloma). Aspergillomas are often asymptomatic and most commonly occur in the upper lobe, the site most frequently cavitated by healed pulmonary tuberculosis. Growth of *A. fumigatus* within the body occurs only in the presence of oxygen. The aspergillomas are brownish yellow or green in colour and bounded by a fibrous wall.

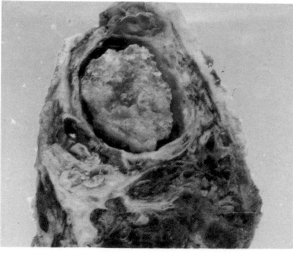

355 Aspergilloma. It consists of a mass of mycelium lying within a pulmonary cavity.

356 Aspergilloma (mycetoma). Whole lung section showing a large cavity in the upper lobe occupied by a large fungal ball (mycetoma). One of the special features of *A. fumigatus* is that it is able to maintain growth within the lung. The mycelium grows within pre-existing bullae or cavities in areas of destroyed lung.

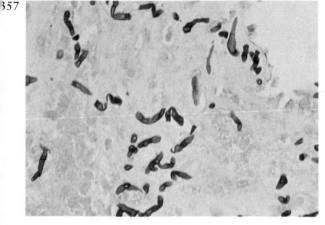

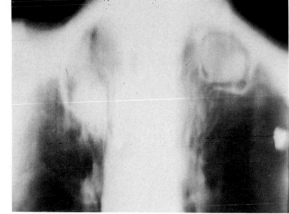

357 Aspergilloma. Fungal hyphae in sputum from a patient with an aspergilloma. Fungal filaments tend to be small and single and the hyphae appear to have abraded ends. (Grocott×140.)

358 Bilateral apical pulmonary aspergilloma. Note the transradiant halo of air surrounding the fungus ball (mycetoma) in this tomogram.

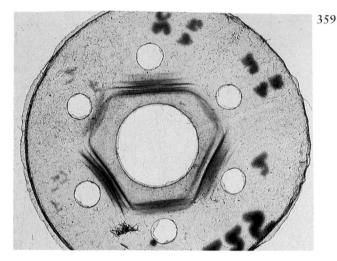

359 Serum antibodies to *Aspergillus fumigatus*. Precipitating antibodies to *A. fumigatus* are present in almost all patients colonised with aspergillus. Multiple precipitin arcs are usually seen. Skin tests for *A. fumigatus* are unlikely to be positive. The immune reaction fades and the precipitins usually become negative when a mycetoma is removed. This test shows five or six precipitin lines directed against four of the aspergillus antigens. (Ouchterlony's method, amido schwartz stain, transmitted light.)

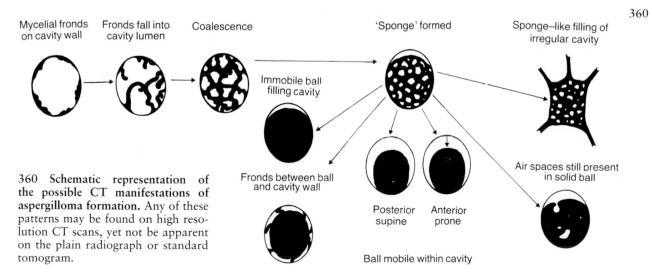

360 Schematic representation of the possible CT manifestations of aspergilloma formation. Any of these patterns may be found on high resolution CT scans, yet not be apparent on the plain radiograph or standard tomogram.

361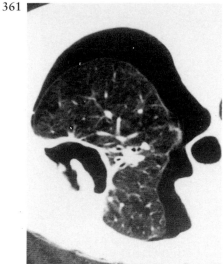

364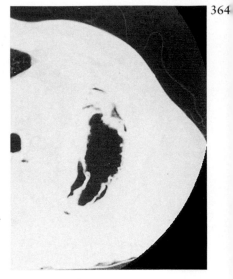

361–363 Mycetoma formation. These three CT scans at adjacent levels show an old tuberculous cavity in the right upper lobe, in which a mycetoma developed. In **361** a mycelial mass projects into the cavity, appearing like a frond or finger. In **362** the mass reaches the opposite wall of the cavity and in **363** it appears as a solid ball of mycelia containing a small transradiancy of enclosed air. The air around the mass will be seen as the halo or air crescent sign on the radiograph. (A shallow pneumothorax is also present on the right.)

364 Mycetoma. There was no evidence of a mycetoma within the large left-sided cavity on the radiograph, although the sputum and precipitins were positive. The CT scan shows the grossly contracted left hemithorax and the very large left upper zone cavity. The cavity walls are lined by a number of irregular sheets of mycelia, invisible by any other non-invasive method of investigation.

365, 366 Mycetoma. A homogeneous rounded opacity lies on the posterior wall of a large cavity in the left upper lobe in the supine CT scan (**365**). By repeating the scan in the prone position (**366**), the mass falls away from the posterior wall to be arrested anteriorly where the cavity is narrower. This degree of mobility is typical of mycetomas (on very rare occasions, intracavity mobility of a mass may be due to carcinoma, haematoma or inspissated pus).

362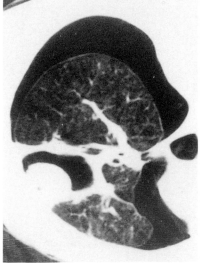

365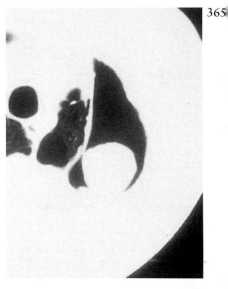

363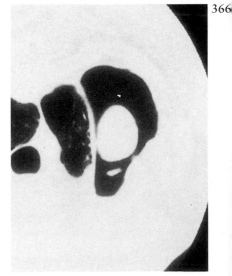

366

Invasive aspergillosis

This is an uncommon but serious form of pulmonary mycosis in which fungal infections spread throughout the lungs, producing granulomata and necrotic and suppurative lesions. Invasive aspergillosis can be rapidly progressive, causing extensive pulmonary damage (necrotising aspergillosis) and death within a few days. Fulminating invasive aspergillosis can be accompanied terminally by blood-borne dissemination.

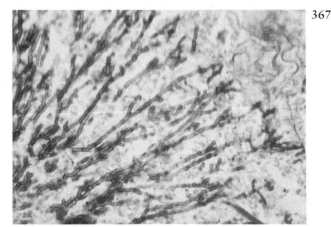

367 Invasive aspergillosis. Microscopic appearance of sputum from patients with invasive aspergillosis, showing an abundance of freely branching luxuriant fungal hyphae.

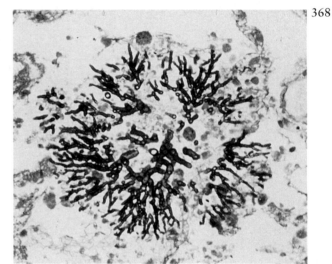

368 Invasive aspergillosis of lung. A profusion of dichotomously branching filaments in the lung, with a characteristic radial or 'sunburst' arrangement of the mycelium. (H & E and GMS×100.)

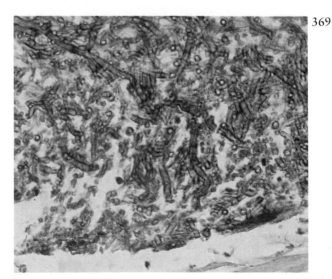

369 Invasive aspergillosis of pleural space. Densely packed branching fungal hyphae occupying multiple abscess cavities and limited inferiorly by the pleura.

Actinomycosis

Actinomycosis is a chronic suppurative infection caused by *Actinomyces israelii* and related anaerobic filamentous bacteria. These organisms are saprophytes which normally reside in the mouth, gastro-intestinal tract and female genital tract. Infection is invariably endogenous and cervicofacial infections are most common but, rarely, the lungs or abdomen may be affected.

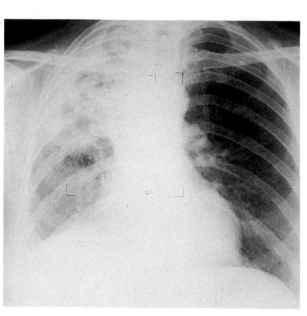

370

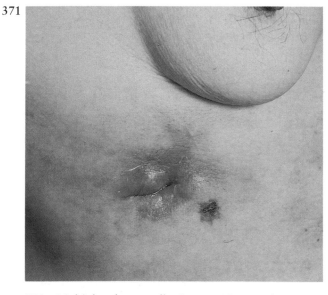

371

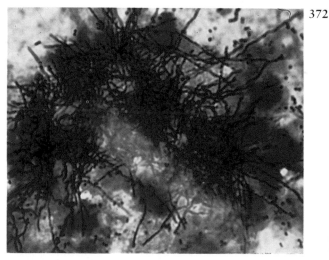

372

370 Pulmonary actinomycosis may follow aspiration of saliva into the lungs. Low-grade pneumonitis develops with fever and a productive cough, followed by spread to the pleura resulting in empyema and sinuses of the chest wall. Cavitating lung disease may occur.

For the development of actinomycosis to take place, two events must occur: tissue damage sufficient to provide a focus of diminished oxidation–reduction potential and inoculation with actinomyces species. *A. israelii* is seldom present as the only pathogen and actinomycotic lesions usually culture a mixture of aerobic and anaerobic bacteria.

371 Multiple chest wall sinuses. Untreated actinomycosis will lead to chronic persistent infection. Periosteal reactions may result in new bone formation on the undersurface of the ribs. Treatment is by surgical drainage of the infection and prolonged intravenous administration of penicillin in high doses for 4 weeks, followed by oral penicillin for up to 6 months.

372 Actinomycosis. 'Sulphur' granules are diagnostic and consist of colonies of Gram-positive mycelial filaments surrounded by eosinophilic 'clubs'. The mycelial filaments often show irregular staining which gives a beaded appearance. The eosinophilic 'clubs' may be antigen–antibody complexes.

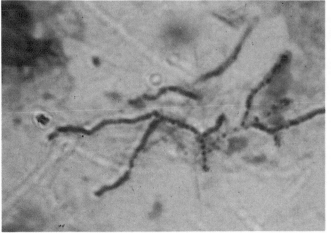

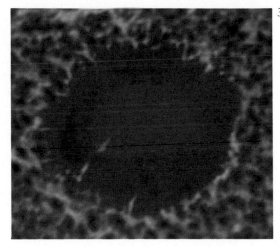

373 Actinomycosis. Gram-positive branching mycelial filaments and pus cells in sputum. Formerly thought to be a fungus, the organism is now classed as a Gram-positive branching anaerobic bacterium. (Gram-stain×960.)

374 A colony of actinomyces in the lung. In the centre is a dense mass of mycelial filaments. The periphery of radially arranged eosinophilic 'clubs' is surrounded by polymorphonuclear leucocytes. (H & E×350.)

Nocardiosis

The nocardia species are aerobic Gram-positive non-capsulated non-motile pleomorphic organisms, varying from bacillary to filamentous saprophytes. Infection may be associated with: pneumonitis; nodular, occasionally cavitating, radiographic opacities with tissue necrosis and abscess formation; pleural disease with effusions; and periosteal reactions with new bone formation and sinuses.

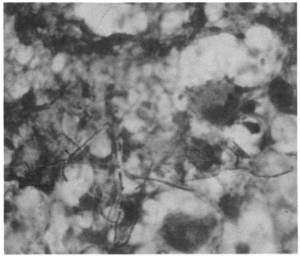

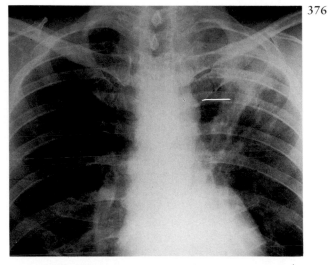

375 *Nocardia asteroides*. Filamentous organisms in pus aspirated from lung abscess (Ziehl–Nielsen stain.) The majority of infections caused by *N. asteroides* are encountered in patients with impairment of cell-mediated immunity.

376 Nocardiosis. Chest radiograph showing cavitating consolidated lesion in the left upper lobe. Tuberculosis was suspected but routine investigations and bronchoscopy failed to provide a diagnosis. Nocardiosis was found at open lung biopsy.

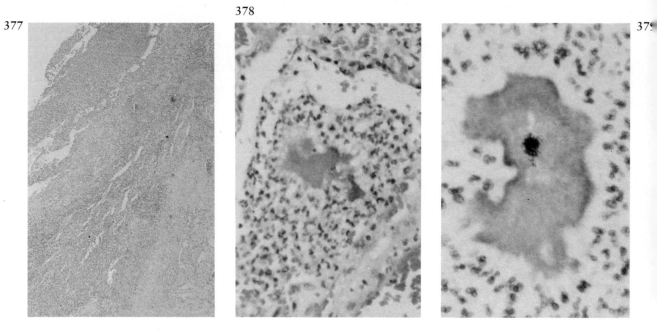

377–379 **Nocardiosis.** Abscess cavity lined by pus and granulation tissue (377), low power. High power showing 'granule' in the lung (378). Gram-positive bacilli-like organisms in 'granules' (379).

18 Parasitic diseases of the lung

Animal parasites, although a major cause of morbidity and mortality worldwide, are rarely direct causes of lung disease. Parasites can affect the lung in four ways:

1 During the migration phase of their lifecycle in the human body.
2 By embolic spread or direct extension.
3 As a primary manifestation.
4 Secondary to systemic disease.

Table 23. Parasites affecting the lung.

Parasite	Distribution	Disease	Pulmonary manifestations
1 Parasites affecting the lung during the migration phase of their lifecycle			
Nematodes			
Ascaris lumbricoides	Southeast Asia, Africa, Central and South America	Ascariasis	Pulmonary eosinophilia (Loeffler's syndrome)
Necator americanus *Ancylostoma duodenale*	Tropical and subtropical Asia and Africa, Middle East	Hookworm disease	
Strongyloides stercoralis	South America	Strongyloidiasis	
Toxocara canis *Toxocara catis*	Worldwide	Toxocariasis (visceral larva migrans)	
Wuchereria bancrofti *Brugia malayi* *Brugia pahangi*	Southeast Asia Indian subcontinent	Filariasis	Tropical pulmonary eosinophilia
Gnathostoma spinigerum	East and Southeast Asia	Gnathostomiasis	Eosinophilia, haemoptysis
Trematodes			
Paragonimus westermani Other *Paragonimus* spp.	East and Southeast Asia, Africa	Paragonimiasis	Mass shadow
Cestodes			
Echinococcus granulosus	Worldwide	Hydatid disease	Mass/cyst
Echinococcus multilocularis	Worldwide		
2 Parasites affecting the lung by embolic spread			
Protozoa			
Entamoeba histolytica	Central America, Middle East, Africa	Amoebiasis	Abscess, empyema
Toxoplasma gondii	Worldwide	Toxoplasmosis	Interstitial pneumonitis (AIDS)
Nematodes			
Trichinella spiralis	Worldwide	Trichinosis	Eosinophilia, muscle weakness
Trematodes			
Schistosoma haematobium	Africa, Middle East	Schistosomiasis	Arteritis, vascular obstruction
Schistosoma mansoni	South America, Africa	Schistosomiasis	
Metagonimus yokogaisai	East Asia	Metagonimiasis	Pulmonary granulomas
Heterophyes heterophyes	Middle East, East Asia	Heterophyiasis	
Arachnids			
Armillifer armillatus *Linguatula serrata*	Africa, South America	Pentastomiasis	Pneumonitis

Table 23. Parasites affecting the lung continued.

Parasite	Distribution	Disease	Pulmonary manifestations
3 Parasites affecting the lung as a manifestation of general disease			
Protozoa			
Pneumocystis carinii	Worldwide	Pneumocystosis	Pneumonia (AIDS)
Plasmodium falciparum	Africa, South America, Southeast Asia, Indian subcontinent	Malignant tertian malaria	Pulmonary oedema
Cryptosporidium	Worldwide	Cryptosporidiosis	Pneumonia (AIDS)

Ascariasis

Ascariasis is caused by the large roundworm *Ascaris lumbricoides* and is the most common soil transmitted intestinal helminthiasis in man. It is responsible for a large number of deaths and much morbidity worldwide. The lifecycle is shown in **380**.

Ascariasis is endemic in many countries in Africa, Asia and Central and South America.

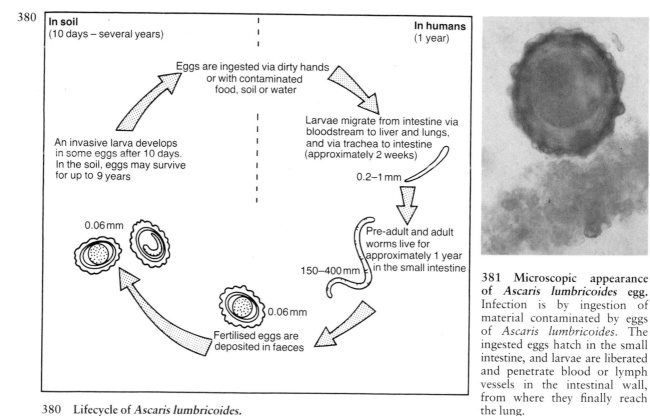

380

In soil
(10 days – several years)

In humans
(1 year)

Eggs are ingested via dirty hands or with contaminated food, soil or water

An invasive larva develops in some eggs after 10 days. In the soil, eggs may survive for up to 9 years

Larvae migrate from intestine via bloodstream to liver and lungs, and via trachea to intestine (approximately 2 weeks)

0.2–1 mm

0.06 mm

Pre-adult and adult worms live for approximately 1 year in the small intestine

150–400 mm

0.06 mm

Fertilised eggs are deposited in faeces

380   Lifecycle of *Ascaris lumbricoides*.

381   Microscopic appearance of *Ascaris lumbricoides* egg. Infection is by ingestion of material contaminated by eggs of *Ascaris lumbricoides*. The ingested eggs hatch in the small intestine, and larvae are liberated and penetrate blood or lymph vessels in the intestinal wall, from where they finally reach the lung.

382 Pulmonary eosinophilia (Loeffler's syndrome). Diffuse peripheral mottling and prominent peribronchial markings concentrated in the perihilar region.

Pneumonitis occurs 4–16 days after infection, with fever, cough, bronchospasm, expectoration, eosinophilia and pulmonary infiltration. Larvae of human or animal ascarides may be found in the sputum, and growing larval worms are sometimes expelled from the nose. The diagnosis is usually made by finding the characteristic eggs in the faeces or spontaneously expelled adult worms. Symptoms and physical signs usually disappear in a few days.

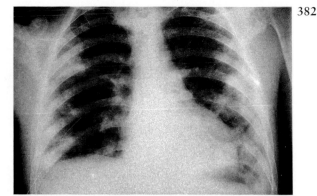

382

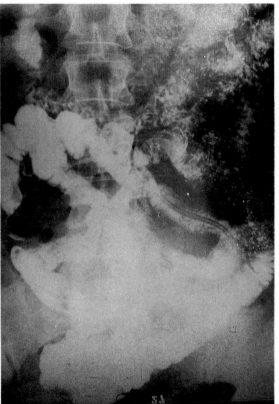

83

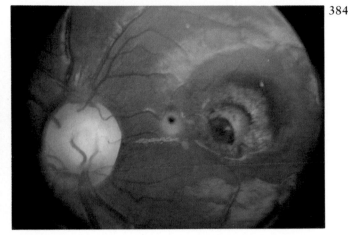

384

384 *Ascaris lumbricoides* larva lying in the fundus. Ingested eggs hatch, releasing larvae which migrate through the intestine to enter the venules or lymphatics. The larvae eventually pass into the pulmonary capillaries where they migrate into the bronchioles, reach the pharynx, and are swallowed again to reside in the intestine. As larvae migrate through the lungs, itching, wheezing, dyspnoea and angioneurotic oedema may occur. Some migrating larvae may escape the pulmonary capillary bed and reach the systemic circulation to be scattered throughout the body.

383 *Ascaris lumbricoides*. Small bowel barium contrast study showing large adult worm. Eggs are found in the stool when the larvae become adult, some 6–8 weeks after infestation.

Tropical pulmonary eosinophilia (filariasis)

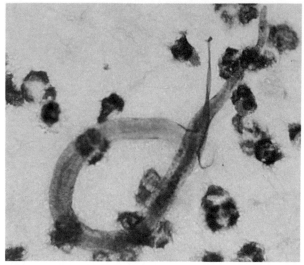

Wuchereria bancrofti and *Brugia malayi*, as well as filarial worms of animal origin, may give rise to a syndrome known as tropical pulmonary eosinophilia. Both of these parasites are borne by mosquito vectors. *W. bancrofti* occurs most frequently in India, Southeast Asia, Africa and the Pacific Islands, as well as arising in pockets of infection in the Caribbean, Egypt and South America. *B. malayi* is restricted to South India, Southeast Asia, the Philippines, China and South Korea.

The clinical features are of asthma with eosinophilia and diffuse bilateral reticular nodular shadowing in the lungs.

385 Microfilaria blood film. Microfilaria are seldom demonstrated in the blood of patients with tropical eosinophilia; the diagnosis is suggested by the clinical features and by the presence of complement-fixing antibodies for filaria and good response to antifilarial medication. The response to diethyl-carbamazine is dramatic. (May–Grunewald–Giemsa×175.)

Pulmonary dirofilariasis

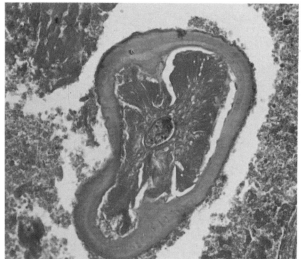

Some animal filariae occasionally infect humans, notably certain species of *Dirofilaria*. These pneumato parasites are normally found in animals including dogs, cats, rabbits, kangaroos, monkeys and racoons. The most common species, *D. immitis*, is a frequent parasite of dogs in tropical and subtropical regions; it is found in the chambers on the right side of the heart and in the pulmonary arteries and is transmitted by mosquito and, possibly, flea vectors. Humans occasionally harbour the adult filaria, but prove unsuitable hosts and the parasite soon dies. Dead worms, found in the pulmonary artery, excite thrombosis leading to infarct of the lung. Dirofilariasis may present as an asymptomatic pulmonary nodule or with chest pain, cough and haemoptysis. Subcutaneous or ocular lesions inciting a granulomatous or eosinophilic reaction may occur.

Human pulmonary dirofilariasis occurs mainly in southeastern states of the USA, Japan and Australia.

386 *Dirofilaria immitis.* Open lung excised biopsy specimen of a suspicious pulmonary nodule.

Hydatid disease

Hydatid disease is a zoonosis caused by various species of the tapeworm *Echinococcus*, the normal lifecycle of which involves carnivores and their prey. Two species commonly infect man: *E. granulosus* and *E. multilocularis*. The lifecycle is summarised in **387**. Humans are usually infected by handling dogs, and the disease is most common in sheep-rearing countries.

Pulmonary hydatid cysts may be detected by chance or with features of a lung abscess. Rarely, hydatids may rupture with acute expectoration of salty hydatid cyst fluid containing scolices.

The radiographic appearance varies. Some cysts appear as single or multiple rounded well-defined, dense masses, while in others a crescent of air is visible between the hydatid and the compressed surrounding lung – the 'pulmonary meniscus' sign. If the cyst ruptures, the radiograph may show a fluid level in the lesion, sometimes with the membrane floating on the surface – the 'water lily' sign.

When hydatid pulmonary disease is suspected, an intradermal Casoni test can be performed, although immunoelectrophoresis or enzyme immunoassay test for a specific circulating antigen are more satisfactory.

Surgery is required when symptoms occur, often supplemented by medical treatment with mebendazole or albendazole for 8–12 weeks. Cure rates are low, although a majority show some improvement.

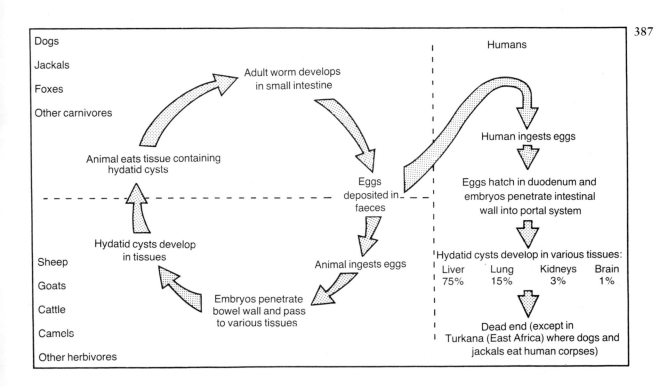

387

387 **Lifecycle of *Echinococcus granulosus*.** The lifecycle of *E. multilocularis* is similar, but the eggs are usually ingested by rodents.

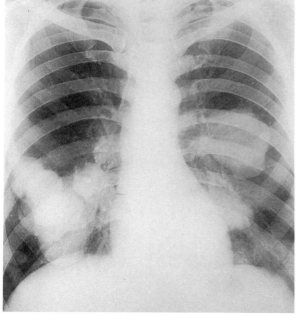

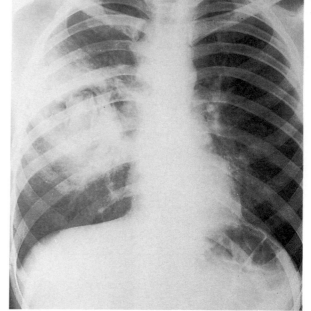

388   Multiple hydatid cysts. No complication is present. The cysts are usually smooth and spherical, but superimposition or distortion by adjacent structures may give a false impression of nodulation or other irregularity (calcification of hydatid cysts within the lung parenchyma is rare).

389   Hydatid cyst. The right-sided cyst has ruptured into a bronchus, causing detachment of the ectocyst from the adventitia. The two layers are separated by a crescent of air. The lung parenchyma is infected and there is consolidation adjacent to the upper and lower poles of the cyst.

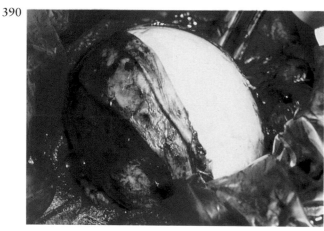

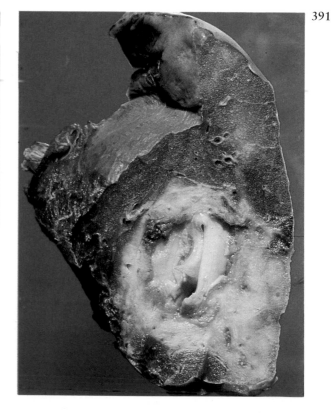

390   Surgical enucleation of a large hydatid cyst from the right lung. Simple cysts may be removed along with the adventitial membrane. During surgery it is important to protect the pleura from contamination by spilled cyst fluid. Larger or complicated cysts may require segmental or lobar resection.

391   Lobectomy specimen showing a large hydatid cyst. Note the thin, white adventitial layer of cyst and the surrounding pneumonia.

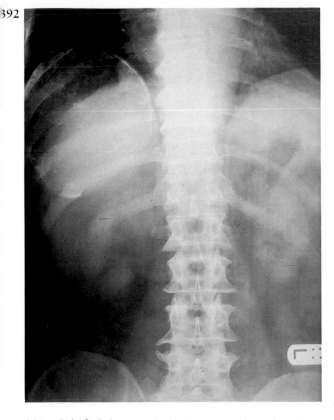

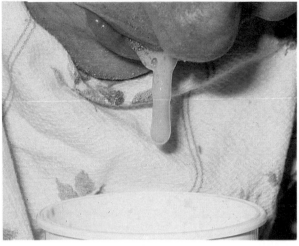

393 Cholangiopulmonary fistula. Yellow, frothy bile-stained fluid from a ruptured hepatic hydatid cyst has drained through the diaphragm, pleura and lung.

392 Calcified hepatic hydatid cyst. When the chest physician suspects pulmonary hydatid disease, a liver ultrasound scan is worthwhile because these cysts are multisystemic.

Amoebiasis

Amoebiasis is caused by *Entamoeba histolytica*, a protozoan with a cystic and a trophozoite stage.

E. histolytica has a worldwide distribution but is more prevalent in the tropics. The disease is usually transmitted by excreted cysts in the faecally contaminated material. Ingested cysts release trophozoites in the small intestine to be carried in the faecal stream into the caecum. The initial lesion is a small focus of necrosis in the large intestine, which develops into a characteristic undermined sharply defined ulcer. The crater of the ulcer contains trophozoites, which may metastasise to the liver, lung and other extraintestinal sites.

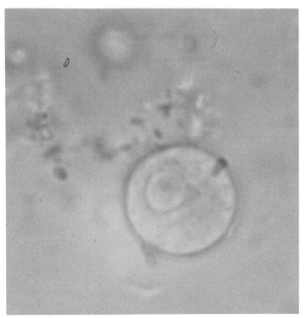

394 *Entamoeba histolytica.* Excreted cysts.

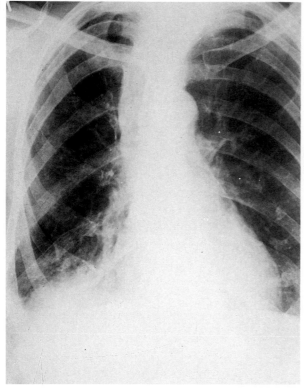

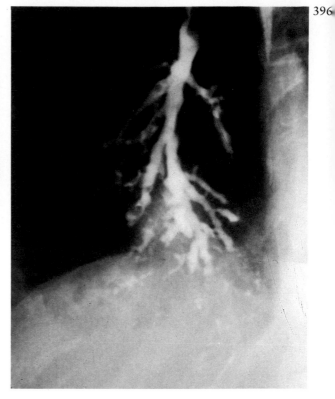

395 Pleuropulmonary amoebiasis. Cholangiopulmonary fistula. Typically, an amoebic hepatic abscess ruptures into the pleura (causing an amoebic pleural effusion) or into the lung (resulting in a hepatobronchial fistula with expectoration of amoebic 'anchovy paste' pus).

396 Pleuropulmonary amoebiasis. Radio-opaque dye demonstrating an amoebic hepatic abscess and broncho-pleural fistula.

Schistosomiasis

Schistosomiasis (bilharziasis) comprises a group of diseases that may affect the genitourinary and gastro-intestinal systems and are caused by trematodes of the genus *Schistosoma*. The three most common species that infect man are *S. haematobium S. mansoni* and *S. japonicum*. The lifecycles of the three species are similar (**397**). Humans are the definitive host and are infected by contact with fresh water containing schistosome cercaria. Cases are reported mainly in Egypt and South America. Most adult *S. haematobium* live in the bladder, prostatic and uterine plexus of veins; *S. mansoni* inhabit tributaries of the inferior mesenteric veins; and *S. japonicum* inhabit venules of the superior and inferior mesenteric veins.

Infection may be considered as:

Stage 1. Primary infection. Itching, with an erythematous papular rash, may develop at the time of the skin penetration by the cercaria (swimmers' itch).

Stage 2. Acute schistosomiasis (Katayama fever) after approximately 4–6 weeks, characterised by fever, severe toxaemia, cough, arthralgia, hepato-splenomegaly and eosinophilia.

Stage 3. The effect of the lesions and resulting complications caused by a host reaction to the eggs in the urinary bladder, intestines, liver, lungs and other systems of the body appear 3 months to several years after infection. The eggs reach the pulmonary circulation as emboli, obstruct the small arterioles and pass through their walls to lie immediately outside them. The resulting reaction around the eggs forms the characteristic schisto-somal granuloma. The types of lesion produced are arterial and parenchymatous.

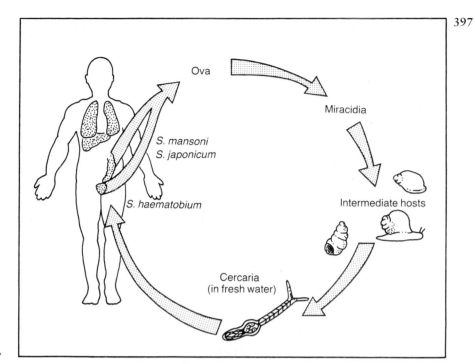

397 Lifecycle of *Schistosoma*.

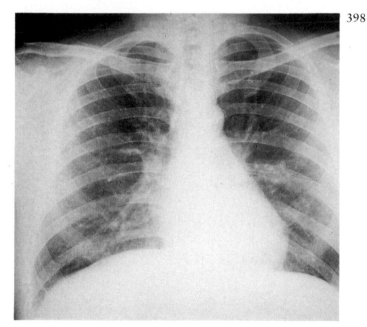

398 Pulmonary schistosomiasis chest x-ray. Progressive diffuse interstitial pulmonary fibrosis, with slight prominence of the pulmonary artery indicating pulmonary hypertension.

Eggs reach the pulmonary circulation either through the portosystemic collateral circulation in *S. mansoni* and *S. japonicum* infections, or through anastomosis between the vesical plexus of veins and the inferior vena cava in *S. haematobium* infections.

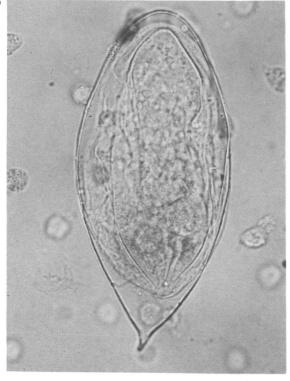

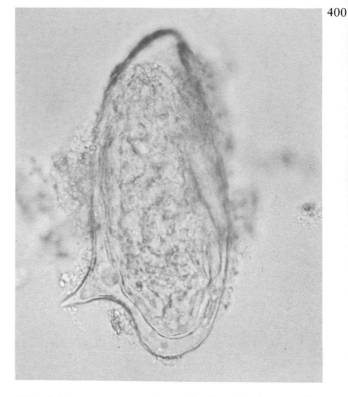

399 *Schistosoma haematobium* **egg.** Confirmation by finding terminally spined eggs in the urine.

400 *Schistosoma mansoni* **egg.** Confirmation by detecting laterally spined eggs in the stool.

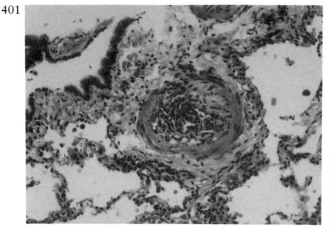

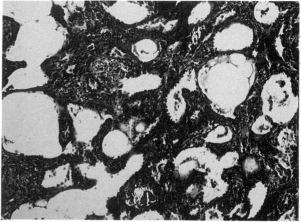

401 Pulmonary schistosomiasis. Arterial lesion in a small branch of the pulmonary artery showing fibroelastosis and surrounding chronic inflammatory cell infiltration. The passage of eggs causes necrosis of the arterial walls. This is followed by healing with thickening, narrowing and, finally, occlusion of the vessels, with restriction of the capacity of the pulmonary vascular bed. Consequently, the pulmonary pressure rises and eventually the pulmonary artery dilates and may reach aneurysmal size (schistosomal cor pulmonale).

402 Pulmonary schistosomiasis, parenchymatous lesions. Extravascular granulomas form around eggs lying close to the bronchioles and alveoli. Much granulomatous tissue may cause extensive lung scarring. These patients may present with bronchial asthma, bronchitis, bronchiectasis or pulmonary emphysema.

Malignant tertian malaria

Infection with *Plasmodium falciparum* may cause a severe and potentially fatal form of malaria. Dramatic deterioration due to the very high number of parasites in the blood may result in pulmonary oedema, anaemia and renal failure. Pulmonary and cerebral oedema are invariably present in fatal cases of *P. falciparum* malaria. The neutrophils are sequestered in pulmonary capillaries, probably triggering increased vascular permeability which is severe enough to cause pulmonary oedema resembling the adult respiratory distress syndrome.

Symptoms are caused only by asexual infection of red cells. The intraerythrocytic parasite may differentiate into sexual parasites: the gametocytes which, if ingested by the mosquito, may transmit the infection to others; and merozoites which go on to infect circulating red cells. Symptoms usually appear 7–14 days after an infecting bite, but may be delayed for up to 6 months.

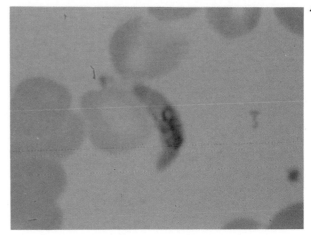

403 *Plasmodium falciparum* gametocyte in blood film. The crescent or banana shape is characteristic.

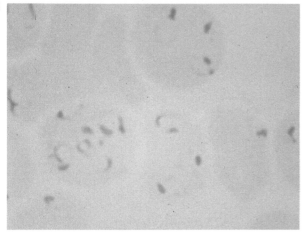

404 *Plasmodium falciparum.* Multiple intraerythrocytic parasites (ring forms).

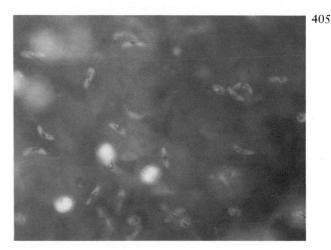

405 *Plasmodium falciparum* granulocytes in Buffy coat (acridyl orange fluorescent stain).

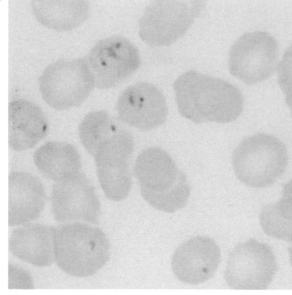

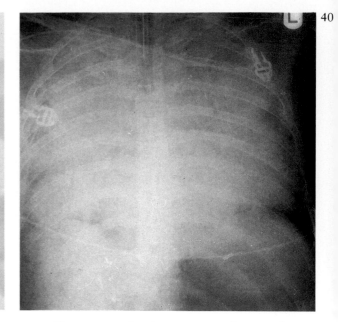

406 *Plasmodium falciparium* showing the heavy intra-erythryocytic parasitaemia and banana-shaped gametocytes.

407 **Chest x-ray showing acute respiratory distress syndrome** with florid pulmonary oedema in a fatal case of *P. falciparum* malaria.

19 HIV and immunocompromised respiratory disease

Opportunistic infections

T cells, B cells, phagocytes and complement work together in the body, combining natural and adaptive immunity mechanisms to provide a versatile and durable defence in depth against bacterial and viral infections. Deficiency in these body defence mechanisms may result in chronic or recurrent infections, infections with unusual organisms, or an unsatisfactory response to therapy. It is therefore no longer sufficient to recognise the causal organisms of a respiratory infection without assessing those background factors that allow the infection to become established. Resistance to infection may be impaired

Table 24. Some opportunistic infections in the immunocompromised.

Mechanism	Defect	Type of Infection
Poor T cell mediated immunity	Renal transplant recipients	Pneumocystis Mycobacterium tuberculosis
	Bone marrow transplant recipients	Atypical mycobacterium (MAIS) Cytomegalovirus (CMV)
	Neoplasia treated with chemotherapy	Herpes Varicella-zoster
	Hodgkin's disease	Epstein–Barr virus Candida albicans
	Prolonged corticosteroid immuno-suppressive therapy	Toxoplasma Aspergillus Legionella
	Acquired immune deficiency syndrome (AIDS)	
	Elderly, alcoholic, diabetic	
Poor humoral immunity Ineffective B cells	Hypogammaglobulinaemia	Herpes zoster, mycoplasma, Giardia
	Myelomatosis Leukaemia	Campylobacter Pneumococcus Aspergillus, Pseudomonas, Pneumocystis, Phycomycetes
	Sickle-cell disease	S. paratyphi
	Splenectomy	Pneumococcus
Poor phagocytosis	Chronic granulomatous disease of childhood	S. aureus Gram-negative enteric bacilli
	Neutropenia	Pseudomonas
	Anaplastic anaemia	
Poor local macrophage function	Cystic fibrosis	Pseudomonas S. aureus
	Alveolar proteinosis	Nocardia asteroides
	Pneumoconiosis	Atypical mycobacteria
	Assisted ventilation and nebulisers	Pseudomonas, Serratia, Flavobacterium

by a local failure of lung defence mechanisms (defective mucociliary clearance or bronchial obstruction from malignancy), or impoverished by congenital or acquired poor cellular (T cell) or humoral (B cell) immunity, or by defective neutrophils and macrophages.

Impaired cell-mediated immunity

The number of immunocompromised individuals is increasing as programmes of chemotherapy for malignant disease and organ transplantation advance and as infection with the human immunodeficiency virus (HIV) spreads. In world terms, acquired immune deficiency syndrome (AIDS) is numerically the largest cause of respiratory illness due to a cell-mediated immune deficiency and is illustrated in the following section. The reader is reminded that these conditions are not unique to AIDS and that other causes of T cell suppression will result in the same spectrum of opportunistic infections.

Pulmonary manifestations of HIV infection (acquired immune deficiency syndrome)

The causative virus responsible for AIDS was identified in 1983 and is now called the human immunodeficiency virus (HIV). Following infection and seroconversion, the patient is asymptomatic for a latent period which may last for many years. The virus infects CD4 antigen bearing cells, leading to both a reduction in the number and impairment in function of these cells.

The primary target for the virus is the helper–inducer subset of CD4 lymphocytes. As the CD4 cell count falls the risk of infection increases (Table 25). The proportion that will develop HIV-related disease is unknown. In those who go on to develop clinical manifestations of HIV infection, the lungs are involved in up to two-thirds of patients, with a wide variety of pathogens, many of which may co-exist. Up to 15% of the pulmonary complications are non-infectious in aetiology, including Kaposi's sarcoma and lymphoma. AIDS is diagnosed when HIV seropositive patients develop one of the opportunistic infections detailed (Table 26).

Table 25. AIDS and opportunistic infections and the CD4 lymphocyte cell count.

Years after onset	CD4 (Normal 1000/mm³)	Infection
7	400	Bacterial pneumonia
7.5	300	Herpes, oral candida
8	>200	Tinea, tuberculosis
9	≤200	Pneumocystis Coccidioidomycosis Histoplasmosis Cryptococcus Toxoplasma Cryptosporidium
10	<200	Cytomegalovirus (CMV) M. avium–intracellulare
10	0	Death

Table 26. Pulmonary complications of HIV infection

Opportunistic infections diagnostic of AIDS
  Pneumocystis carinii pneumonia
  Pulmonary toxoplasmosis
  Extraintestinal (e.g. pulmonary) strongyloidiasis
  Bronchopulmonary candidiasis
  Pulmonary cryptococcosis
  Disseminated histoplasmosis
  Disseminated *Mycobacterium avium-intracellulare* or *M. kansasii*
  Cytomegalovirus pneumonia
  Herpes simplex pneumonia

HIV-related pulmonary infections
  Tuberculosis
  Nocardiosis

Presumed HIV-related pulmonary disorders
  Pyogenic bacterial pneumonia, *S. pneumonia*, *S. aureus*, Gram-negative organism
  Mycobacterium tuberculosis
  Lymphoid interstitial pneumonitis (diagnostic of AIDS in HIV seropositive children less than 13 years of age)

AIDS-related pulmonary neoplasia
  Kaposi's sarcoma
  Non-Hodgkin's lymphoma

Pneumocystis carinii pneumonia (PCP)

Pneumocystis carinii pneumonia is the respiratory infection most frequently associated with AIDS.

Patients typically present with an insidious onset of pyrexia, night sweats, dry cough and exertional dyspnoea accompanied by significant weight loss. The most important clinical sign is tachypnoea at rest. Purulent sputum, haemoptysis and chest pain are not usually associated with PCP. HIV infection is suggested by the presence of oropharyngeal candidiasis, generalised lymphadenopathy or Kaposi's skin lesions.

Pneumocystis carinii infection is usually seen in patients with CD4 cell counts of $200 \times 10^9/l$ or less, the low count indicating significant immunosuppression.

Early diagnosis of PCP is important, as hypoxic respiratory failure with rapid life-threatening deterioration is common. Investigations will usually entail examination of induced sputum, bronchoalveolar lavage or transbronchial lung biopsy (**Table 27**).

Pneumocystis carinii is distributed worldwide. The organism is a multiflagellate protozoan, similar to *Toxoplasma gondii*. Three forms of the organism are recognised: trophozoite, cyst and sporozoite. The lifecycle is not well understood but it is believed that sporozoites emerge from the cysts and develop into trophozoites, which in turn mature to form new cysts by asexual or sexual intermediate stages.

The key to a successful outcome is early treatment which should be commenced empirically while awaiting the results of induced sputum or BAL cytology and culture. The following acute treatment regimens may be employed:

- Trimethoprim 15–20 mg per kg body weight per day, with sulphamethoxazole 75–100 mg per kg body weight per day, plus folinic acid 15 mg per day.
- Dapsone 100 mg per day, with trimethoprim 10–15 mg per kg body weight per day, plus folinic acid 15 mg per day.
- Pentamidine 4 mg per kg per day intravenously (usually given over 6 hours).

After commencing therapy some patients continue to deteriorate for the first 48 hours and significant clinical improvement is delayed for 5–7 days. Treatment is given for about 21 days and may be complicated by toxic drug reactions, especially skin rashes, mucocutaneous ulceration and blood dyscrasias. In severe PCP accompanied by arterial hypoxia, adjuvant high dose corticosteroids may be beneficial.

For patients who survive the first episode, up to 50% suffer a recurrence. The attack rate can be reduced with prophylactic therapy. Treatment with zidovudine may help to maintain the CD4 count and specific PCP prophylaxis with trimethoprim – sulphamethoxazole or dapsone–trimethoprim taken by mouth three times a week or twice monthly nebulised pentamidine reduces recurrence.

Table 27. Diagnostic investigations in HIV pulmonary disease.

Investigation	Method	Analysis
Induced sputum	3–5% saline via ultrasonic nebuliser with postural drainage (less sensitive than bronchoscopy and often poorly tolerated by patients)	Stain for *P. carinii* trophozoites with Giemsa Stain for *P.carinii* cysts with methenamine silver Stain and culture for mycobacteria, fungi and pyogenic bacteria
Broncho-alveolar lavage	180–360 ml buffered isotonic saline to give more than 100 ml aspirate	As above

Transbronchial lung biopsy		Touch preparation
		  Stain for *P. carinii*
		Transbronchial biopsy
		  Haematoxylin and eosin Gram stain for bacteria
		  Stains for *P. carinii*
		  Stain/culture for mycobacteria/ fungi
		  Culture for viruses

Open lung biopsy		As above To exclude Kaposi's sarcoma or lymphoma

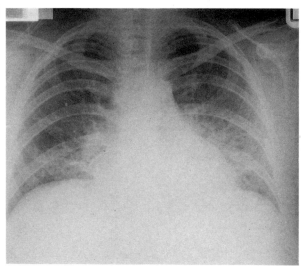

408

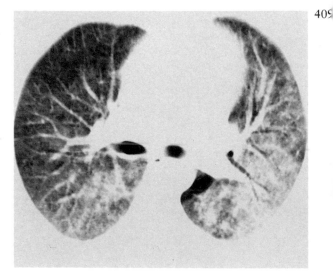

409

408 *Pneumocystis carinii* pneumonia. Chest radiograph showing bilateral reticulogranular perihilar infiltration, coalescing to give an alveolar pattern of homogeneous proximal air space shadowing with peripheral and basal sparing. A high index of suspicion is required, for the early radiographic changes are slight, with equivocal blurring of vascular pattern which may then progress to the characteristic 'ground glass' perihilar infiltrate. Atypical chest radiograph features, such as hilar adenopathy or pleural effusion suggest the presence of an additional pathological process.

409 *Pneumocystis carinii* pneumonia. CT scan revealed extensive bilateral infiltration becoming confluent on the left side. Note the left lung air bronchogram and unsuspected localised hypertransradiant space lying in the left paravertebral recess. (Same patient as in **408**, who presented after a 6-week illness with breathlessness, fever and significant hypoxia. The arterial oxygen tension was 6.7 kPa (50mm Hg).)

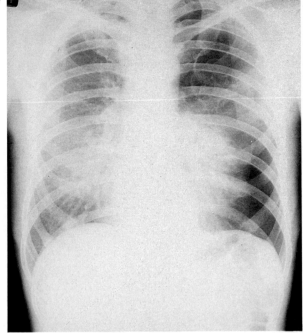

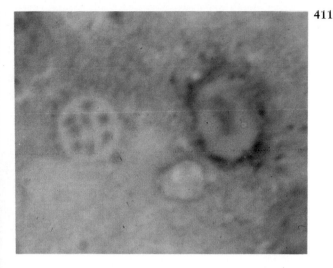

411 *Pneumocystis carinii* **pneumonia.** Transbronchial biopsy. Cysts approximately 5μm in diameter containing up to eight oval bodies called sporozoites are diagnostic.

410 *Pneumocystis carinii* **pneumonia.** Chest radiograph. Classic appearance of perihilar shadowing accentuated on the left side by the partial collapse of the lung due to a spontaneous pneumothorax, a recognised complication of PCP.

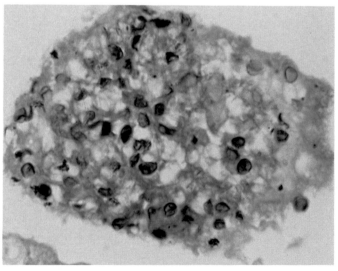

412 *Pneumocystis carinii* **pneumonia.** Transbronchial lung biopsy specimen showing amorphous background material and black-staining thick-walled cysts of *P.carinii* within the alveoli. (Grocott×350.)

413

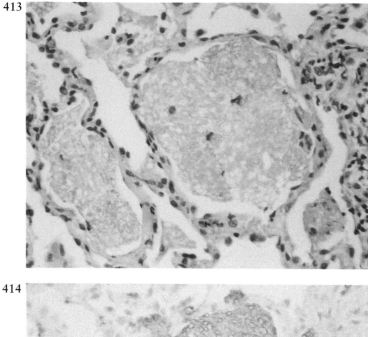

413 *Pneumocystis carinii* **pneumonia.** Transbronchial lung biopsy. The alveoli contain a foamy amorphous exudate and are infiltrated with organisms and chronic inflammatory cells. (H&E×100.)

414

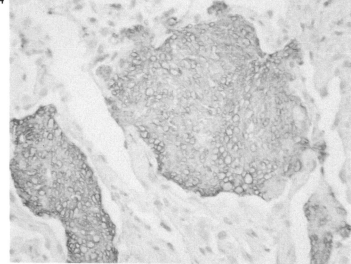

414 *Pneumocystis carinii* **pneumonia.** Transbronchial lung biopsy. The same section (**413**) stained with monoclonal antibodies. The foamy amorphous exudate is now shown to contain innumerable cysts and trophozoites of PCP. (Immunoperoxidase monoclonal antibody stain ×100.)

415

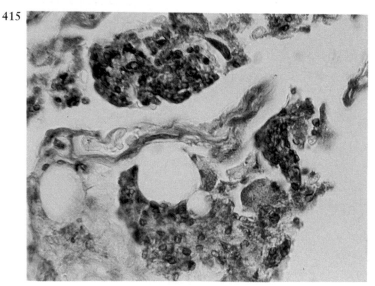

415 *Pneumocystis carinii* **pneumonia.** Transbronchial lung biopsy specimen showing clusters of thick-walled, black-staining cysts in the foamy exudate and alveolar lung tissue. (Methenamine silver staining ×350.)

Cytomegalovirus (CMV) in AIDS

Cytomegalovirus, a DNA virus indistinguishable from herpes simplex, is a major cause of morbidity and mortality in HIV positive patients. It is a common infection with worldwide distribution, present in the white blood and other body cells in infected individuals. Congenital infection may result in the death of the foetus *in utero* and it is estimated that 1 in every 1,000 infants is retarded by CNS damage. Silent infection in children and young adults is common and CMV antibody titres are frequently elevated. 2% of young adults, 10% of pregnant women and 50% of immunosuppressed renal transplant patients excrete cytomegalovirus. CMV pneumonia or hepatitis occurs in immunosuppressed patients. Latent infection may be re-activated or new infection may be acquired from transplants or blood transfusions.

Diagnosis may be made serologically by detecting specific IgM to CMV (indicating active infection) or by finding rising titres of IgG antibody. CMV may be detected after 24 hours of tissue culture by the use of monoclonal antibodies to viral antigens expressed on the infected culture cells (detection of early antigen by fluorescence (DEAF) test). CMV intranuclear inclusion bodies, if present, provide firm evidence of infection. In AIDS patients with suspected CMV infection, the finding of co-incident retinitis, hepatitis or colitis is a helpful diagnostic pointer.

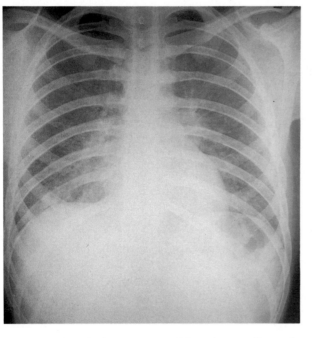

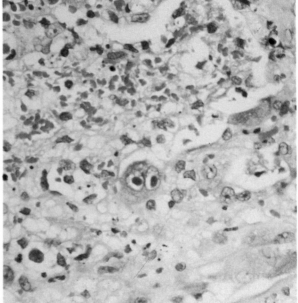

416 Cytomegalovirus pneumonitis. Chest radiograph showing perihilar infiltration. Pulmonary CMV frequently occurs in association with PCP, and the clinical and radiographic patterns of these two infections are indistinguishable. Ganciclovir or foscarnet are the only available treatments, both of which require lifelong administration and intravenous access.

417 Cytomegalovirus pneumonitis. Prominent intranuclear inclusion bodies in the alveolar wall on transbronchial lung biopsy diagnostic of CMV infection. CMV virus particles accumulate within the nucleus of an infected cell to produce a single dense inclusion. The space between the nuclear membrane, together with the encircling cytoplasm, gives rise to the characteristic 'owl's eye' appearance. (H & E × 160.)

Mycobacterial infection in AIDS

In the course of HIV infection, *Mycobacterium tuberculosis* usually precedes PCP, whereas non-tuberculous mycobacterial infections (MAIS complex) occur later when there is severe immuno-suppression. MAIS complex produces an illness very different from *M. tuberculosis*. It is characterised by systemic symptoms with fever and weight loss. Blood cultures are commonly positive. Pulmonary involvement is less common. MAIS complex is resistant to most drugs used to treat tuberculosis and therefore therapy is difficult and seldom effective.

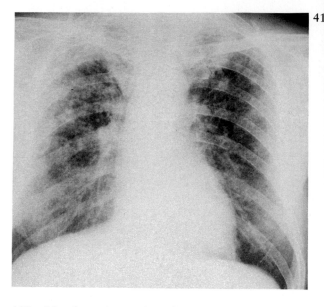

418 *Mycobacterium tuberculosis* in an HIV-positive patient. Chest radiograph with widespread pulmonary infiltration. There is a wide range of possible radiographic presentations. Cavitating disease is unusual and extrathoracic dissemination is common. Patients with PCP and CMV pneumonitis seldom produce sputum, but a productive cough often accompanies tuberculosis. The sputum smear and subsequent culture were positive for *M. tuberculosis*, and the patient responded to standard antituberculous chemotherapy.

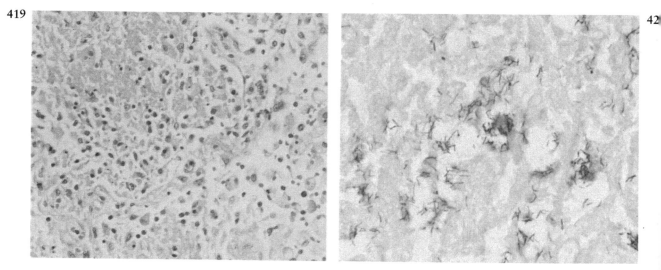

419, 420 Non-tuberculous mycobacterial lung infection. Lung biopsy (**419**) showing a paucity of granuloma in a severely immunocompromised AIDS patient. (H&E×40.) Abundant acid-fast bacilli are present (**420**), identified as *M. avium–intracellulare* (same section as in **419**). (Ziehl–Nielsen stain × 40.)

Atypical mycobacteria are often highly resistant to antituberculous drugs, even to those to which they show *in vitro* sensitivity.

Toxoplasmosis in AIDS

Toxoplasmosis occurs worldwide and is caused by *Toxoplasma gondii*, a protozoan obligate intracellular parasite that is transmitted exclusively by cats to humans, animals and birds.

Acquired infection is common and seldom causes symptoms. In Britain about a fifth of young adults and half of all 70-year-olds show serological evidence of previous infection. Disease in AIDS patients is commonly due to reactivation rather than to newly acquired infection. Patients will usually have a low titre of anti-toxoplasma antibodies from previous infection, but are unable to mount an IgM response or an increase in IgG level. Negative toxoplasma serology would make the diagnosis unlikely.

In individuals with impaired cell-mediated immunity the intracellular parasites persist and may cause life-threatening pneumonitis, almost invariably accompanied by CNS disease. The diagnosis is suggested by the clinical features, supported by CT scanning of the brain (demonstrating 'ring-enhancing' lesions due to abscess formation) and by appropriate serology, and confirmed on tissue biopsy.

Treatment followed by lifelong prophylaxis with pyrimethamine and sulphamethoxazole may be life saving.

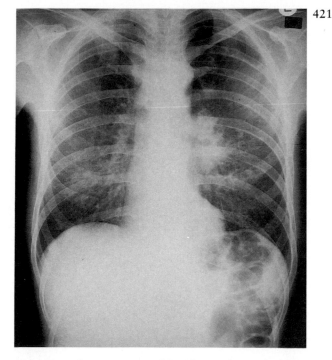

421 Toxoplasma pneumonitis. Chest radiograph showing diffuse interstitial infiltration and hilar adenopathy. This is an unusual opportunistic infection in the lung, even in AIDS, and there are no characteristic chest radiograph features.

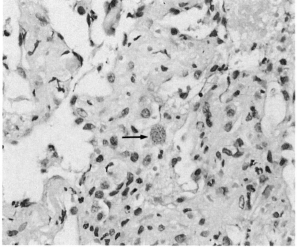

422 Toxoplasma pneumonitis. Lung biopsy with cysts containing sporozoites in the tissues (arrowed).

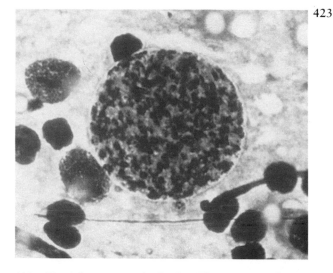

423 Toxoplasma cyst in brain. The cysts are large, about 200 µm in size, and contain up to 3,000 slowly dividing trophozoites. Confirmation by brain biopsy is potentially hazardous, but may be considered should there be no response to a trial of anti-toxoplasma therapy. A presumptive diagnosis may be made in the presence of enhancing mass lesions on cerebral CT scan.

Cryptococcosis in AIDS

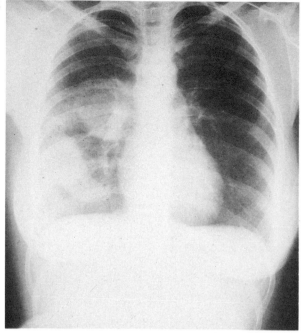

424

Cryptococcus neoformans is an encapsulated yeast that occurs worldwide and is particularly found in soil contaminated by pigeon droppings. The organism is acquired by inhalation. The pattern of pulmonary disease is very variable, ranging from life-threatening pneumonia with acute respiratory distress in the immunocompromised host to the chance finding of a 'coin lesion' on chest x-ray in an otherwise symptom-free individual. A subacute course with fever, pleurisy, effusions and single or multiple nodular radiographic deposits is common Although acquired by inhalation, the organism may disseminate and typically presents with pyrexia, headache and mental changes due to chronic meningitis. In patients with normal host defences, spontaneous regression of the clinical and radiographic manifestations is expected, although stable chronic infection may occur. In the immunocompromised patient and those with AIDS, progression is common and the response to antifungal therapy uncertain. Cryptococcosis occurs in about 10% of AIDS patients.

424 **Cryptococcosis.** Chest radiograph with infiltration of right middle and lower lobes and associated pleural reaction. Patient with normal immune status.

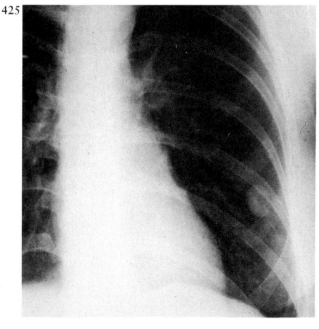

425

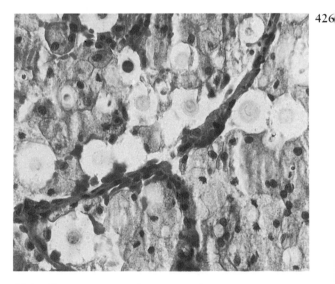

426

425 **Cryptococcosis.** Chest radiograph with subpleural 'coin lesion' due to an isolated cryptococcal granuloma (cryptococcoma). Carcinoma was suspected. Wedge resection of the mass was diagnostic. Asymptomatic patient with normal immune status.

426 *Cryptococcus neoformans* in a lung biopsy specimen. Granulomatous pneumonia. The clear spaces within the alveoli are the encapsulated fungal cells. (Alcian blue and haematoxylin×400.)

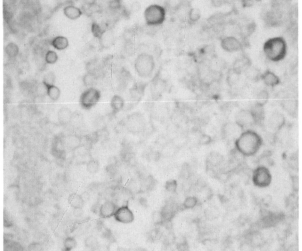

427 *Cryptococcus neoformans* in lung nodules. Numerous fungal cells are demonstrated. (PAS×360.)

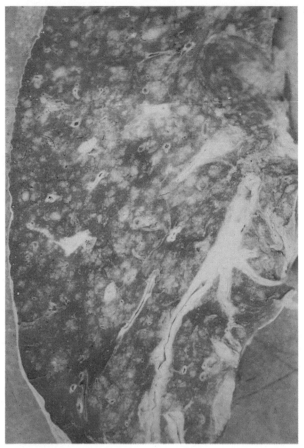

428 *Pulmonary cryptococcosis.* Postmortem whole lung specimen showing fatal multiple cryptococcal abscesses in an immunosuppressed patient with AIDS. Pulmonary cryptococcosis is commonly associated with disseminated infection and meningitis.

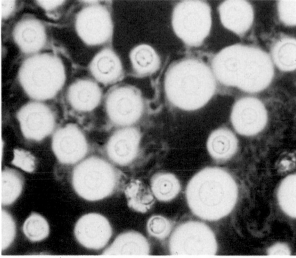

429 *Cryptococcus neoformans* meningitis. India ink 'negative' stain of cerebrospinal fluid sediment. This patient experienced a chronic, fluctuating, eventually fatal course. Treatment with amphotericin B or fluconazole may be life savings.

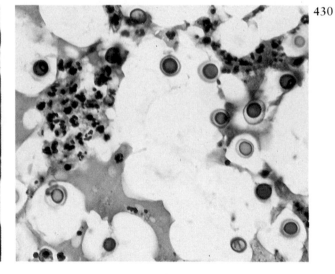

430 *Cryptococcus neoformans* meningoencephalitis. Necropsy specimen of brain tissue with numerous oval or round thin-walled fungal cells seen in circular clear spaces. The spaces represent the capsule polysaccharide that lacks affinity for the stain. (Alcian blue and haematoxylin×400.)

Kaposi's sarcoma (KS)

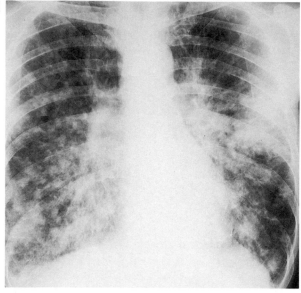

Approximately one-third of AIDS patients develop KS lesions, often of the skin (especially the face), the oropharynx, genitalia, gastrointestinal tract and lungs. Lymphatic involvement may produce gross oedema of affected areas.

Pulmonary involvement by KS commonly presents with dyspnoea, cough and haemoptysis. Bronchoscopy may show cherry-red slightly raised mucosal lesions, which may bleed excessively if biopsied. The histology is often inconclusive. The radiographic abnormalities include nodular pulmonary infiltrates mimicking PCP, adenopathy and blood-stained pleural effusion.

431 Kaposi's sarcoma. Chest radiograph. Note that the interstitial shadowing is a little coarser than that seen in PCP and CMV pneumonitis. Patients with pulmonary KS usually have cutaneous KS lesions.

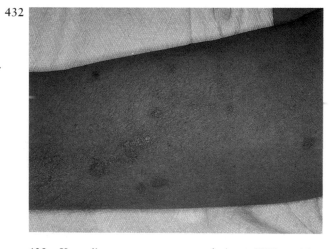

432 Kaposi's sarcoma cutaneous lesions. HIV positive patient with aggressive KS. In AIDS the distribution of KS can be classic, with initial lesions appearing on the lower legs. Lesions can also be scattered widely over the body with a predilection for the face, especially around the eyes and the tip of the nose.

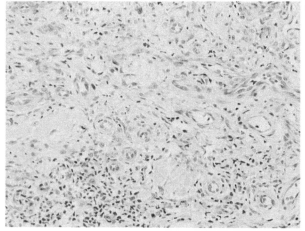

433 Kaposi's sarcoma. Histology of a cutaneous lesion. The tumour nodule consists of a mass of spindle cells with poorly developed vascular channels formed from atypical endothelial cells, some of which contain red blood cells and deposits of haemosiderin. (H & E ×25.)

Lymphoma in HIV infection

Non-Hodgkin's B cell lymphoma is frequently found in association with AIDS. The majority of patients have extranodular disease involving the gut, liver, central nervous system, soft tissue and bone marrow.

Pulmonary involvement is present in about a fifth of those who develop non-Hodgkin's lymphoma. Presentation is with pulmonary parenchymal nodules, pleural effusion and mediastinal adenopathy, often in association with peripheral node enlargement. Treatment is difficult and the prognosis poor.

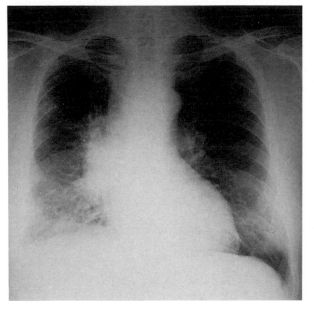

434 Pulmonary non-Hodgkin's lymphoma. Chest radiograph showing mediastinal adenopathy and nodular infiltration.

435 Mediastinal non-Hodgkin's lymphoma. High grade large cell B cell lymphoma. (H & E × 100.)

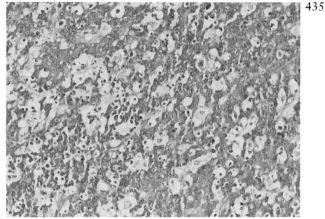

Chronic mucocutaneous candidiasis

This appears to be due to a restrictive defect of T cell function, with an inability to mount a protective immune response to *Candida albicans* and related fungi. The condition may be familial and associated with autoimmune endocrine disorders.

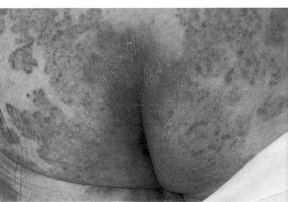

436 **Chronic mucocutaneous candidiasis** involving the skin over the buttocks. The condition typically commences as persistent oral candidiasis, with involvement of the nails and adjacent skin.

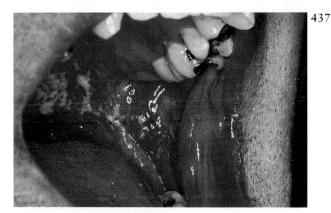

437 **Chronic mucocutaneous candidiasis** with oral chronic hyperplastic candidiasis.

Impaired humoral immunity

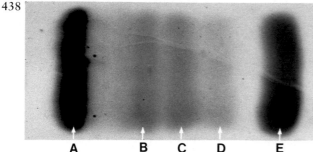

There is an increased susceptibility to infection associated with depression of normal serum immunoglobulin levels and a defective antibody response. Pneumococcal and Gram-negative infections predominate.

438 Multiple myeloma. Cellulose acetate electrophoresis showing a band of abnormal globulin. (A = multiple myeloma, B = β, C = α_2, D = α_1, E = albumin.)

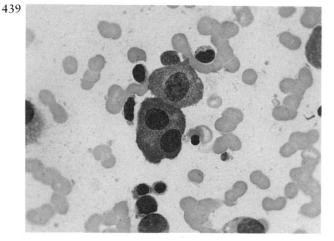

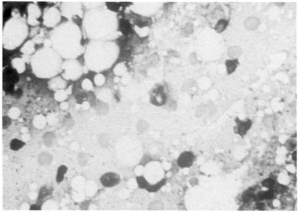

439 Multiple myeloma. Abnormal plasma cells in peripheral blood film.

440 Multiple myeloma. Bone marrow infiltrated by abnormal plasma cells.

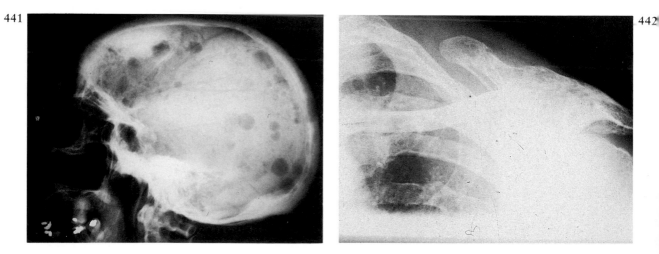

441, 442 Multiple myelomatosis with 'punched out' lytic bone cysts in the skull and clavicles. The clue to diagnosis was recurrent chest infections caused by humoral depression.

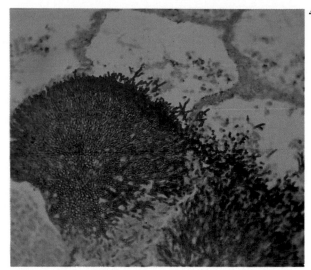

443 **Invasive pulmonary aspergillosis.** This patient was receiving cytotoxic chemotherapy for acute leukaemia. Fatal dissemination to the meninges and other organs may occur. (Silver staining.)

Impaired phagocytosis

Patients, especially young children, who have undergone surgical or autosplenectomy are at risk of serious, overwhelming infections. Defective splenic reticuloendothelial clearance of encapsulated organisms may allow enough organisms to divide and so overwhelm the humoral defence mechanism.

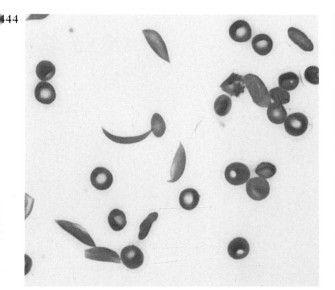

444 **Sickle-cell disease.** Autosplenectomy caused by recurrent splenic infarction is associated with *S. pneumonia* septicaemia and *Salmonella* osteomyelitis due to bone infarction. (Leishman stain×1000.)

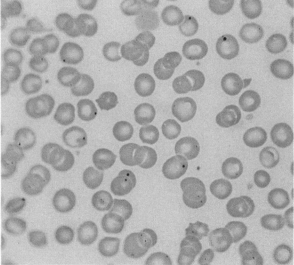

445 **Howell–Jolly bodies** (DNA fragments) present in the circulating red cells are characteristic of absent splenic function. (May-Gruenwald-Giemsa×175.)

Staphylococcal lung abscesses

 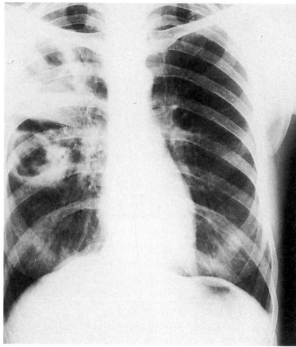

 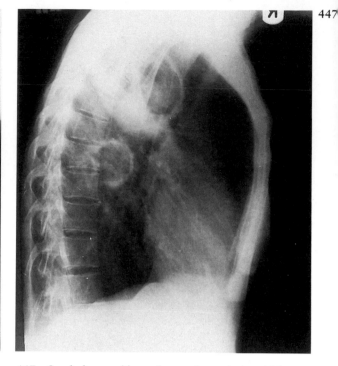

446 Staphylococcal lung abscess. Two large cavities are present in the right lung. This heroin addict presented with a cough, chest pain and fever. The sputum was purulent.

447 Staphylococcal lung abscess. Lateral view 446.

 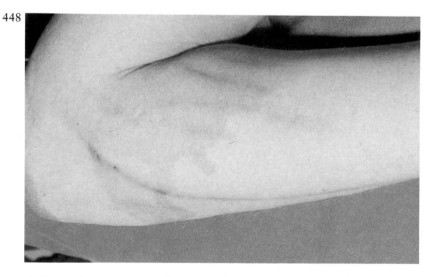

448 Staphylococcal lung abscess. Multiple injection sites were present over all accessible veins. Intravenous drug abusers are at risk notably from bacterial septicaemia, but also from viral hepatitis and HIV transmitted by syringes and needles contaminated with infected blood.

20 Immunological lung injury

Certain respiratory disorders and their systemic counterparts can be explained by classic types I, II, III or IV reactivity (**Table 28**). However, it is increasingly recognised that some respiratory diseases are caused by a complex interplay of more than one of these mechanisms. In these types of lung injury there is growing acknowledgement of the part played by T and B cells.

Table 28. Gell–Coombs' types of mechanisms of lung injury.

Immune type	I	II	III	IV
Alternative name	Immediate hypersensitivity	Cytotoxic antibody	Antigen–antibody immune complex	Delayed type cell-mediated
Cell types involved	B Mast cell Basophil Eosinophil	B or K Macrophage	B Polymorphs Platelets	T Macrophage Giant and epithelioid
Immunoglobulin	IgE	IgG, IgM	IgG	
Clinical disorder – respiratory	Asthma Hay fever Rhinitis	Goodpasture's syndrome	Sarcoidosis Erythema nodosum Rheumatoid lung Rheumatopneumo-coniosis Fibrosing alveolitis	Sarcoidosis Nitrofurantoin lung Allergic alveolitis Bronchopulmonary aspergillosis Wegener's granulomatosis Churg–Strauss syndrome
– systemic	Conjunctivitis Urticaria	Glomerulonephritis	Serum sickness Systemic lupus erythematosus Uveitis, scleritis Retinal vasculitis Behçet's syndrome	Graft rejection Contact dermatitis Phacoantigenic uveitis Phylctenular conjunctivitis Interstitial keratitis
Diagnostic measurements	Immediate skin tests Raised blood and mucosal IgE	Immunofluorescence reveals linear IgG in alveolar and renal basement membrane	Circulating immune complexes Complement conversion High ESR Immunofluorescence	Skin tests Lymphocyte transformation Macrophage migration inhibition Cell-mediated cytotoxicity Colony inhibition
Treatment – steroids	Yes	Yes	Yes	Yes
– other	Sodium cromoglycate	Plasmapheresis	Immunosuppressives and immunostimulants	Immunosuppressives

TYPE I. Immediate hypersensitivity

449

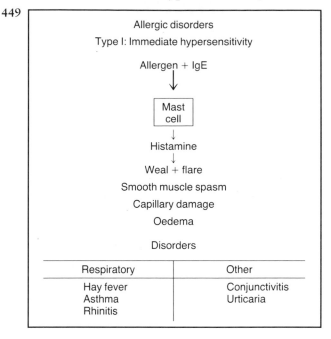

449 **Type I.** Intermediate hypersensitivity.

Bronchial asthma

Asthma is a common and treatable condition. Although there is no universally accepted definition, bronchial asthma may be defined as 'a disorder of function that is characterised by dyspnoea caused by widespread narrowing of peripheral airways in the lungs, varying in severity over short periods of time, either spontaneously or with treatment'. Asthma is frequently underdiagnosed and even when recognised is often undertreated.

Although asthma is usually considered in terms of wheeze, chest tightness and dyspnoea, there are some patients in whom cough, which may be productive, is predominant. This overlap between bronchitic symptoms, with chronic airflow obstruction, and chronic bronchial asthma remains an intractable diagnostic problem. The reported prevalance of asthma varies worldwide. There is good evidence that asthma is most common in developed countries, and in the UK and USA it afflicts about 10% of children.

Whereas relatively little is known about the factors, genetic or otherwise, that predispose certain subjects to develop asthma, much more is known of the many influences which may provoke an attack in asthmatic subjects (**Table 29**).

Table 29. Factors which may provoke asthma.

Exercise
Cold air
Inhaled airborne allergens
   seasonal pollens
   airborne fungi/moulds
   house dust mite
   household pets
Inhaled gaseous chemicals
Respiratory tract infections
Drugs
   beta-blocking drugs
   aspirin and analogues
Menstruation
Pregnancy
Climate and air pollution
Ingested allergens
   alcoholic drinks
   colouring agents
   sulphur dioxide
Sleep
Non-specific inhaled irritants
   smoke/fumes
Emotion

Clinically, it is convenient to divide asthmatics into two major subgroups:

1 *Extrinsic asthma*. This usually begins early in life, especially affecting males. Patients demonstrate positive immediate hypersensitivity to skin prick tests and also show a high incidence of seasonal rhinitis and flexural eczema.

2 *Intrinsic asthma*. Found in middle-aged adults, especially females. Recognisable allergic features are absent.

Patients in either group may be susceptible to the same aggravating factors and may respond to the same treatment.

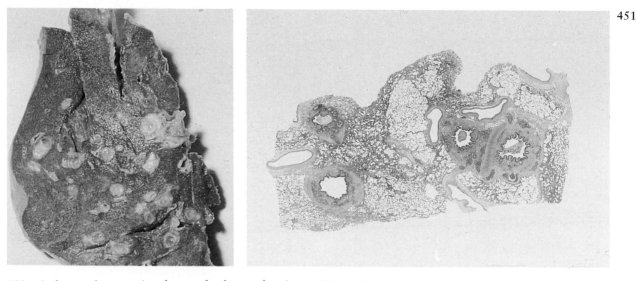

450 Asthma – lung section from a fatal case showing plugs of very viscid mucus projecting from some of the sectioned large airways. The mucous plugs are present between attacks and can be detected at bronchoscopy.

451 Asthma – lung section from a fatal case showing generalised plugging of small and medium-sized bronchi. The lungs were hyperinflated and the large airways appeared normal. The lumen of the plugged airways was occluded by a mixture of mucous and proteinaceous exudate. (H&E.)

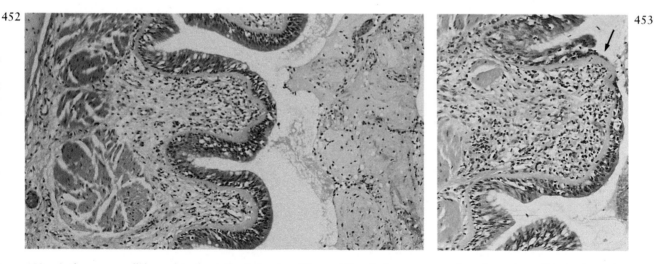

452 Asthma – small bronchi, about 3mm in size. The folded undulating shape of the surface epithelium reflects the severe bronchospasm causing significant airway narrowing. There is marked basement membrane thickening and moderate metaplasia of goblet cells. Also note the proteinaceous secretions and cellular debris plugging the airway (right side of picture). (H&E.)

453 Asthma – mucosal surface of small bronchus. This shows an area of recent mucosal desquamation (arrow) with early epithelial regeneration. This is a common feature in severe asthmatic attacks. (H&E.)

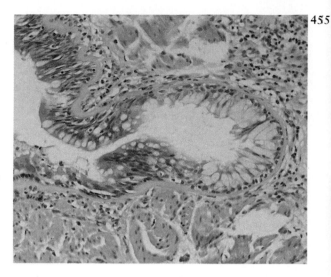

454 Asthma – small bronchiole. The bronchial mucosa has been thrown into folds by the smooth muscle constriction and mucosal oedema. There is a cellular infiltrate. The alveoli appear enlarged in the hyperinflated lung tissue. (H & E.)

455 Asthma – mucosal surface of a bronchiole with mucous plugging, a marked reduction in diameter, and loss of ciliated epithelium, which is replaced by a large number of goblet cells. There is a patchy eosinophilic infiltrate in the submucosa. (H & E.)

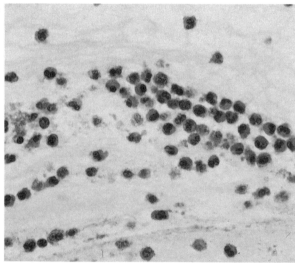

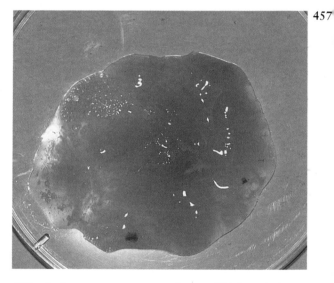

456 Asthma – eosinophilic infiltrate in mucous plug. In addition to eosinophils, plugs contain an admixture of protein and desquamated bronchial cells.

457 Asthma – sputum specimen. Thick gelatinous sputum containing eosinophils and other cell debris in inspissated mucous plugs.

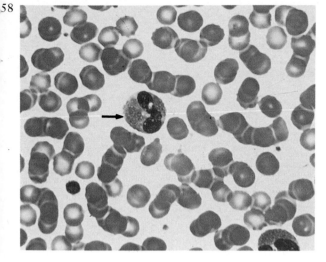

458 Asthma – blood eosinophilia. Circulating blood eosinophilia (arrow) is a common but not unique finding with asthma, especially in allergic bronchopulmonary aspergillosis and allergic granulomatosis.

459 Asthma – Charcot–Leyden crystals in sputum. Needle-like bodies, some 20–40 µm in length, formed by the aggregation of the basic protein derived from the eosinophil cell membrane. They are a common finding in asthma or other lung conditions associated with eosinophilic inflammation, accumulating in mucus and mucous plugs.

460 Asthma – bronchiolar casts (Curshmann's spiral) in a sputum cytological specimen. These are spirals of condensed mucinous material, arranged around a central thread, which form in the peripheral airways. (Methylene blue stain.)

Immunological mechanisms

The pathogenesis of asthma is not well understood, but it is evident that in some way it is related to inflammation of the airways. The inflammation is multifactorial due to a complex interplay of neural responses, inflammatory cell infiltration and the release of chemical mediators.

Table 30. Mast cell derived mediators of inflammation.

Preformed
Histamine
Eosinophil chemotactic factor
Neutrophil chemotactic factor
Neutral proteases
Acid hydrolases
Heparin proteoglycans

Membrane derived
Leukotrienes
Prostaglandins
Thromboxanes
Platelet activating factor

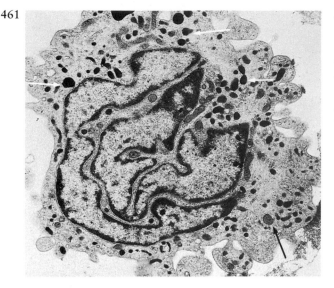

461 Mucosal mast cell obtained by broncho-alveolar lavage from an asthmatic patient. Note the prominent lysosomal dense bodies (arrow) containing secretory granules and the peripheral pseudopodia. From studies in animals and in humans it is widely recognised that type 1 hypersensitivity reactions occur through an interaction of allergen with IgE on the surface of the mast cell. These cells are present throughout the airways, being localised to the bronchial epithelium and mucosa.

Mast cells lavaged from the airways of patients with atopic asthma exhibit increased immunologically mediated and spontaneous responsiveness leading to histamine release. (Transmission electron micrograph.)

Some triggering factors

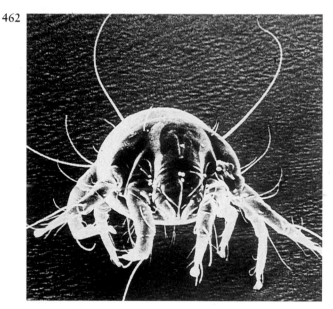

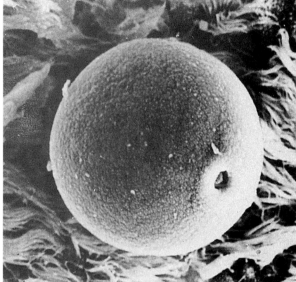

462 The house dust mite (*Dermatophagoides pteronyssinus*). Two main species are responsible for allergic symptoms: *D. pteronyssinus* in Europe, and *D. farinae* in the Middle East and North America. The mite survives upon sequestrated human skin scales in moist temperate environments. Mattresses and bed linen are often infested and provide the link between mite allergy and nocturnal symptoms in the sensitive individual. The allergic symptoms are most severe from November to January, when mite activity is most intense. The mite faecal pellets are the major source of allergen. (Electron micrograph photograph.)

463 Grass pollen grain against a background of ciliated epithelium of rat. The severity of rhinitis, hay fever and grass pollen asthma is related to the quantitative seasonal counts of pollen grains in the atmosphere. The most common varieties of grass pollen are the crested dog's tail, fescue, meadow rye, timothy, cocksfoot and brome.

The nature of the pollen varies with geographical regions and farming practice; pollens from the rag weed in the USA, the *Prosopis* species of tree in the Middle East, and the mulberry or olive along the Mediterranean coasts are especially common causes of allergy.

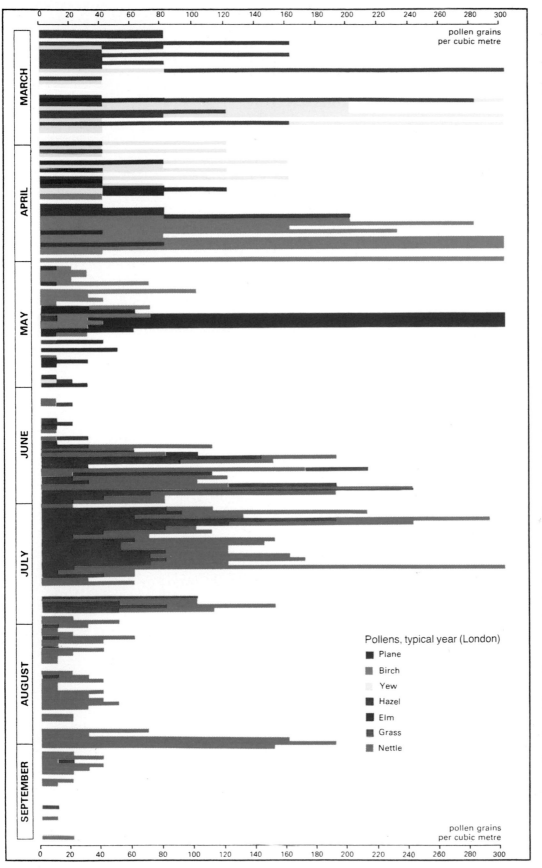

464 Summer pollen chart. The pollen count is obtained by sampling air sucked through a special chamber that deposits the pollen grains on to a sticky glass plate. The plate is examined after 24 hours and the count of pollen grains is expressed as the number of grains per cubic metre of air. A count of 50 pollen grains per cubic metre of air can cause discomfort to sensitised individuals.

Different plants produce pollen at different times of the year. Symptoms are most commonly caused by the airborne pollens liberated from trees, grasses and nettles.

Pollens, typical year (London)

- Plane
- Birch
- Yew
- Hazel
- Elm
- Grass
- Nettle

pollen grains
per cubic metre

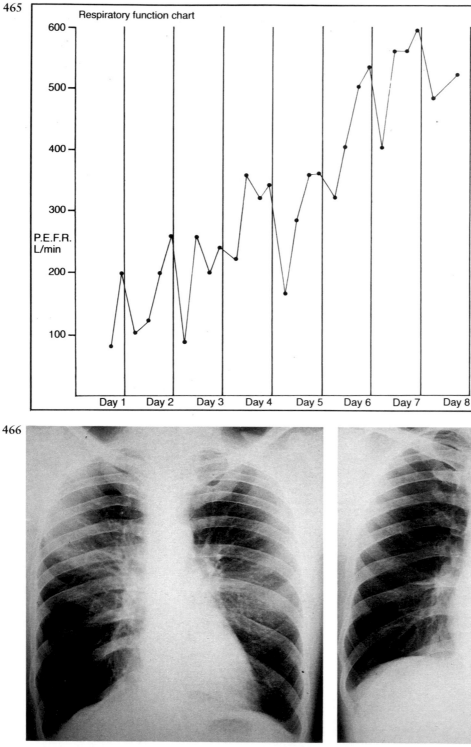

466

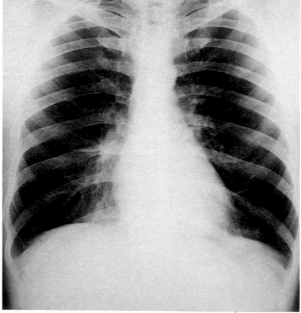

467

466 Acute attack of asthma. The radiological signs at presentation are those of hyperinflation. The rib cage silhouette is square and the sides of the thorax are parallel. The diaphragms at the mid-clavicular point are depressed and cross the anterior ends of the seventh ribs, the muscle reflections of the right diaphragm are visible and the upper lobe blood vessels are distended.

467 Asthma. The same patient as in **466**, on the eighth day of treatment. The rib cage silhouette is normal. The peak expiratory flow chart shows improvement with treatment.

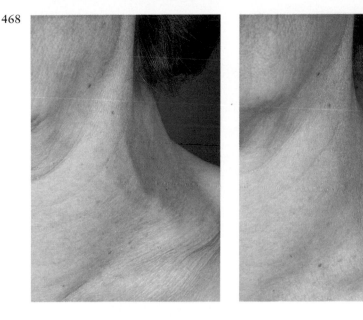

468, 469 Asthma – the jugular venous pulsation. The large intra-thoracic pressure swings seen in severe asthma cause corresponding variations in the venous pressure.

The jugular venous pressure is high during expiration (**468**), with filling of the neck veins. On inspiration the neck veins empty (**469**).

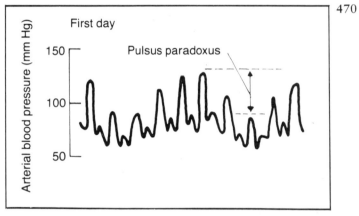

470 Pulsus paradoxus. The arterial pressure trace shows a variation in pressure of 30 mmHg between inspiration and expiration.

Pulsus paradoxus is defined as a more than 10% or 10 mmHg fall in systolic pressure with inspiration. It is an exaggeration of the normal finding of decreased arterial pressure with inspiration.

This sign reflects large expiratory pressures found in both severe asthma and severe fixed airflow obstruction.

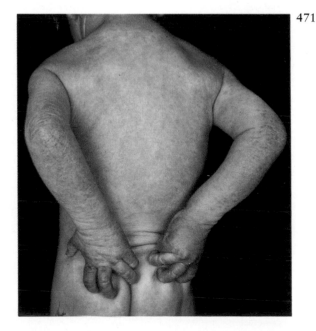

471 Childhood eczema. Itchy eczematous lesions on the hands and trunk, which become excoriated and secondarily infected. A family history of atopy is common and eczema may precede or accompany extrinsic asthma or rhinitis.

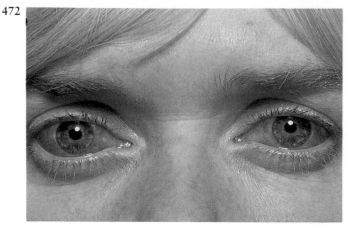

472 Grass pollen allergy. Conjunctivitis in a young atopic asthmatic who experienced severe summer asthma and hay fever.

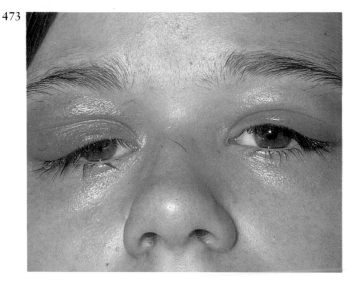

473 Aspirin sensitivity. Periorbital angioedema accompanied by wheezing and urticaria 2 hours after ingestion of aspirin. This response can be life-threatening and is most common in non-atopic asthma sufferers, especially those with nasal polyps.

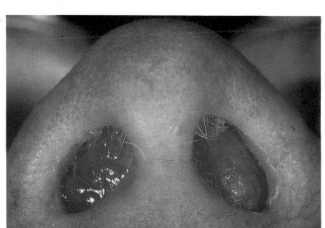

474 Asthma and nasal polyps. Bilateral nasal polyposis. Polyps are more common in asthmatics than in normal controls. Nasal polyps and aspirin sensitivity are most common in intrinsic female, middle-aged asthmatic patients. The polyps may be single or multiple.

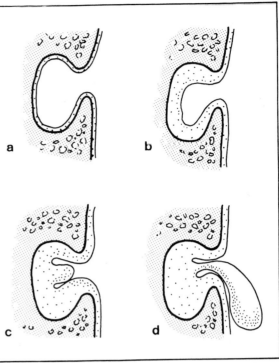

475 Development of nasal polyp. Increasing swelling of the mucosal lining of a small bone-lined air space or sinus (a–c) ultimately leads to the prolapse of a tongue of evaginated mucosa which forms the polyp (d).

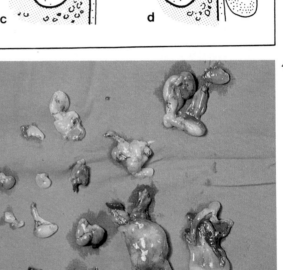

476 Multiple nasal polyps. All were removed from an aspirin-sensitive chronic rhinitis sufferer.

477 Large single posterior nasal polyp. These result from prolapse of the mucosa lining the sinuses (usually the ethmoid) into the nasal cavity.

Polyps consist of swollen mucous membrane, the spaces being filled by fluid containing lymphocytes, plasma cells and strikingly large numbers of eosinophils.

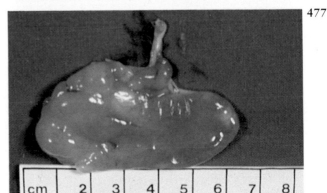

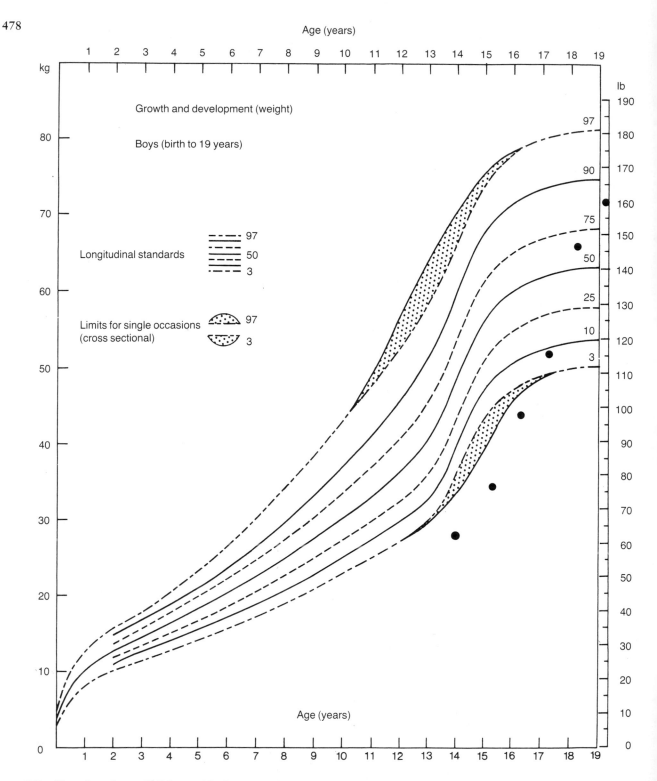

478 Chronic asthma. Children with chronic asthma tend to be thin and below average in both height and weight. The 14-year-old boy with perennial asthma, illustrated in **479**, suffered retardation of growth. Effective treatment with corticosteroids resulted in satisfactory growth (**480**). The points on the growth velocity chart (●) show a significant 4-year delay in growth at presentation, which was corrected by the age of 18. Height (not shown) at age 18 lay on the 75th centile.

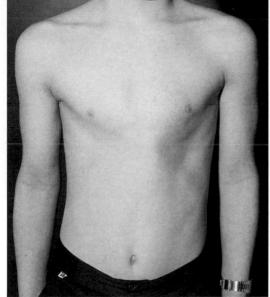

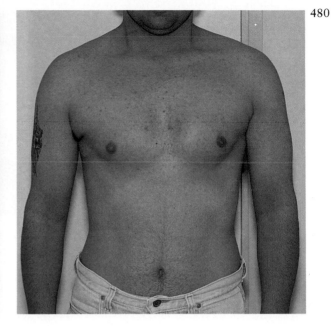

479 Chronic asthma. Poorly controlled asthma in childhood may result in delayed growth. Chest deformity is here seen in a 14-year-old boy with a history of severe untreated asthma throughout childhood. There is overinflation with prominence of the upper central part of the chest ('pigeon chest'), and deep sulci extend laterally from the xiphisternum (Harrison's sulci). (Same patient as in **478**.)

480 Chronic asthma. The same patient as in **479**, now aged 23. His asthma was well controlled but still required oral maintenance corticosteroids.

Skin prick tests for allergy

Skin prick testing (SPT) with common inhaled allergens is a simple, safe and rapid way of identifying atopic individuals. Positive skin tests indicate the presence of specific IgE in the blood and the size of the reaction correlates closely with the total serum IgE level.

The choice of SPT antigen depends upon the purpose of skin testing in the individual patient. If the intention is solely to confirm atopy, testing with grass pollen, house dust mite, animal furs and controls will identify the great majority of atopic individuals.

Table 31. Commonly used skin prick test solutions.

Saline negative control
Histamine positive control
House dust extract
Dermatophagoides pteronyssinus
Grass pollen mix
Early/late tree pollens
Weed/shrub pollens
Alternaria, Cladosporium
Aspergillus fumigatus
Cat dander
Dog fur
Horse hair
Other relevant environmental allergens
    Bermuda grass (Middle East)
    olive pollen (Mediterranean)
    rag weed (USA)

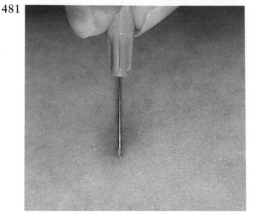

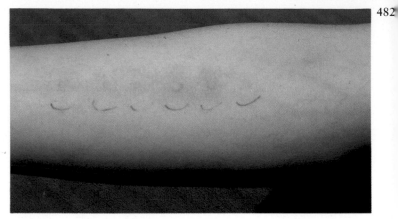

481 The technique of skin prick testing for allergy. The point of a fine-gauge needle is passed through a drop of allergen-containing solution into the superficial layers of the skin, introducing about 10^{-6}ml of liquid. This is a painless and bloodless procedure.

482 Immediate skin prick test reactions showing weals, pseudopodia and surrounding flares. The allergen reacts with a specific class of antibody bound to mast cells or circulating basophils, which leads to the release of vasoactive amines. The reaction is maximal at 15–20 minutes and fades in 60–90 minutes. The responses to skin tests are measured as the maximum diameter of the weal – a reaction larger than 3mm in diameter is usually significant. Controls are essential for proper interpretation, the saline diluent serving as a negative control and a dilute histamine phosphate solution as a positive control.

Eosinophilic pneumonia

Pulmonary disease associated with either blood or tissue eosinophilia embraces a wide group of conditions. In some the cause is well established, such as drug reactions, parasite infestations, asthma and allergic bronchopulmonary aspergillosis. A tentative association may be assumed with microfilaria infection in some cases of tropical pulmonary eosinophilia, but in the remainder the cause is obscure.

The immunological mechanism may not be a type I reaction, but as these conditions often present with asthmatic symptoms they are best considered with asthma.

Eosinophilic pneumonia is characterised by transient non-segmental radiographic shadows, accompanied by a moderate blood eosinophilia. Symptoms vary in severity, but can be mild and may even be absent.

Table 32. Classification of pulmonary eosinophilia.

Simple pulmonary eosinophilia (Loeffler's syndrome) (page 187)
Asthmatic pulmonary eosinophilia (ABPA) (page 136)
Drug-induced pulmonary eosinophilia
Tropical pulmonary eosinophilia (page 148)
Hypereosinophilic syndrome
Chronic pulmonary eosinophilia
Churg–Strauss syndrome

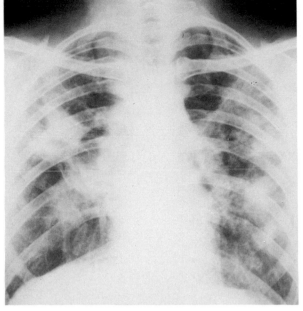

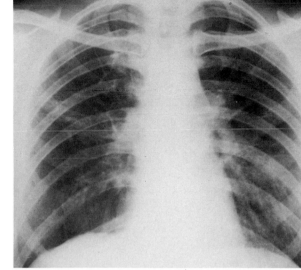

483 Eosinophilic pneumonia (Loeffler's syndrome). Non-segmental scattered soft densities in the right perihilar region and peripherally. The total white cell count was $10500 \times 10^9 l$ with 1600 (15%) eosinophils. The patient complained of cough, malaise, fever and wheezing.

484 Eosinophilic pneumonia (Loeffler's syndrome). Spontaneous clearing usually occurs within a month. In this case corticosteroids were given, with prompt remission of the shadowing seen in **483**. Typically, symptoms are mild and settle spontaneously. The illness is due to the passage of parasitic larvae, most commonly *Ascaris lumbricoides*, through the lung.

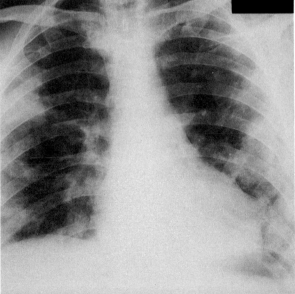

Table 33. Some drugs causing pulmonary eosinophilia.

Aspirin and analogues
Penicillamine
Sulphasalazine
Carbamazepine
Phenytoin
Nitrofurantoin
Sulphonamides
Penicillin
Tetracycline
Methotrexate
Bleomycin
Chlorpromazine
Chlorpropamide
Sodium cromoglycate

485 Pulmonary eosinophilia caused by drugs. This eosinophilic pulmonary infiltrate developed during para-amino salicylic acid therapy for tuberculosis. The infiltrate is typically peripheral and fleeting, resolving to be replaced by other shadows on the same or opposite side. The shadowing clears when the medication responsible for the reaction is discontinued, recurring if the patient is re-challenged with it. A number of drugs may be implicated (**Table 33**).

Chronic (cryptogenic) pulmonary eosinophilia

This is a condition with persistent eosinophilic infiltration, variable blood eosinophilia and systemic symptoms, with cough, dyspnoea, weight loss, fever, night sweats and, sometimes, lymphadenopathy and hepatomegaly. Asthma is not a constant feature and in the majority of cases serum immunoglobulin IgE levels are normal or only slightly elevated.

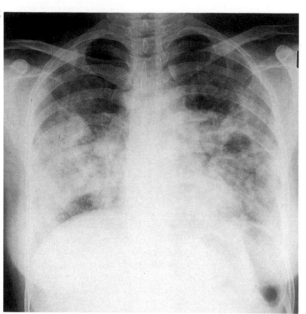

486

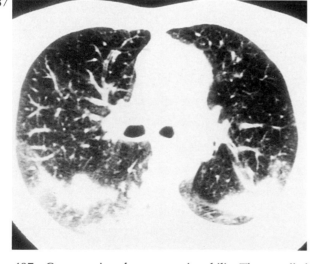

487

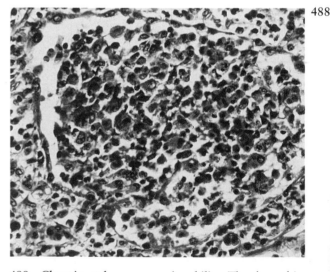

488

486 Chronic pulmonary eosinophilia. This extensive shadowing cleared with corticosteroid drugs. The typical pattern of 'reversed pulmonary oedema' is more usual. Blood eosinophilia may be increased, but in a third of cases it is normal. Eosinophils may be seen in the sputum.

487 Cryptogenic pulmonary eosinophilia. The so-called 'reversed bat's wing' appearance on the radiograph is seen to be due to well-defined dense crescent-shaped opacities lying posteriorly in both upper lobes away from the midline. The remaining lung fields are almost normal. This appearance is seen in approximtely 50% of cases and has not been recorded in other conditions.

488 Chronic pulmonary eosinophilia. The lung biopsy shows infiltration of the alveolar walls by eosinophils and histiocytes. The alveolar space is filled by an exudate containing eosinophils.

TYPE II. Cytotoxic antibody-mediated lung injury

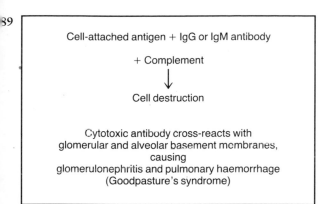

Cell-attached antigen + IgG or IgM antibody

+ Complement

↓

Cell destruction

Cytotoxic antibody cross-reacts with
glomerular and alveolar basement membranes,
causing
glomerulonephritis and pulmonary haemorrhage
(Goodpasture's syndrome)

489 Type II. Cytotoxic antibody-mediated injury.

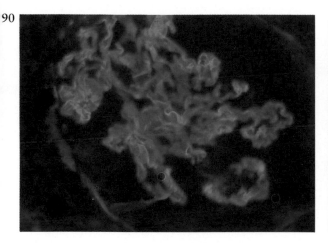

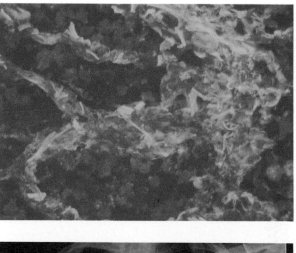

490, 491 Goodpasture's syndrome. Renal (490) and lung biopsy (491) specimens showing linear fluorescence of the basement membrane due to deposition of IgG antibasement membrane antibodies. (Antihuman IgG labelled fluorescein isocyanate preparations.) This disease is characterised by alveolar haemorrhage, haemoptysis, anaemia and proliferative glomerulonephritis. Haemosiderin-laden macrophages are present in the sputum.

The antigen to which the antibody is directed is located in type IV collagen and the immune reaction damages the renal and pulmonary capillary bed. The absence of vasculitis and necrotic respiratory tract lesions distinguishes it from Wegener's granulomatosis.

Treatment includes corticosteroids, immunosupressives and plasmapheresis to remove the circulating antibody.

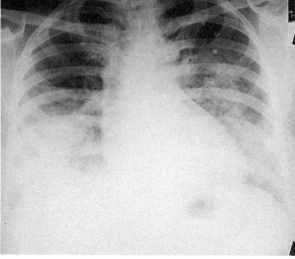

492 Goodpasture's syndrome. Chest radiograph of acutely dyspnoeic patient showing extensive bilateral consolidation with an air bronchogram due to alveolar haemorrhage.

TYPE III. Immune complex lung injury

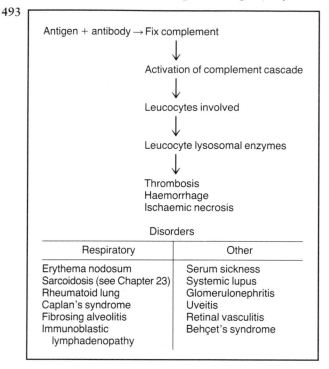

Antigen + antibody → Fix complement
↓
Activation of complement cascade
↓
Leucocytes involved
↓
Leucocyte lysosomal enzymes
↓
Thrombosis Haemorrhage Ischaemic necrosis

Disorders

Respiratory	Other
Erythema nodosum	Serum sickness
Sarcoidosis (see Chapter 23)	Systemic lupus
Rheumatoid lung	Glomerulonephritis
Caplan's syndrome	Uveitis
Fibrosing alveolitis	Retinal vasculitis
Immunoblastic lymphadenopathy	Behçet's syndrome

493   Type III. Immune complex lung injury.

Respiratory associations of connective tissue disorders

Pulmonary manifestations occur frequently in the multisystem connective tissue diseases (**Table 34**). The patient's soil or terrain plays an important part in moulding the onset and progression of the disease, and there are many influencing factors. Vasculitis is a dominant but ill-understood feature of some connective tissue disorders. As its name suggests, it is characterised by inflammation of blood vessels ranging from large muscular arteries, to medium-sized and small arteries, arterioles, capillaries, venules and veins. Vessel size is one method of classifying these overlapping syndromes (**494**). Fibrinoid necrosis involving the whole vessel wall is a conspicuous feature.

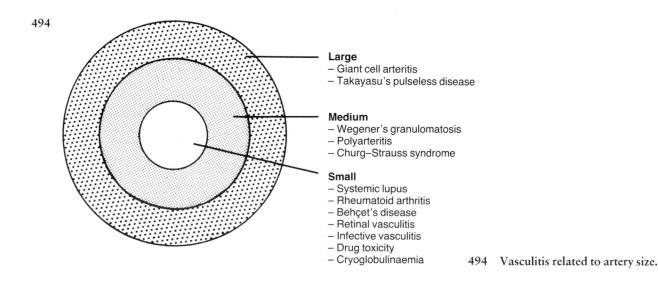

Large
– Giant cell arteritis
– Takayasu's pulseless disease

Medium
– Wegener's granulomatosis
– Polyarteritis
– Churg–Strauss syndrome

Small
– Systemic lupus
– Rheumatoid arthritis
– Behçet's disease
– Retinal vasculitis
– Infective vasculitis
– Drug toxicity
– Cryoglobulinaemia

494   Vasculitis related to artery size.

Rheumatoid arthritis

A wide range of pleuropulmonary complications are described, although all are rare except for lung fibrosis and pleural effusion. Respiratory infections, bronchitis, bronchiectasis, lung nodules, apical fibrosis, fibrosing alveolitis, pleural effusions, pleural thickening, relapsing polychondritis, obliterative bronchiolitis and amyloidosis may occur. Cryoglobulinaemia and serum Ciq binding activity are negative in uncomplicated rheumatoid arthritis, but positive in three-quarters of those with extra-articular disease including lung involvement.

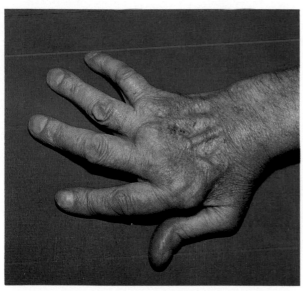

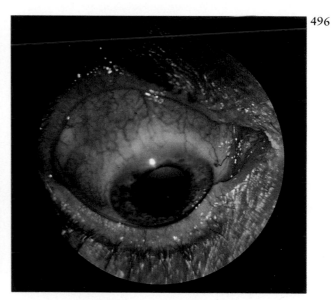

495 Rheumatoid arthritis. The hands at a late stage of the disease, showing the typical deformity.

496 Rheumatoid arthritis. Episcleritis indicates activity of the rheumatoid process.

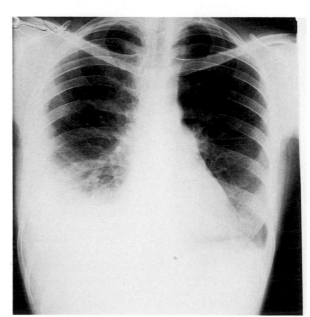

497 Rheumatoid pleural effusion. This is the most common respiratory manifestation. It is usually asymptomatic and occasionally precedes joint symptoms. The fluid is characteristically an exudate with low glucose concentration, raised lactate dehydrogenase, low complement, raised cholesterol and high titre of rheumatoid factor. Pleural biopsy typically shows chronic inflammation with no specific features.

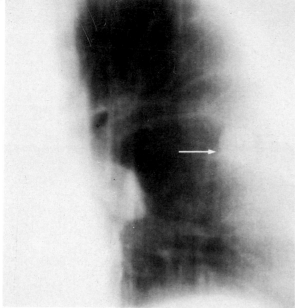

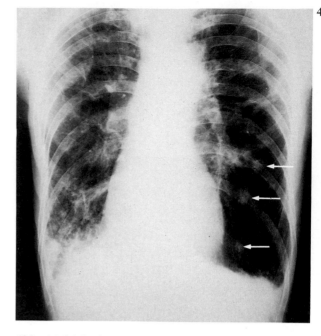

498 Rheumatoid pulmonary nodules. Usually subpleural and more common in men. Occasionally, they cavitate and may be associated with haemoptysis. Biopsy of solitary nodules may be necessary to exclude malignancy.

499 Multiple rheumatoid nodules.

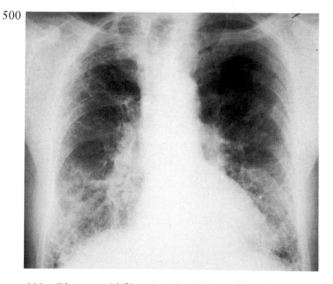

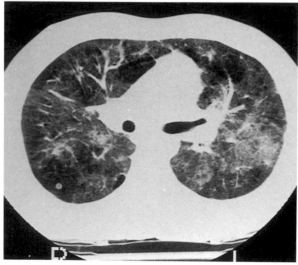

500 Rheumatoid fibrosing alveolitis. Diffuse lower zone shadowing. Typical clinical features include fingernail clubbing, central cyanosis and bilateral end inspiratory basal crackles. The radiograph shows predominantly basal distribution of reticular nodular shadowing. Lung function testing shows decreased compliance, restricted lung volumes and a reduced carbon monoxide transfer factor. The overall appearances are identical to those seen in 'lone' cryptogenic fibrosing alveolitis. The pathogenesis is uncertain.

501 Rheumatoid fibrosing alveolitis. Peripheral and central changes are present throughout both lung fields, being more marked on the left than on the right. On the left a fine interstitial fibrosis is mixed with an 'air space' semi-confluent background. On the right the areas of linear fibrosis are coarser and distort the lung architecture. Rheumatoid alveolitis can look identical to fibrosing alveolitis from other causes, but pleural thickening and localised areas of linear fibrosis and collapse are more common than in cryptogenic fibrosing alveolitis.

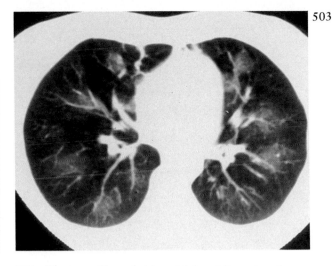

502 Rheumatoid fibrosing alveolitis – lung biopsy. Histology reveals thickened alveoli, fibrosis and disorganisation of the lung architecture leading to honeycombing.

503 Rheumatoid arthritis. Adult obliterative bronchiolitis (10 mm slice width CT). Patches of high and low attenuation of varying size are scattered throughout both lung fields with no evidence of volume loss. This is a common finding in obliterative bronchiolitis and, although it is not diagnostic, it is more commonly seen in this condition than in other conditions associated with narrowed airways and air trapping. Thick (10 mm) sections are more valuable in this condition than high resolution scans.

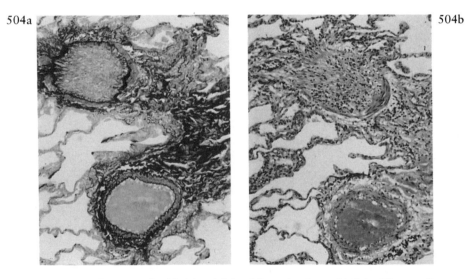

504a, b Rheumatoid arthritis. Adult obliterative bronchiolitis. The small airways are narrowed or obliterated by chronic inflammatory cells and fibrotic scar tissue. The accompanying bronchiolar artery is disrupted and infiltrated by inflammatory cells. Progressive breathlessness may lead on to respiratory failure. On auscultation, widespread crackles are accompanied by mid or late inspiratory high pitched squeaks. (Stained for elastin Van Gieson stain (a) and H&E (b).)

Table 34. Connective tissue disorders with a respiratory component.

Disorder	Features Respiratory	Features Other	Pathology	Autoantibodies	Immune Complexes	HLA
Rheumatoid arthritis	Pleural effusion Cavitating necrobiotic nodules Alveolitis Fibrosis Obliterative bronchiolitis	Synovitis Caplan's syndrome	Rheumatoid necrobiotic nodules	Rheumatoid factor ANA/DNA Antiperinuclear	IgG, RF IgM, RF	DR4/1
Systemic lupus erythema-tosus	Pleurisy + effusion Pericarditis Infarcts Alveolitis Shrinking Lung	Rash Nephritis Psychosis Arthritis	Vasculitis Deposition of immune complexes	Lupus coagulant Rheumatoid factor ANA, DNA Anti erythrocyte	+++	DRW
Sjögren's syndrome	Dry naso-pharynx Bronchitis Infiltrates Granuloma Pseudolym-phoma	Dry eyes Enlarged parotids Arthritis CREST	Plasma cell infiltration Lymphoepithelial exocrine gland lesions	Salivary duct and thyroid Rheumatoid factor SS-A (Ro) SS-B (La); ANA		B8 DR3
Progressive systemic sclerosis	Alveolitis Interstitial fibrosis Pulmonary hypertension Honeycombing	CREST	Intimal thickening – infarcts Collagen deposition	ANA Anticentromere		A1 B8 DR3 DR5
Mixed connective tissue disease	Pulmonary hypertension Pleurisy Abnormal lung function	Polyarthritis Raynaud's pheno-menon Sclero-dactyly Nephritis	Intimal proliferation Interstitial mononuclear infiltrates Hyaline deposition	ANA Rheumatoid factor Nuclear RNP		
Wegener's granuloma-tosis	Cavitating nodules	Nasopharyn-gitis Uveitis Nephritis Skin vasculitis Polyarthritis	Granulomatous angiitis	Rheumatoid factor Antibody to neutrophil cytoplasmic antigen (Anca)	+++	
Lymphomatoid granuloma-tosis	Cough Dyspnoea Haemoptysis	Arthralgia Renal vasculitis	Necrotising vasculitis			
Churg–Strauss allergic granuloma-tosis	Asthma Pleurisy Pericarditis Pneumonia	Skin vasculitis	Eosinophilic granulo-matous vasculitis			
Polyarteritis nodosa	Asthma Flitting infiltrates	Nephritis Mesenteric occlusion Polyneuritis Skin vasculitis	Eosinophilic vasculitis HBsAg positive			

Table 34. Connective tissue disorders with a respiratory component continued.

Disorder	Features Respiratory	Other	Pathology	Autoantibodies	Immune Complexes	HLA
Fibrosing alveolitis	Dyspnoea Cyanosis Fibrosis Pulmonary hypertension Haemosiderosis	Clubbing Hyper- trophic pulmonary osteoarth- opathy	Mononuclear cell infiltrate Alveolar wall thickening Hyponatremia	ANA Rheumatoid factor Mitochondrial	+++	B8

Systemic lupus erythematosus (SLE)

Widespread inflammatory changes occur in connective tissue, blood vessels and serosal surfaces. Pleuropulmonary involvement is common and more frequent than in any other collagen disease. The cause is unknown. It affects females nine times more frequently than males, occurring at any age, but most commonly arising in those between 20 and 40 years of age. Circulating immune complexes deposit in the lungs and kidneys producing a granular deposition pattern. Pleurisy is associated with effusions and with polyarthritis, 'butterfly' facial skin eruptions, nephritis, neuropsychiatric manifestations, pericarditis or Raynaud's disease. Necrotising renal and cerebral vasculitis carry a poor prognosis. Pulmonary vasculitis is rare.

B cells are overactive, producing autoantibodies, whereas T cells are underactive and fail to suppress B cells. The disease occurs particularly in HLA-DRW2 and HLA-DRW3 individuals.

A variety of pleuropulmonary abnormalities may occur:

- Pleurisy and effusions.
- Acute lupus pneumonia.
- Atelectasis.
- Shrinking lungs and diaphragmatic dysfunction.
- Fibrosing alveolitis.
- Alveolar haemorrhage.

Table 35. Pleural effusion in SLE.

1 Yellow exudate
2 ANF positive
3 LE cells present
4 Complement level low
5 Glucose level high

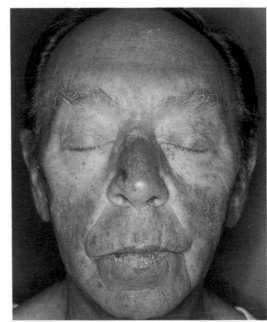
505

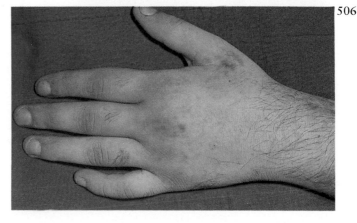
506

505 Systemic lupus erythematosus. The facial butterfly rash is a feature of discoid lupus and is present in about 50% of patients with systemic lupus.

506 Systemic lupus erythematosus. Petechial eruption with vasculitis may be caused by tissue deposition of circulating immune complexes.

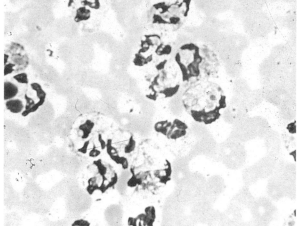

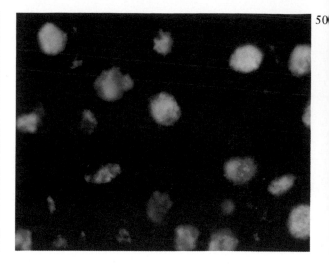

50

507 Lupus erythematosus cells (LE cells) showing inclusions of nuclear material within the cytoplasm of a polymorphonuclear leucocyte. LE cells are found in 90% of cases of SLE. DNA antibodies are found in 75% and their presence is used as a supporting diagnostic test for SLE. The LE cell is produced *in vitro* by the phagocytosis by neutrophils of nuclear fragments with antinuclear antibodies. *In vivo*, LE cells may form in the bone marrow, synovial cerebrospinal or pleurocardial fluids.

508 Antinuclear antibody (ANA). Indirect immuno-fluorescence using rat liver tissue and fluorescein-conjugated antihuman IgG. The fluorescein shows a diffuse distribution staining the whole nucleus. These are present in 90% of cases of SLE, but provide less specific diagnostic information than DNA binding antibodies. Other serological characteristics include rheumatoid factor, circulating immune complexes and hypocomplementaemia.

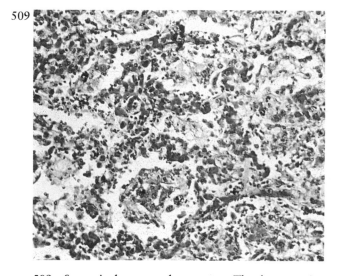

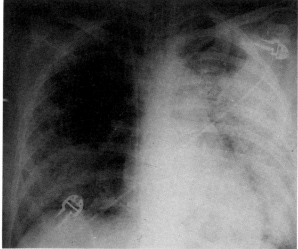

51

509 Systemic lupus erythematosus. The lung section shows a mixed cellular infiltrate and mild interstitial fibrosis. Pulmonary involvement includes pleurisy with a friction rub or effusion, shifting pulmonary infiltrates, plate atelectasis and interstitial lung disease; these all lead to hyperventilation, impairment of diffusion capacity and a restrictive pattern of respiration. The lungs, like the kidneys, are vulnerable to immune complex injury.

510 Systemic lupus erythematosus. Chest radiograph of a patient receiving assisted ventilation who presented with life-threatening dyspnoea, respiratory failure and haemoptysis. Intrapulmonary haemorrhage is an unusual presenting feature. The widespread pulmonary infiltrations and confluent shadowing in the left lung are caused by blood in the alveoli and air spaces due to intrapulmonary haemorrhage.

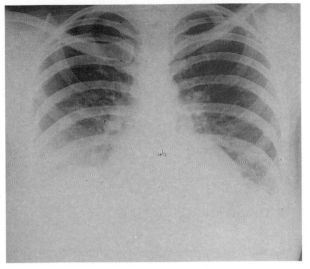

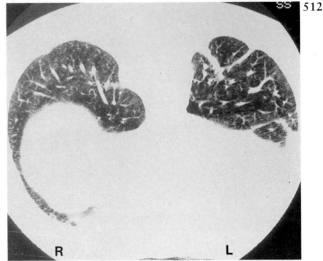

511 **Systemic lupus erythematosus.** Chest radiograph of dyspnoeic patient showing elevation of the diaphragm due to impaired diaphragmatic muscle function. The appearance may be described as 'shrinking' or 'vanishing' lung.

512 **Systemic lupus erythematosus.** High resolution CT (HRCT) scan of thorax (prone). Irregular bands of density (fibrosis and atelectasis) extend from the pleural surface into the lung parenchyma. There are no characteristic features of SLE on HRCT, but it is common to find pleural thickening or fluid, irregular areas of fibrosis or collapse, and atypical areas of irregular consolidation. Fibrosing alveolitis is rarely seen.

Pulmonary vasculitis in Behçet's disease

Behçet's disease was originally described as a triad of oral and genital ulceration with relapsing uveitis, but is now recognised as a multisystem disease (513). The syndrome is rare in the UK but more common in Turkey, the Middle and Far East and Japan. The pathology is a vasculitis principally involving the veins. Pulmonary vasculitis may occur as a result of the deposition of circulating antigen–antibody complexes. Cryoglobulins of IgM or IgG class are present in 75% of cases. The patient may present with dyspnoea, pleuritic chest pain, cough and haemoptysis, and the chest radiograph with patchy infiltrates, effusions or pulmonary fibrosis. Rarely, necrotising pulmonary vasculitis with life-threatening haemoptysis may occur.

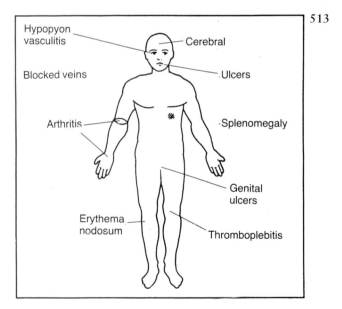

513 Clinical features of Behçet's disease.

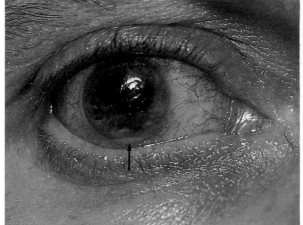

514

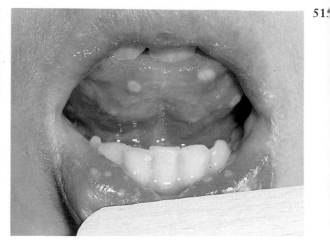

515

514 Uveitis. Hypopyon with fluid level, keratic precipitates and posterior synechiae. Ocular involvement is more frequent in HLA-B5 patients.

515 Recurrent aphthous stomatitis is most frequent in HLA-B12 patients. Ulceration of the mouth is virtually a constant feature and similar ulcers may involve the alimentary tract mucosa.

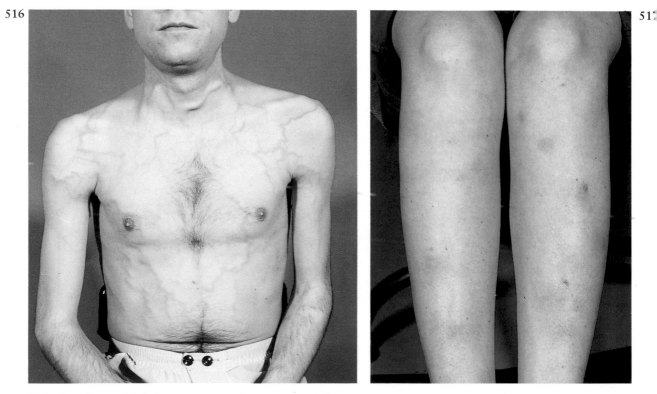

516

517

516 Superior and inferior vena cava obstruction in Behçet's disease.

517 Erythema nodosum. Chronic erythema nodosum may be found in 80% of cases of Behçet's disease.

518 Chronic genital ulceration. Ulceration of the scrotum, penile shaft and perineum or haemorrhagic lesions of the glans penis, labia and vaginal mucosa are common.

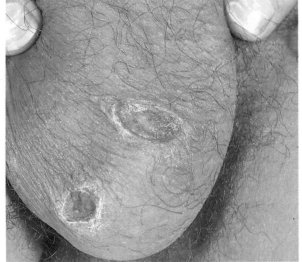

518

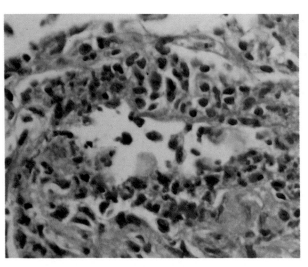

519 Behçet's disease. A small pulmonary vein disrupted and infiltrated by polymorphonuclear leucocytes and mononuclear cells. (H&E×445.)

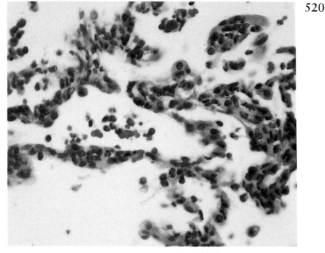

520

520 Behçet's disease. The interalveolar septums are infiltrated by polymorphonuclear leucocytes. (H&E×225.)

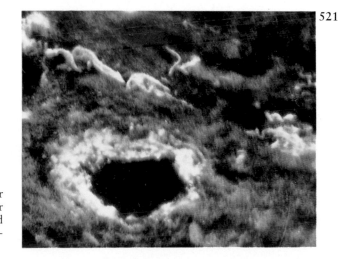

521

521 Behçet's disease. Prominent granular staining for C3 complement in the wall of a small vein. Similar staining for fibrinogen in the wall of a small vein and adjacent perivascular tissue was demonstrated. (Immunofluorescence microscopy.)

TYPE IV. Cell-mediated lung injury

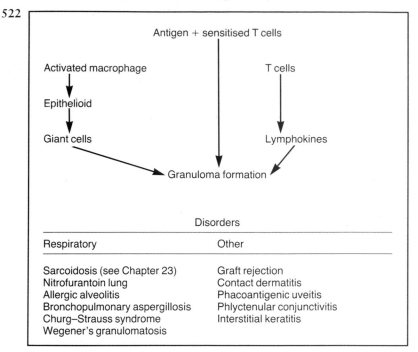

Antigen + sensitised T cells

Activated macrophage

T cells

Epithelioid

Giant cells

Lymphokines

Granuloma formation

Disorders

Respiratory	Other
Sarcoidosis (see Chapter 23)	Graft rejection
Nitrofurantoin lung	Contact dermatitis
Allergic alveolitis	Phacoantigenic uveitis
Bronchopulmonary aspergillosis	Phlyctenular conjunctivitis
Churg–Strauss syndrome	Interstitial keratitis
Wegener's granulomatosis	

522 Type IV. Cell-mediated injury.

Extrinsic allergic alveolitis (hypersensitivity pneumonitis)

The repeated inhalation of various organic dusts (and certain low molecular weight chemicals) (**Table 36**) causes a hypersensitivity granulomatous pneumonitis, reflecting Type IV cell-mediated re-activity which predominantly involves the peripheral gas-exchanging parts of the lung. There is also evidence of Type III reactivity with delayed-type skin tests and precipitating antibodies. Initially, repeated inhalation of the offending antigen leads to the production of circulating precipitating antibodies and to circulating immune complexes (Type III), but sufficient antigen invasion also leads to macrophage activation and to epithelioid cell granuloma formation (Type IV).

The syndrome of hypersensitivity pneumonitis covers a range of reactions. The classic acute presentation with chills, dry cough and influenzal symptoms develops 4–9 hours after heavy exposure. The main clinical findings are tachypnoea and mid to late inspiratory crackles. Repeated exposure may result in irreversible lung fibrosis and respiratory impairment. Finger clubbing is not a feature at any stage.

An insidious chronic onset is the usual response to budgerigar (parakeet) antigen. Patients present with malaise, dyspnoea, unproductive cough and sometimes weight loss, often over months or even years.

Table 36. Nature and sources of organic dust antigens in extrinsic allergic alveolitis.

Disease	Dust exposure	Nature of antigen to which precipitin is shown
Farmers' lung	Mouldy overheated hay	Thermophilic actinomycetes *Micropolyspora faeni* *Thermoactinomyces vulgaris*
Fog fever in cattle	Mouldy hay	*Micropolyspora faeni*
Bagassosis	Mouldy overheated sugarcane bagasse	*Thermoactinomyces sacharii*
Mushroom workers' lung	Mushroom compost dust and spores	Thermophilic actinomycetes (see farmers' lung)
Maltworkers' lung	Mouldy barley or malt	*Aspergillus fumigatus* *Aspergillus clavatus*
Bird fanciers' lung	Pigeon and budgerigar droppings Wax coating feathers – 'pigeon bloom'	Avian serum protein antigens (probably IgA)
Pituitary snufftakers' lung	Powder of porcine and bovine posterior pituitary extract	Serum protein and pituitary antigens
Wheat weevil disease (Millers' lung)	Infested wheat flour	*Sitophilus granarius*
Maple strippers' lung	Maple bark	*Cryptostroma (Coniosporium) corticale*
Sequoisis	Mouldy redwood sawdust	*Aureobasidium (Pullularia) pullulans graphium*
Suberosis	Oak bark, cork, dust	Mouldy oak bark *P. frequentans*
Woodworkers' lung	Sawdusts of oak, cedar, etc.	Sawdust extracts
Summer pneumonitis		*Trichosporon cutaneum*
Wood pulp workers' lung	Mouldy soft woods	*Alternaria* species
Cheese washers' lung	Moulds on cheese	*Penicillium casei*
New Guinea lung	Mouldy thatch dust	Extracts of thatch
Smallpox handlers' lung	Smallpox scabs	
Paprika splitters' lung	Mouldy paprika pods	*Mucor stolonifer* and species
Humidifier or forced air conditioner system lung	Fungal spores in air conditioning ducts and in home humidifiers	Thermophilic actinomycetes
Washing powder lung	Biological powders	*Bacillus subtilis*
Poultry handlers' lung	Poultry feathers and products	Turkey and chicken proteins
Isocyanate alveolitis	Printing, electronics, paint	Isocyanates

Diagnosis of extrinsic allergic alveolitis

- Identification of potential source of antigen in the patient's home or work environment.
- Characteristic clinical, radiological or functional changes of the disease.
- Demonstration of precipitating antibodies to the causal agent in the patient's serum. However, precipitins may be found in healthy exposed subjects with no lung disease and may disappear quite quickly when exposure ceases in patients with irreversible lung disease.

Farmers' lung

This is due to the inhalation of spores of thermophilic actinomycetes, filamentous bacteria that grow in hay or damp organic matter. The spores are liberated when mouldy hay is fed to cattle, usually in the winter.

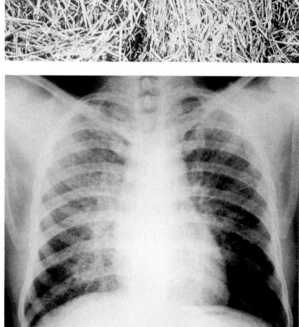

523

523 Farmers' lung. The mouldy hay (right) contrasts with that which has been freshly stored (left). The principal organism responsible for farmers' lung is *Micropolyspora faeni* (85% of cases), but other thermoactinomyces species are also important. When stored with a water content above 30%, the hay, grain or other vegetable matter becomes heated as a result of the metabolism of rapidly multiplying thermophilic organisms. This is the best recognised example of extrinsic allergic alveolitis in the UK. The prevalence of farmers' lung is related to local rainfall and to farming methods and can be prevented by adequate drying of crops before storage.

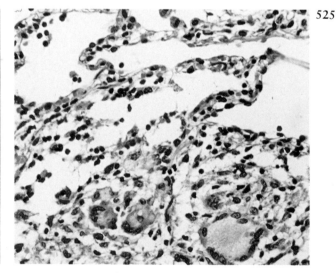

525

524 Acute farmers' lung. Fine nodular mid-zone proximal shadows are visible. Recurrent breathlessness, dry cough, influenza-like symptoms of malaise, fever and limb pains occur at an interval of six hours after heavy exposure to mouldy hay. In mild attacks there may be no lung function abnormality. Severe attacks show a restrictive defect.

525 Farmers' lung. Focal granulomatous lesions, together with a diffuse interstitial chronic inflammatory cell infiltrate of histiocytes and plasma cells, are centred on the small bronchi. The non-caseating granulomata often contain characteristic clefts and doubly refractile foreign material of vegetable origin, which distinguishes them from sarcoid lesions.

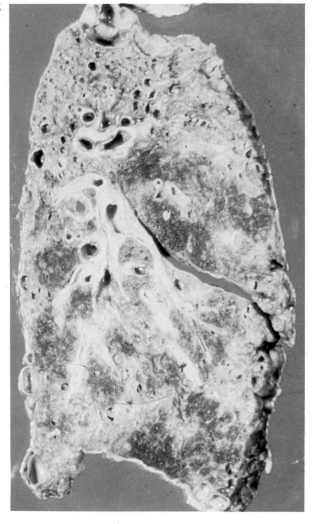

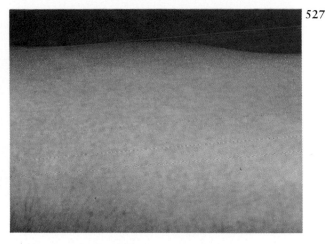

527 Farmers' lung. A late skin reaction (Type III) to *M. faeni* was observed six hours after an intradermal injection of 0.1 ml of test solution. Complement and IgG are classically involved and in most subjects specific precipitating antibody is present. Some late reactions may be mediated by IgE antibodies alone.

526 Whole lung section of extrinsic allergic alveolitis due to chronic farmers' lung. Diffuse interstitial fibrosis causing contraction and distortion of the lung parenchyma with honeycombing and cyst formation. The changes are predominantly in the upper lobes and involve central areas of the lung in contrast to the characteristic basal and peripheral fibrosis in cryptogenic fibrosing alveolitis.

528 Bronchial challenge test to *M. faeni* (diagrammatic). Late asthmatic reaction (Type III) accompanied by moderate systemic symptoms maximal at eight hours after challenge with *M. faeni*.

The other causes of extrinsic allergic alveolitis may produce similar bronchospasm on provocation testing.

The safety of bronchial provocation tests is often questioned. They should only be performed under medical supervision with facilities available to treat bronchospasm. Skin and bronchial challenge tests are complementary in sorting out the specificity of antigens suspected to be the cause of extrinsic alveolitis.

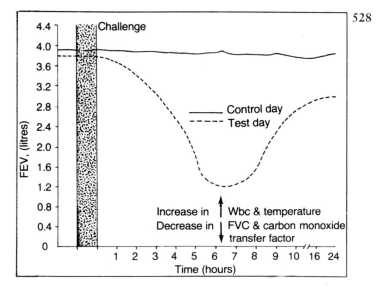

Bird fanciers' lung

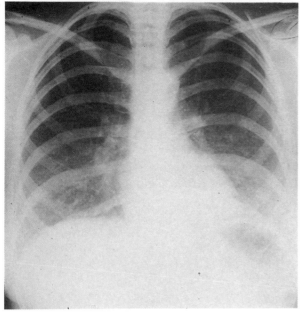

Bird fanciers' lung is caused by inhaled avian serum proteins present in the dry dust of excreta and in the bloom present on the feathers. At least in pigeons, IgA seems to be the most important antigen present in the bloom that covers and imparts a gloss to the feathers. Pigeon fanciers whose exposure occurs intermittently when cleaning the loft often present with acute symptoms. Budgerigar fanciers are constantly exposed to birds kept indoors and more often present with chronic insidious lung disease. The estimated incidence of lung disease among budgerigar owners lies between 0.5 to 7.5%.

Evidence of sensitisation to pigeon protein is found in 35% of all pigeon breeders and it is likely that about 15% of fanciers experience hypersensitivity reactions.

529 Bird fanciers' lung. Acute extrinsic allergic alveolitis in a young budgerigar fancier with diffuse lower zone nodular shadowing. At this stage, the patient's only symptoms were an irritating cough and vague malaise.

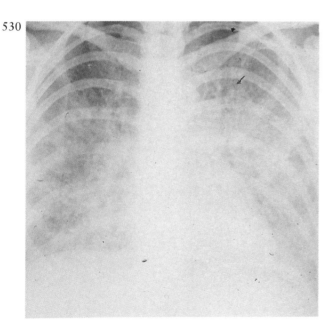

530 **Bird fanciers' lung.** Acute extrinsic allergic alveolitis. Fine, widely disseminated nodular shadows ('ground glass'), in association with severe dyspnoea, rigors and fever, followed continuing heavy exposure to birds. Lung volumes were greatly reduced. Fine inspiratory crackles were heard throughout both lung fields. Same patient as shown in 529, seven weeks later.

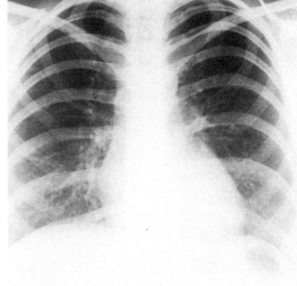

531 **Bird fanciers' lung.** Complete reversal of the symptoms and the radiographic shadowing occurred after removal from contact with the allergens. (Same patient as shown in 529.)

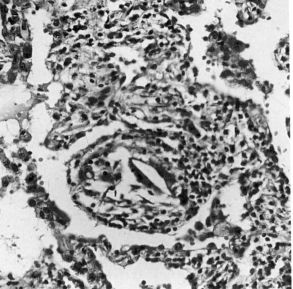

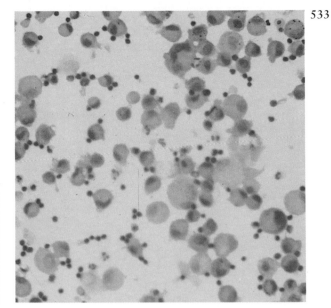

532 Acute bird fanciers' lung – lung biopsy. Interstitial alveolar wall infiltrate of lymphocytes, plasma cells, foamy histiocytes and 'clefted' granuloma are present. Unlike sarcoidosis the granulomata contain doubly refractive organic material, are not present in the lymph nodes and resolve rapidly without hyalinisation. (H& E×100.)

533 Acute allergic alveolitis. Bronchoalveolar lavage cytological specimen showing a large number of lymphocytes with macrophages. Typically, the proportion of lymphocytes in the recovered cell total is greatly increased and their presence gives further support to the diagnosis of extrinsic allergic alveolitis.

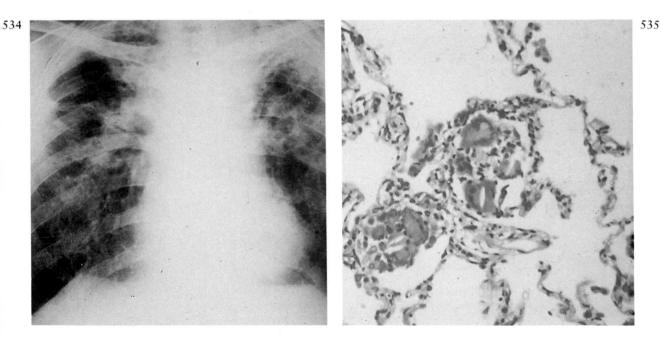

534 Chronic bird fanciers' lung. Upper lobe fibrosis and cavitation leading to a permanent severe ventilatory restriction and diffusion defect.

535 Chronic bird fanciers' lung with extensive fibrotic scarring, disorganisation of the normal alveolar structure and development of honey-combing.

Wegener's granulomatosis

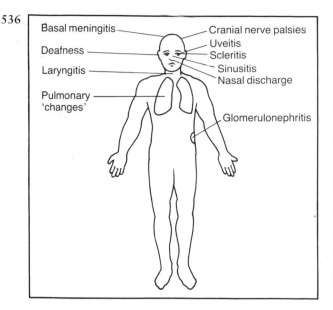

536

Basal meningitis
Deafness
Laryngitis
Pulmonary 'changes'

Cranial nerve palsies
Uveitis
Scleritis
Sinusitis
Nasal discharge

Glomerulonephritis

536 Clinical features of Wegener's granulomatosis.

In this multisystem disorder the classic presentation is with a granulomatous angiitis involving the upper and lower airways and the kidney, resulting in necrotising granulomatous vasculitis of the airways, focal glomerulonephritis and disseminated vasculitis. Characteristically, the onset is insidious and occurs during the fourth or fifth decade. The course is progressive and results in intractable sinusitis, nodular pulmonary lesions and terminal renal involvement. Biopsy shows ulcerating granulomatous angiitis in which pulmonary vessels are especially involved. This suggests Type III injury. The disease may be localised to the lungs or widely disseminated.

The term 'limited Wegener's granulomatosis' was introduced to describe lung and possibly extrathoracic Wegener's in the absence of glomerulonephritis. This limited form of the disease follows a less aggressive course than classic Wegener's.

The diagnosis is confirmed by finding serum antineutrophilic cytoplasmic antibodies (ANCA).

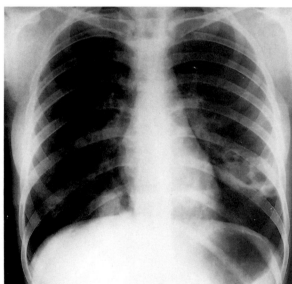

537

537 Localised Wegener's granulomatosis. Multiple nodular lesions are present in both lower zones, with cavitation and an early alveolar infiltrate in the left lower zone.

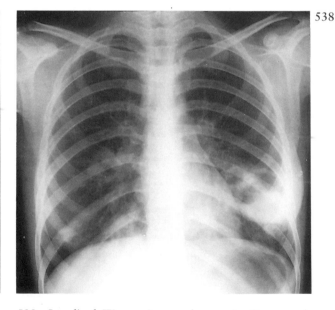

538

538 Localised Wegener's granulomatosis. One month later, cavitation in the left lung has increased as a consequence of vasculitis and gangrene. The alveolar shadowing was due to intrapulmonary haemorrhage. (Same patient as shown in 537.)

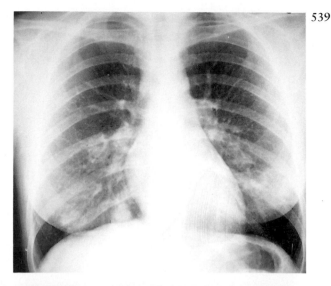

539

539 Localised Wegener's granulomatosis. Improvement was seen after two months of immunosuppressive therapy with cyclophosphamide and prednisolone. (Same patient as shown in 537.) Lung involvement is present in 95% and can manifest as cough, haemoptysis, dyspnoea or chest radiograph abnormality in an asymptomatic patient.

540

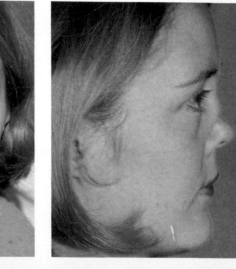

541

540, 541 Wegener's granulomatosis – upper respiratory tract lesion. Collapsed and ulcerated nose. Invasive granulomatous tissue extending through the nasal cartilage and subcutaneous tissues has produced a 'saddle nose' deformity. Nasal mucosal biopsy may be diagnostic.

542

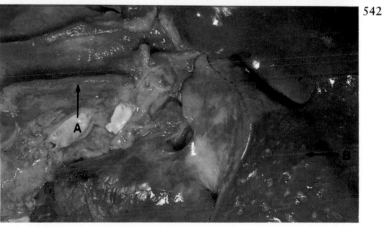

542 Wegener's granulomatosis – lower respiratory tract lesion. Haemorrhagic ulceration of the trachea (arrow A) and proximal bronchi. The cut surface of the lower lobe is haemorrhagic from a terminal infarction (arrow B).

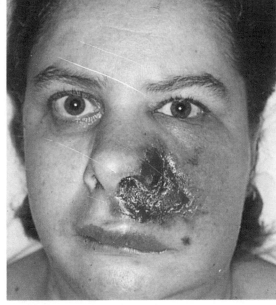

543

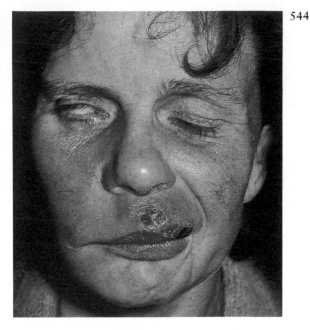

544

543 Wegener's granulomatosis. Pyoderma gangrenosum can occur. This florid ulceration extended into the nostrils. Immunosuppression provides initial rapid improvement. (ANCA positive.)

544 Generalised Wegener's granulomatosis with vascular lesions in the brain, spinal cord, peripheral nerves and kidney, and pulmonary cavitation. This patient had a right seventh nerve cranial palsy. There is also vasculitis of the upper lip. (ANCA positive.)

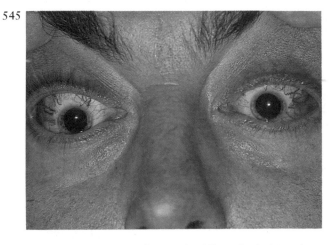

545

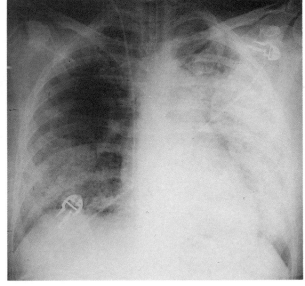

546

545 Wegener's granulomatosis. Bilateral scleritis. There was also underlying iridocyclitis, retinal vasculitis and minimal conjunctivitis. Following treatment, ANCA titre fell.

546 Wegener's granulomatosis. Chest radiograph showing extensive alveolar shadowing due to alveolar haemorrhage. The patient presented with profuse haemoptysis and respiratory failure. Antiglomerular basement membrane antibodies were negative.

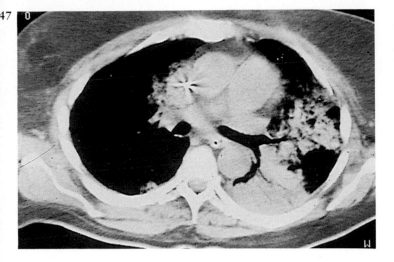

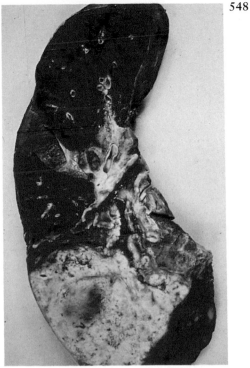

547 Wegener's granulomatosis. CT scan showing extensive lower lobe consolidation with an air bronchogram in the left lower lobe. The appearances are due to a combination of infarction and alveolar haemorrhage. (Same patient as shown in **546**.)

548 Wegener's granulomatosis. Macroscopic lung section. A large creamy-yellow infarcted lesion with necrosis and cavitation involves most of the lower lobe.

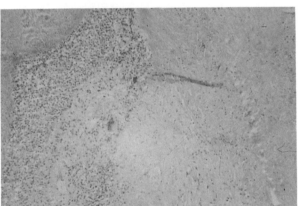

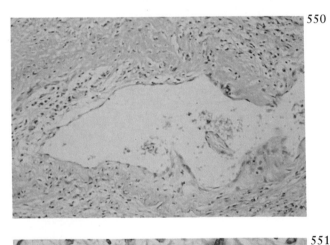

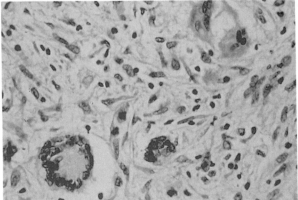

549 Lung biopsy of infarcted lung. An area of necrosis with involvement of the small airways, poorly formed granulomata and serpiginous areas of necrosis surrounded by chronically inflamed tissue in which there is a suggestion of pallisading. (H & E × 25.)

550 Wegener's granulomatosis. A vessel is partially obliterated by fibrous tissue in which there are chronic inflammatory and sparse giant cells. The normal vascular wall is destroyed. The surrounding tissue contains lymphocytes and plasma cells.

551 Wegener's granulomatosis. A later stage than that shown in **550**, with a healing granuloma, fibroblast proliferation and multinucleated giant cells. (H & E × 100.)

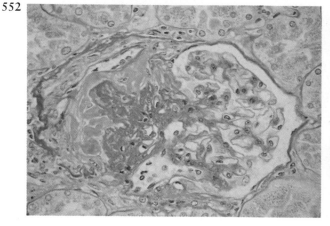

552 **Wegener's granulomatosis.** Glomerular involvement with characteristic histological findings of necrosis and angiitis in the capillary tuft, and eosinophilic fibrinoid degeneration. Renal involvement is seen in 85% of patients.

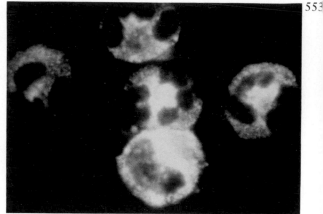

553 **Wegener's granulomatosis – ANCA test.** Antineutrophilic cytoplasmic autoantibodies (ANCA) identified in serum by immunofluorescence microscopy using alcohol-fixed human neutrophils. A positive test indicates activity.

Polyarteritis nodosa

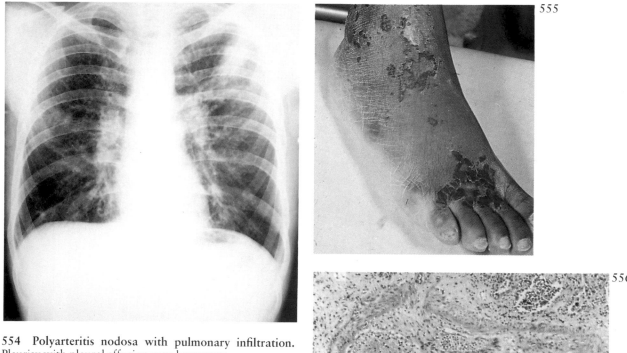

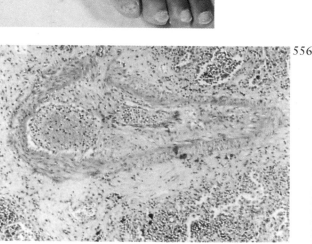

554 **Polyarteritis nodosa with pulmonary infiltration.** Pleurisy with pleural effusion may be present.

555 **Polyarteritis nodosa.** Mononeuritis with vasculitis.

556 **Polyarteritis nodosa.** Arteritis usually begins in the media and extends to the outer coats of the arterial wall; necrosis, inflammatory cell infiltration and eventual healing with fibrosis then follow. The vessel wall is partially destroyed and the lumen occluded by thrombosis.

Polyarteritis nodosa (PAN) is a collagen disease characterised by inflammatory and necrotising lesions in all three layers of small arteries and arterioles, leading to aneurysm, thrombosis and infarction. Men are affected four times more frequently than women. Clinical features include a rapid deterioration with unexplained fever, weight loss, a high sedimentation rate, hypertension and glomerulonephritis, neurological involvement, arthritis and abdominal pain. Lung involvement presents with a cough, haemoptysis, pneumonia and asthmatic symptoms. A very high blood eosinophilia points to the diagnosis, which may be confirmed by finding arteritic lesions in skin or muscle biopsy, or visceral aneurysm on angiography. Apart from a strong association with hepatitis B antigen, only minor immunological abnormalities are found in PAN

The Churg–Strauss syndrome of eosinophilic granulomatosis is delineated as a variant of PAN because of asthma, granuloma formation and generalised vasculitis. Visceral angiography reveals aneurysms. Raised IgE levels and possible immune complex and cell-mediated granulomata all indicate Type I, II and IV lung injury (**Table 28**).

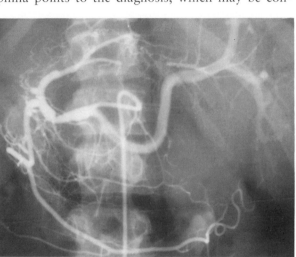

557

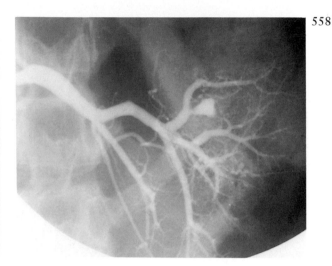

558

557 Visceral angiography. Aneurysms are demonstrated in the splenic artery and left hepatic artery.

558 Visceral angiography. Magnified renal arteriogram demonstrating aneurysms of the renal artery.

Lymphomatoid granulomatosis

This form of angiitis and granulomatosis, first described in 1972, closely resembles localised Wegener's granulomatosis and usually presents in middle age (occurring slightly more often in males) with fever, cough and dyspnoea. The vessels of the lung, skin, kidneys and central nervous system are

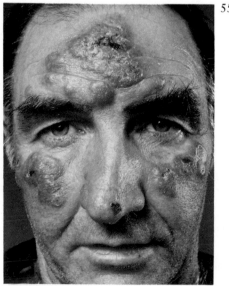

559

559 Cutaneous lymphomatoid granulomatosis with chronic nodular ulcerating lesions. The initial diagnosis was sarcoidosis, but this was later revised to Wegener's granulomatosis when the skin lesion ulcerated and the chest radiograph showed a cavitating lower lobe lesion.

211

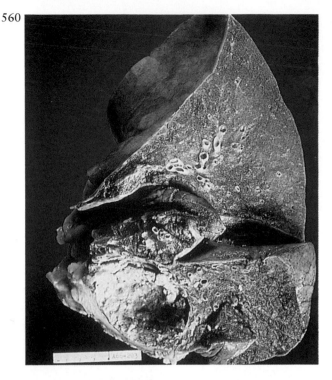

560

most often involved. Extrapulmonary manifestations include a raised erythematous skin rash that resembles erythema nodosum but affects the trunk, skin nodules, central nervous system involvement with cranial nerve palsies, peripheral neuropathy, hepatosplenomegaly or peripheral lymphadenopathy. The prognosis is poor. Some develop T-cell lymphomas and may succumb to sepsis or haemoptysis.

560 Pulmonary lymphomatoid granulomatosis. Extensive necrosis with cavitation of a large nodular lesion in the left lung.

561 Pulmonary lymphomatoid granulomatosis. Bilateral opacities and cavitation in the right mid-zone. The main radiographic features are of multiple bilateral opacities resembling metastases and the absence of hilar adenopathy.

562 Pulmonary lymphomatoid granulomatosis. A highly cellular atypical lymphoreticular infiltrate, rich in mitosis, which often invades or destroys blood vessels.

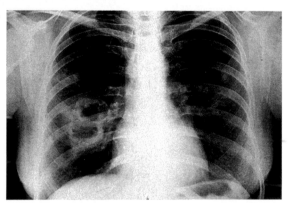

561

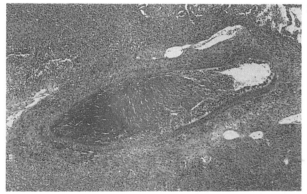

56

Angioimmunoblastic lymphadenopathy

This uncommon condition presents with constitutional symptoms, generalised lymphadenopathy, hepatosplenomegaly, normochromic normocytic anaemia and polyclonal hypergammaglobulinaemia. The diagnosis is made by lymph node biopsy.

563 Angioimmunoblastic lymphadenopathy. The normal lymph node architecture is replaced by a mixed cellular proliferation of immunoblasts and plasma cells, which may also infiltrate the lung. Patients present with fever, lymphadenopathy, anaemia, polyclonal hypergammaglobulinaemia and pulmonary changes reminiscent of Hodgkin's disease. (H & E × 40.)

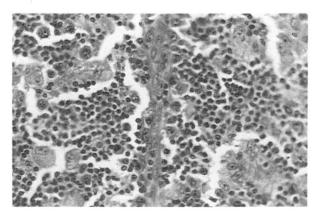

56

21 Occupational lung disease

Pneumoconiosis

The literal meaning of pneumoconiosis is 'dusty lung'. The term is usually taken to mean a permanent alteration of lung structure caused by the inhalation of mineral dust and the tissue reactions of the lungs to its presence (excluding bronchitis and emphysema). The most common pneumoconioses due to fibrogenic dusts are coal workers' pneumoconiosis, silicosis and asbestosis.

Inhaled dust particles are a hazard in certain occupations because, if inhaled, they may reach the terminal bronchioles and alveoli to initiate destructive reactions and fibrosis. The particle size is important: particles in the range 0.5–5 μm may reach the alveoli, especially in the mid-zones of the lungs.

Alveolar macrophages can clear small amounts of dust but, if the clearance capacity is overcome, the macrophages with their retained particles accumulate in the alveoli and respiratory bronchioles. If the dust is not fibrogenic, this accumulation will not impair lung function or shorten life. Alveolar retention of the fibrogenic dust from coal, silica and asbestos impairs lung function and shortens life because of pulmonary fibrosis. Larger particles impact in the proximal airways and are removed by mucociliary clearance. Particles under 0.5 μm behave like a gas and seldom settle in the lungs.

The inhaled non-reactive dusts of tin, iron, barium and antimony may produce extensive shadowing with little if any functional impairment. Coal dust, kaolin and diatomaceous earth may cause moderate functional changes, while severe functional impairment may be caused by the highly fibrogenic dusts of silica, talc and asbestos.

The clinical significance of dust exposure can be difficult to evaluate because of the overwhelming effect of cigarette smoking on lung function.

Table 37. Fibrogenic dusts.

Dust	Pattern of fibrosis	Complications
Coal	Progressive massive fibrosis	
Silica	Nodular fibrosis (silicosis) Progressive massive fibrosis	Pulmonary tuberculosis
Asbestos	Diffuse fibrosis (asbestosis)	Lung cancer

213

Coal miners' pneumoconiosis

The prolonged inhalation of coal dust may lead to three conditions:

1 Coal workers' pneumoconiosis (CWP).
2 Silicosis.
3 Industrial bronchitis.

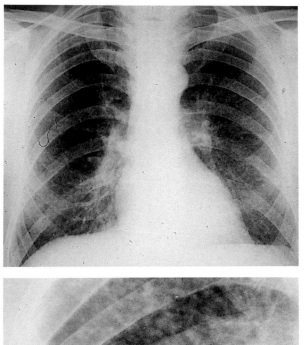

564

564   Simple coal workers' pneumoconiosis. Small round and irregular opacities are scattered throughout both lung fields. The extent of the radiographic abnormality correlates with the coal dust content of the lungs. Simple CWP only progresses with continuing coal dust exposure, has no symptoms and causes no important alteration of pulmonary function.

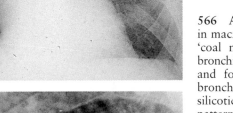

565

565   Simple coal workers' pneumoconiosis. Small rounded regular opacities in the lung fields, measuring 3–10 mm in size. (Category r.)

566   Anthrosilicotic nodule. Accumulation of coal dust in macrophages at the centre of the acinus gives rise to a 'coal macule' in the walls of alveoli and respiratory bronchioles. There is destruction of the bronchiolar muscle and formation of dense collagen that obliterates the bronchiolar lumen and vascular channels. Unlike the true silicotic nodule, the collagen is arranged in an irregular pattern. The process may progress to centrilobular emphysema and fibrosis.

567   Complicated CWP (progressive massive fibrosis). Large fibrotic masses of irregular shape are present in both upper and apical segments of the right lower lobe. Cavitation, when it occurs, is usually due to ischaemic necrosis as the lung masses encroach upon and destroy the adjacent blood vessels and airways. Chronic lung symptoms, significant impairment of pulmonary function and premature death occur.

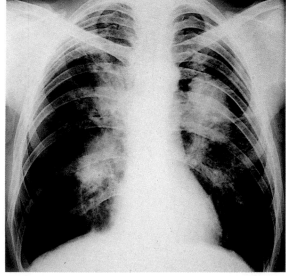

567

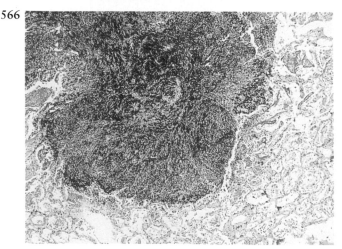

566

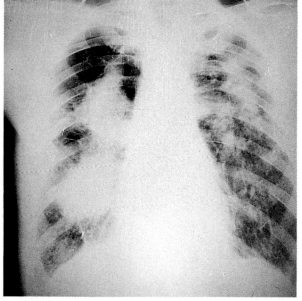

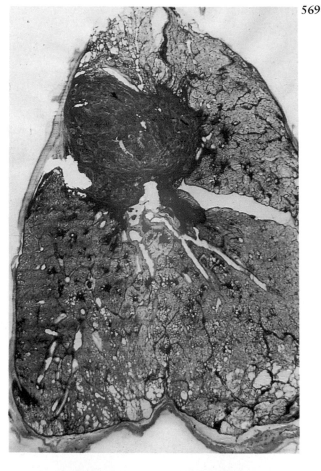

568 Progressive massive fibrosis. Large progressive lesions with considerable distortion of the right lung. Advanced coal workers' pneumoconiosis may terminate in cor pulmonale.

569 Early complicated pneumoconiosis on a background of simple CWP and basal emphysema shown on a large lung section. Characteristic coal macules are present in the lower lung, together with a large anthracotic area of progressive massive fibrosis in the upper lobe. (Gough section.)

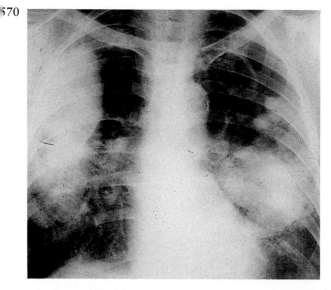

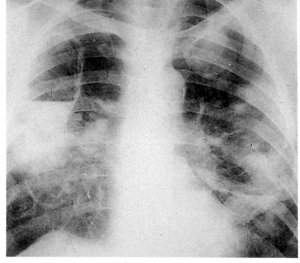

570 Progressive massive fibrosis. The usual discrete x-ray shadows seen in silicosis and coal workers' pneumoconiosis may coalesce to form large masses of collagen, especially in those with rheumatoid arthritis. This example shows unusually large opacities.

571 Progressive massive fibrosis. The centre of the mass may become necrotic and liquefy. Copious black sputum (melanoptysis) was expectorated, leaving these partially fluid-filled cavities. (Same patient as shown in 570.)

Rheumatoid pneumoconiosis (Caplan's syndrome)

Caplan's syndrome (first described in 1953) is the association of rheumatoid arthritis, pulmonary necrobiotic nodules and coal workers' pneumoconiosis. The nodules usually lie at the periphery of the lung fields, are multiple and well circumscribed and range in size from 0.5 to 5 cm. The manifestations of rheumatoid arthritis may be slight or absent, but rheumatoid factor is always present in the serum. Since Caplan's original paper the condition has been described in silicosis, asbestosis and boiler scaler's pneumoconiosis.

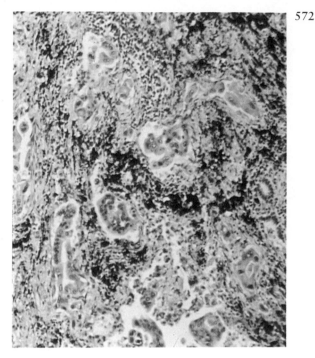

572 Caplan's nodules demonstrate a series of concentric layers, with a centre formed of necrotic tissue surrounded by varying amounts of collagen, coal dust and then a cellular zone of lymphocytes, plasma cells and polymorphs.

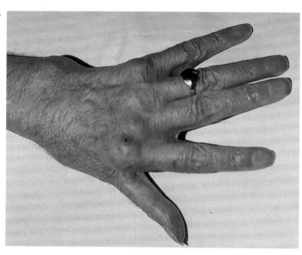

573 Coal miners' tattoo and rheumatoid arthritis alerted the clinician to the possibility of rheumatoid pneumoconiosis in this retired coalface worker. Vasculitis on the knuckle of the first finger is also evident.

574 Caplan's lesions (rheumatoid pneumoconiosis). Lung section showing rheumatoid nodules. These lesions may precede or follow clinical evidence of rheumatoid arthritis. Cellular and necrotising reactions occur at the periphery of silicotic nodules. Concentric calcification and cavitation is common, and pleural effusions may occur.

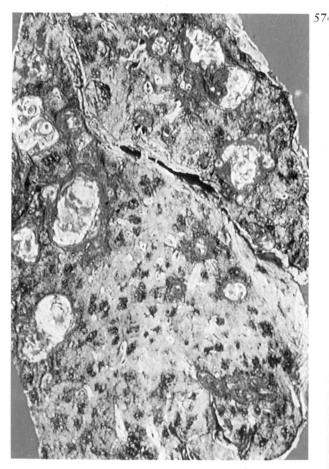

Silicosis

Silicosis is caused by inhalation of fine crystalline silica or silicon dioxide dust (quartz, cristobalite and tridymite). Silicosis occurs in slate and granite quarrying, refractory and foundry work, and in the glass and pottery industries, and abrasive blasting with industrial sand. The pathological changes in the lung are related to the intensity and duration of exposure to silica.

Simple nodular silicosis (575) causes no symptoms. Chronic advanced nodular silicosis with widespread fibrosis may be progressive long after exposure ceases. Accidental heavy short-term exposure may lead to rapidly fatal acute silicosis, with end-stage lung fibrosis in a few months.

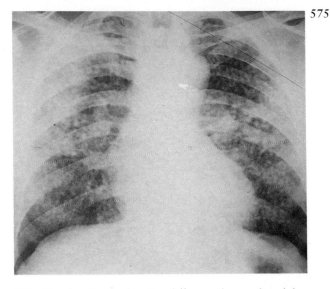

575

575 Simple silicosis showing diffuse widespread nodular lesions, most marked in the mid-zone. The nodules increase in size and coalesce as the disease progresses. Disability is caused by restriction in lung volumes. At a late stage, eggshell calcification of the hilar glands may occur. Simple silicosis describes the x-ray appearance of fine nodulation with no conglomerate nodule greater than 1 cm in diameter.

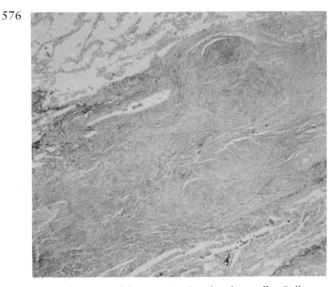

576

576 Silicotic nodules arise in the alveolar walls. Collagen deposited concentrically causes obliterative bronchiolitis. Silica, if present, is found peripherally. In contrast with the lesions in coal pneumoconiosis, the silicotic lesions are proliferative, with an excess of collagen but little silica dust. The inhaled free crystalline silica or silicon dioxide particles are ingested by macrophages and probably converted to salicic acid. The macrophages respond to the 'irritation' by liberating lysosomal enzymes which, it is believed, play an important part in pathogenesis. Relative to the severity of the fibrosis produced, the amount of dust present in the lung is small.

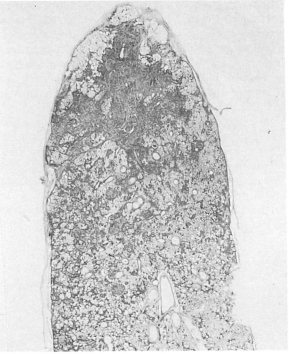

577

577 Conglomerate (massive) silicosis. Lung section showing multiple greyish nodules with aggregation into a large upper lobe conglomerate mass. Except when complicated by tuberculosis, silicotic massive fibrosis almost never cavitates.

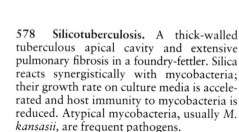

578 Silicotuberculosis. A thick-walled tuberculous apical cavity and extensive pulmonary fibrosis in a foundry-fettler. Silica reacts synergistically with mycobacteria; their growth rate on culture media is accelerated and host immunity to mycobacteria is reduced. Atypical mycobacteria, usually *M. kansasii,* are frequent pathogens.

Asbestos-related disease

The term 'asbestos' is used to describe a number of naturally occurring fibrous mineral silicates which have found widespread commercial use because of the materials' properties of heat, electricity, sound and fire resistance. Asbestos fibres are of two types: serpentine fibres, which are curly and flexible, and amphibole fibres, which are straight and stiff.

Chrysotile (white asbestos), a magnesium silicate, is the most widely used form of asbestos and the only commercially important example of the serpentine group. Commercially important amphiboles include: crocidolite (blue asbestos), an iron magnesium–sodium silicate; amosite (brown asbestos) and anthophyllite, iron–magnesium silicates; and tremolite and actinolite, calcium–iron–magnesium silicates.

The needle-shaped asbestos particles are 20–100 µm long and less than 3 µm in diameter. Chrysotile, because of its curly configuration, has a relatively broad cross-sectional area and penetrates less readily to the periphery than the needle-shaped amphiboles. Inhaled fibres impact in the lower bronchi and alveoli, from where they may reach the pleura, diaphragm or peritoneum.

Most fibres are removed by mucociliary clearance or by the lymphatics after being partially or completely engulfed by macrophages and by epithelial cells lining the airways. Of those fibres that remain in the lungs some become coated with the iron-containing protein ferritin and form asbestos bodies, also known as ferruginous bodies.

Many industrial countries have arrangements for compensation by the state of those workers whose health has been affected by asbestos exposure.

Asbestos-related disease may present as:

1 Diffuse interstitial fibrosis (asbestosis).
2 Asbestos-induced airways disease.
3 Benign pleural disease.
   • Pleural plaques.
   • Pleural effusion.
   • Diffuse pleural thickening.
4 Acute asbestos pleurisy and pleural effusion.
5 Malignant mesothelioma.
6 Lung cancer.

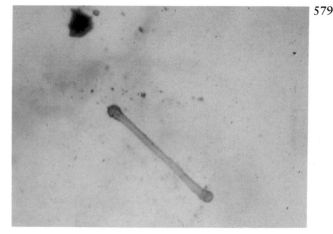

579 Asbestos bodies in the sputum. The asbestos fibre becomes coated with a film of proteinaceous material which is thickened over the sharp ends, giving a bulbous appearance.

Asbestosis

This may be defined as 'fibrosis of the lung caused by asbestos dust, which may or may not be associated with fibrosis of the parietal or pulmonary layers of the pleura'.

The presentation is with shortness of breath on exertion and a cough which is dry or productive of scanty mucoid sputum.

The physical findings are of late inspiratory fine crackles, initially posterolaterally and then becoming more widespread as the disease progresses. Finger clubbing is present in a proportion of cases. Cyanosis and cor pulmonale occur with advanced fibrosis. The interval between the onset of exposure to asbestos and the development of asbestosis with respiratory symptoms is commonly 20 years or longer. The risk of occurrence, severity and speed of onset is broadly related to the intensity and duration of asbestos exposure. During the latent period, inflammatory processes are triggered by the presence of asbestos fibres, resulting in peribronchiolar and alveolar fibrosis and leading eventually to obliteration of the alveolar architecture and extensive fibrosis.

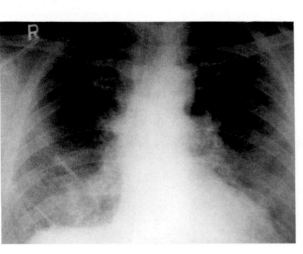

580 Asbestosis. Chest x-ray showing lower zone streaky fibrosis and diffuse haziness, giving the cardiac silhouette a 'shaggy' appearance in a 60-year-old male who, during his working life, spent ten years as an asbestos cement pipe lagger.

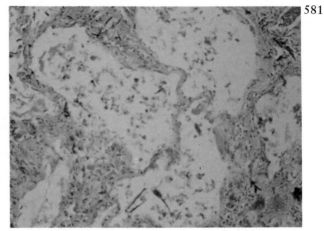

581 Asbestosis. Histological section showing fibrous thickening of the alveolar septa and interstitial fibrosis with obliteration of alveolar spaces that contain asbestos bodies. These gradually shrink, sometimes leaving dark granules of iron oxide.

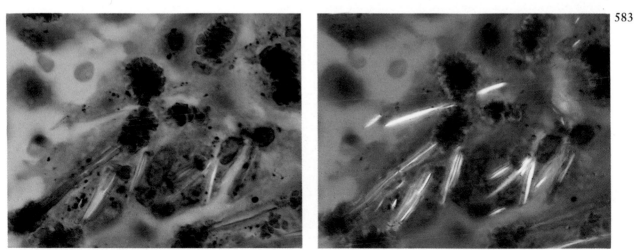

582, 583 Asbestos (ferruginous) bodies. Lung biopsy specimen. The asbestos fibre has become coated with the iron-containing protein ferritin. The tendency to become coated varies with fibre type and size, being greatest for the larger amphibole fibres and least for chrysotile. (H & E×250; **582** normal light, **583** three-quarters polarised light.)

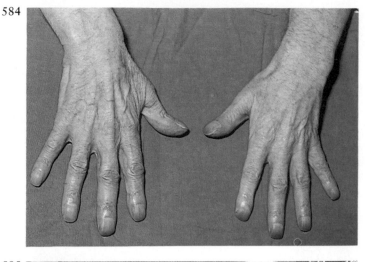

584 Asbestosis. Cyanosis and finger clubbing signify a late stage of asbestosis. The most common complaint is of exercise-induced breathlessness. Auscultation of the chest usually reveals loud inspiratory crackles, best heard at the lung bases. Finger clubbing is present in a third of cases. Asbestosis causes a restrictive respiratory defect and shortens life; 20% will die from respiratory failure.

585

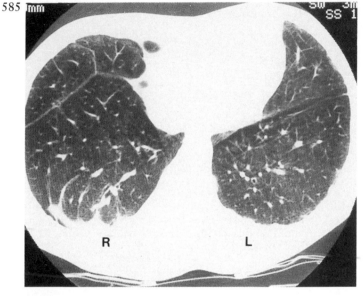

585 Asbestosis. CT scan. Pleural thickening is present posteriorly in both lower zones and is associated with linear and reticular changes in the lung parenchyma. On the right, coarse curved linear densities in the lower lobe merge with thickened pleura and almost certainly represent the formation of an area of rounded atelectasis (the pseudo-tumours of asbestosis). On the left, small linear reticular and branched opacities are caused by thickening of the secondary interlobular septa. Similar, lesser changes are visible in the right middle lobe and lingula anteriorly.

586

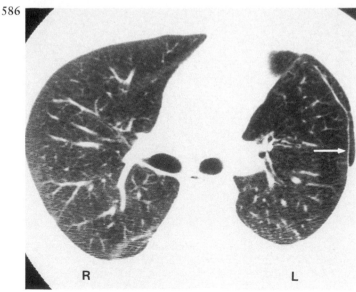

586 Asbestosis. CT scan. The characteristic subpleural line is clearly visible on the left anterolaterally (arrowed). It is usually due to compressed fibrotic alveoli. Similar curved linear densities may be seen in other causes of fibrosing alveolitis, but they are usually not as dense, linear and 'pencilled' in appearance. The subpleural line of asbestosis is frequently bilateral and usually posterior in position. The stretched appearance of the vessels in the lung and the subpleural linear densities are due to a fine interstitial fibrosis.

Benign pleural disease - pleural plaques

These are discrete raised areas, usually situated on the parietal pleura of the chest wall, diaphragm, pericardium and mediastinum. Plaques are composed of featureless hyalinised fibrous tissue, which often calcifies, and their presence is associated with occupational or environmental asbestos exposure.

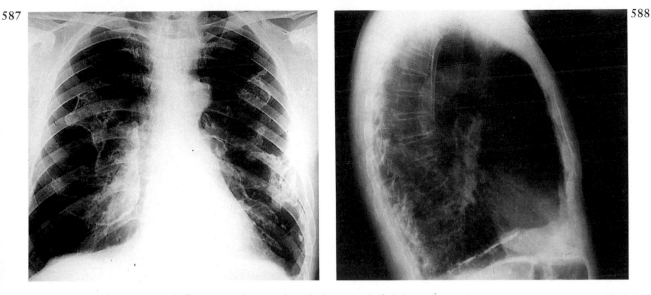

587, 588 Diaphragmatic calcification. Asbestos pleural plaques calcify bilaterally on the diaphragm and lower half of the parietal pleura. This dock worker had unloaded raw asbestos.

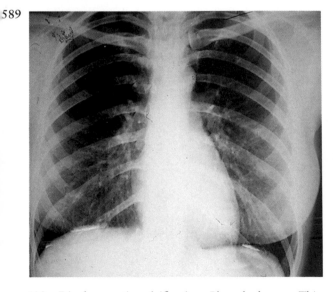

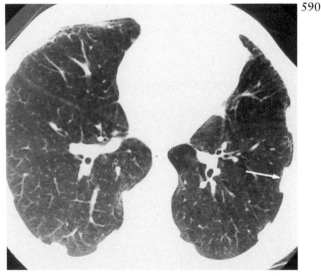

589 Diaphragmatic calcification. Pleural plaques. This dock worker's daughter was 'indirectly' exposed to asbestos from her father's clothing. Pleural plaques reflect asbestos exposure and are associated with an increased risk of developing asbestos and asbestos-related malignant disease.

590 Asbestosis and pleural plaques. The plaques are seen as short well-defined raised areas, giving rise to a turreted appearance (arrow). There is no associated parenchymal change (as in 585). There is pleural thickening anteriorly on the right, with associated irregularity of the lung parenchyma. Branched linear densities are widespread, indicating fibrosis and thickening in the secondary interlobular septa.

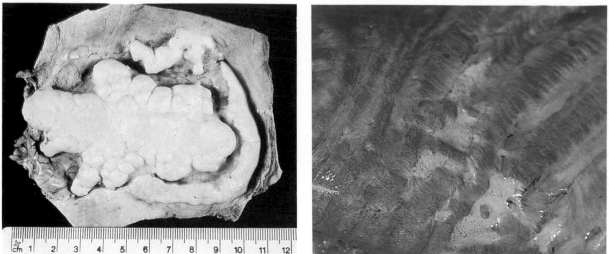

591, 592 Parietal pleural plaques are localised thickenings of the parietal pleura which may be visible on the chest radiograph if large and dense due to calcification.

Plaques are usually bilateral and occur most commonly over the middle and lower posterolateral chest wall and central portion of the diaphragm. Only 15% are detectable in life. They do not significantly interfere with lung function unless the pleura is extensively thickened. The calcified plaque in **591** was visible on the chest radiograph.

Benign pleural disease – acute asbestos pleurisy and pleural effusion

Acute asbestos pleurisy may follow soon after exposure to respirable asbestos fibre. It presents with pleuritic pain, accompanied by breathlessness if an effusion is present, can be recurrent and results in increasing diffuse pleural thickening. Spontaneous resolution is usual. Pleural aspiration reveals an exudate that may be blood-stained and pleural biopsy reveals non-specific pleural inflammation and fibrosis.

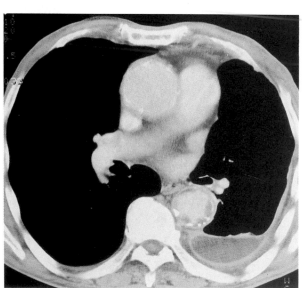

593 Asbestos-related pleural effusion. CT scan. A benign encysted pleural effusion is present on the left posteriorly. Contrast enhancement outlines the covering pleura, which is thickened and extends over the lateral chest wall on this side.

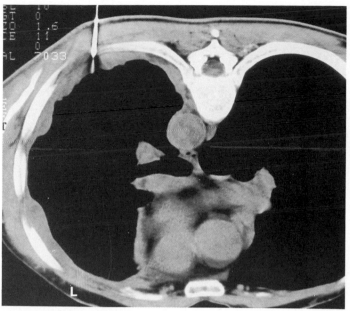

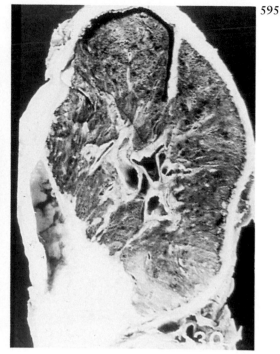

594   **Pleural thickening** (prone scan) caused by asbestos exposure. There is widespread thickening of the parietal pleura in the left hemithorax. The pleura covers the mediastinum and the inner chest wall, but shows no evidence of invasion. A biopsy needle is in position posteriorly.

595   **Benign pleural disease.** Diffuse pulmonary disease (asbestosis) and pleural disease usually occur together after prolonged and substantial asbestos exposure. The lung is encased by thickened pleura and the lung structure is distorted by fibrosis. Lung function tests showed greatly reduced lung volumes (left lung section).

Malignant mesothelioma

This is a tumour which arises from mesothelial cells or, possibly, a more primitive submesothelial cell. The tumour can arise from either pleural layer and in the early stage it is often associated with an effusion.

The risk of mesothelioma increases with the dose of asbestos, and the incidence increases with the time lapse since first exposure.

Inhaled asbestos fibres are deposited preferentially in the peripheral parts of the lung tissue, penetrate the visceral pleura and reach the parietal pleural surface indirectly via the pulmonary lymphatics or by direct transmission from the visceral to parietal pleura.

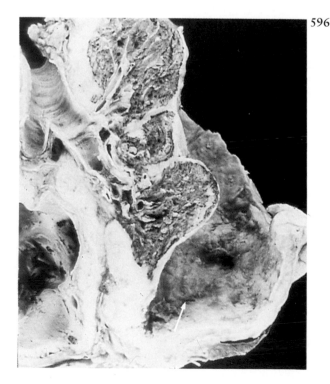

596   **Pleural mesothelioma and diffuse pleural disease.** The mesothelioma (arrowed) is infiltrating the pleura and displacing adjacent lung. The time interval can be short but, typically, there is a latent period of 20 years or more between first exposure to asbestos and the development of mesothelioma. The present evidence suggests that any heavy asbestos exposure, but particularly to crocidolite (blue), may cause a malignant mesothelioma.

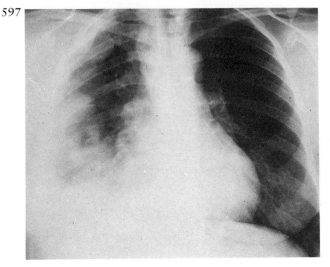

597 **Pleural mesothelioma.** Irregular protuberant pleural opacities give rise to blood-stained effusions. Symptoms are of breathlessness, weight loss, persistent localised aching discomfort and pleurisy.

598 **Mesothelioma.** A uniform 'spindle cell' or sarcomatous appearance is most usual on histology. In some cases, the appearance mimics adenocarcinoma and confident diagnosis is established only at necropsy.

599 **Mesothelioma.** Epithelial cell type consisting of adenopapillary structures.

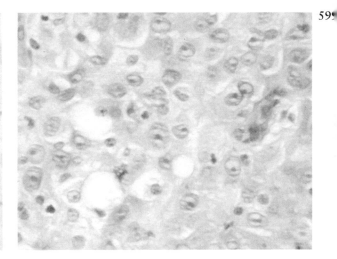

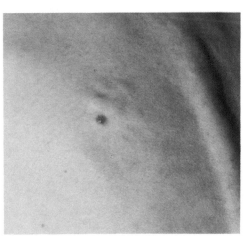

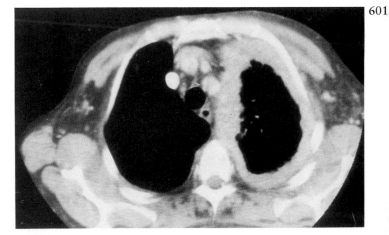

600 **Mesothelial tumours** spread locally and grow along needle and incision tracks.

601 **Mesothelioma.** CT scan. The left lung is surrounded by a thick 'rind' of tumour tissue, causing compression of the lung and centripetal drag on the mediastinum from the chest wall. There is no evidence of infiltration into the lung parenchyma.

Lung cancer and asbestos exposure
There is an increased risk of lung cancer in asbestos workers, with an approximately linear relationship, between dose and mortality. The risk is multiplied in asbestos-exposed smokers.

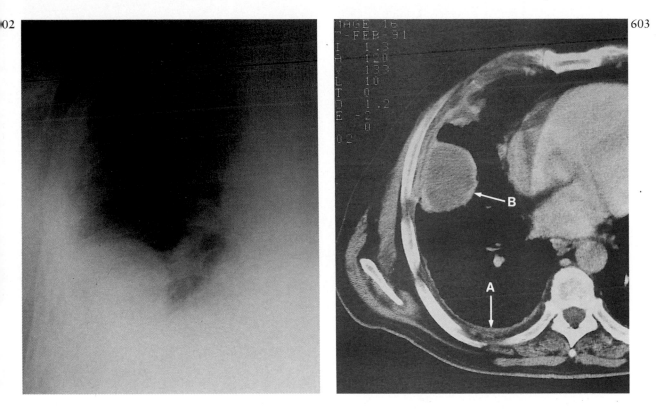

602, 603 Lung cancer and asbestos exposure. Pleural thickening (arrow A) and a cavitating peripheral squamous cell carcinoma (arrow B) in a retired bronchitic cigarette smoker previously exposed to asbestos in lagging materials. He had smoked 40 cigarettes per day for 30 years. The posteroanterior chest radiograph shows pleural thickening and a right basal mass (**602**) localised by the CT scan (**603**).

Mixed mineral dust pneumoconiosis

This is a convenient term used to include pneumoconiosis occurring in workers exposed to respirable crystalline silica (quartz) dust contaminated with carbon, iron haematite or feldspar. Foundry workers (especially fettlers), haematite miners, shale miners and slate cutters are particularly at risk. The pathological consequences depend upon the constituents of the dust. In general the greater the silica content, the more closely does the lung disease resemble silicosis.

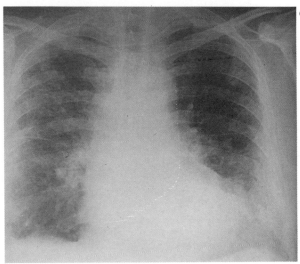

604 Mixed mineral dust pneumoconiosis in a middle-aged man whose previous occupations had included the cleaning of castings in an iron foundry and the manufacturing of reinforced rubber hose pipes, with exposure to industrial grade talc (hydrated magnesium silicate).

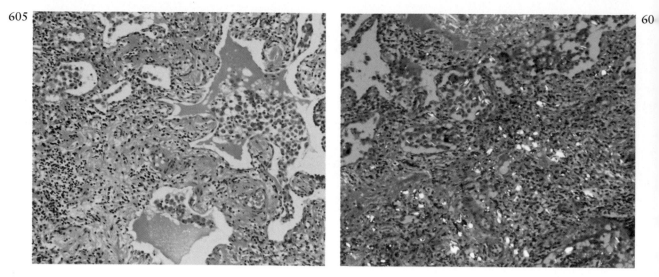

605, 606   Mixed mineral dust pneumoconiosis. Open lung biopsy specimen. Generalised fibrosis with obliteration of the airways (**605**). Polarised light demonstrates the presence of mixed dust particles responsible for lung fibrosis (**606**). (H&E×25.)

Hard metal lung disease

Hard metals used for cutting and grinding are manufactured by hot compression moulding of tungsten carbide, sometimes with tantalum or titanium carbide, in a matrix of cobalt with chromium or nickel. Workers exposed to hard metal dust produced by mixing, shaping and grinding may suffer from asthma, alveolitis and pneumonitis or disabling pneumoconiosis with interstitial lung fibrosis.

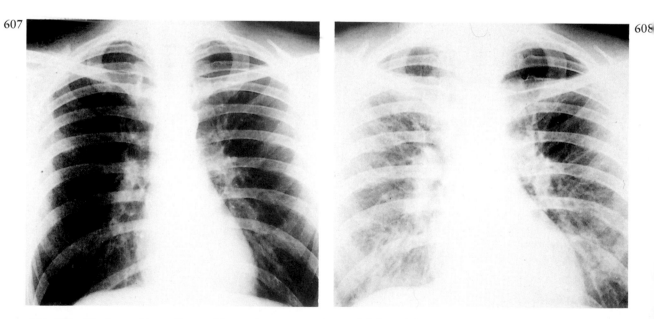

607, 608   Hard metal lung disease. The patient presented complaining of dyspnoea after ten years' exposure to hard metal dust from tool sharpening. The presentation chest radiograph (**607**) was normal but the second, taken eight years later (**608**), shows diffuse interstitial fibrosis.

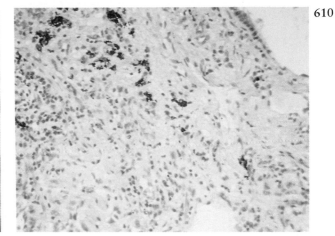

609 Hard metal lung disease. Bronchoalveolar lavage. Alveolar macrophages intermingled with neutrophils and giant cells; the latter are characteristic of hard metal lung disease. (Papanicolaou, original magnification ×100.)

610 Hard metal lung disease. Open lung biopsy. Dense diffuse fibrosis with foci of cellular inflammation and dust pigment deposition. (H & E × 100.)

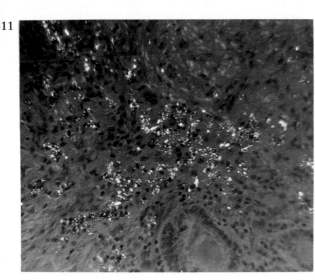

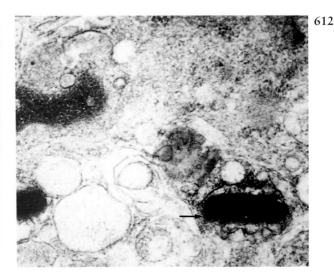

611 Hard metal lung disease. Open lung biopsy. Doubly refractile particles, due to dust pigment deposition seen on polarised light.

612 Hard metal lung disease. Open lung biopsy. Polygonal crystalloid bodies probably due to tantalum present in mitochondrial phagolysosomes (arrow). Multi-element neutron activation analysis (NAA) showed high tungsten, cobalt and tantalum concentrations in the lung biopsy tissue. The characteristic histological appearances with collections of giant cells in lung tissue are now thought to be an allergic reaction to cobalt. (Transmission electron microscopy. Uranyl acetate–lead citrate, original magnification×9,100.)

Beryllium disease

Beryllium disease (berylliosis) affects those working with beryllium metal or soluble beryllium compounds. The ore, beryl, is harmless because it is insoluble.

Inhalation of fumes from molten beryllium or high beryllium–copper alloy causes acute alveolitis (similar to that caused by cadmium), which may be fatal or cause permanent lung fibrosis. Subacute and chronic berylliosis can result from extremely low levels of exposure. Individual susceptibility is an important factor because only 2% of those at risk develop chronic berylliosis. Because beryllium salts are absorbed through the respiratory tract and distributed via the circulation, exposure causes a systemic disease. Chronic berylliosis is characterised by non-caseating granulomata in lung, lymph node, liver, spleen, adrenal gland and kidney. Granulomata in the skin are due to direct exposure.

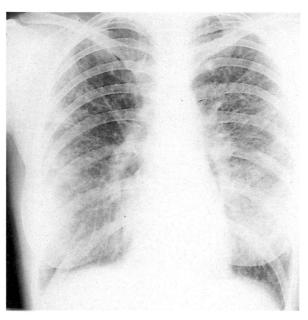

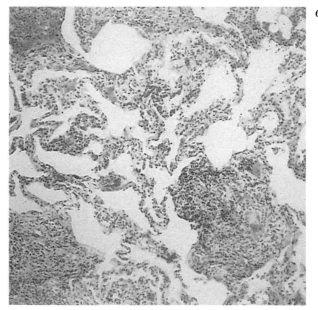

613 Chronic beryllium disease showing pulmonary infiltration resembling sarcoidosis, with fine nodulation distributed in the lungs and bilateral symmetrical enlargement of the hilar nodes. Without corticosteroid treatment, there is relentless progression, with interstitial fibrosis leading to pulmonary hypertension and right heart failure. Corticosteroids ameliorate the condition.

614 Beryllium disease showing 'sarcoid' granulomata with fibrosis. A history of exposure to beryllium, a negative Kveim test, normal serum angiotensin converting enzyme and the presence of beryllium in the tissue or urine confirm the diagnosis.

Benign non-fibrotic pneumoconioses

These are recognised by the presence of multiple small dense opacities on the chest x-ray, which are caused by perivascular collections of dust with an increase in reticulin fibres but no collagen. Lung function is unchanged and there are no symptoms. The dusts responsible include iron dust (siderosis) from mining and processing iron ore and steel, oxides of iron from welding, barium sulphate (baritosis), antimony, tin and chromate dusts.

Organic dust diseases – byssinosis

Byssinosis is a disease of the airways caused by occupational exposure to dust from raw cotton and also from flax, hemp and sisal. After prolonged exposure the worker becomes breathless at work on re-exposure. This 'Monday feeling' may improve as the week progresses but, eventually, constant symptoms of cough, sputum production and breathlessness are indistinguishable from chronic bronchitis.

The raw cotton may be directly antigenic or, alternatively, the symptoms may be caused by the inhalation of large numbers of fungal spores or Gram-negative bacteria contained in the cotton.

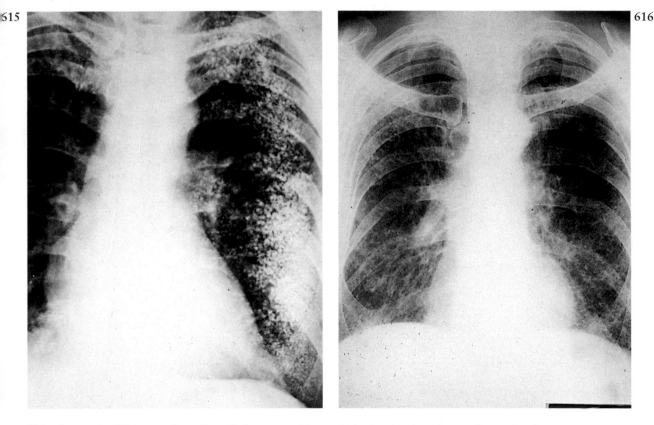

615   Stannosis. Widespread small radiodense opacities caused by retained tin oxide are present. Inhalation of inert tin dust produced by mining, or tin oxide fumes from smelting, have no known effect upon lung function or health.

616   Byssinosis. Chest radiograph of a cotton worker who complained of chest tightness and dyspnoea during the working week. There are no specific x-ray features. The pathological changes are mostly non-specific, with features similar to those found in chronic bronchitis or asthma. The disease is not characterised by alveolitis, lung fibrosis or emphysema. The pathogenesis is not understood, nor is the curious pattern of respiratory reaction which is due neither solely to irritation nor to allergy.

Occupational asthma

The term 'occupational asthma' describes asthma induced by hypersensitivity to an agent encountered at work in a previously healthy individual. Atopic subjects are particularly at risk, but with high levels of exposure non-atopic individuals may become sensitised.

Inhalation of protein-laden dust, complex biological materials or synthetic chemicals in the form of aerosols, dust or fumes may cause an allergic response in the airways if these substances bind to body proteins to act as haptens. Asthma may be the consequence of an IgE dependent response to soluble proteins or chemicals, and insoluble particulate organic dust may cause an alveolitis due to a T lymphocyte granulomatous response.

The major concern with both occupational asthma and allergic alveolitis is the development of chronic damage to the lungs. Therefore, the diagnosis of occupational asthma is important and can be made from the history of asthmatic symptoms related in time to periods at work.

There are many causes of occupational asthma (**Table 38**). In some countries, industrial benefit payments may be made to workers suffering from work-related asthma. In the UK, prescribed occupational exposure includes contact with those materials shown in **Table 39**.

Table 38. Materials causally linked to asthma in the workplace.

Vegetable	Animal	Plastic or chemical
Grain dust	Danders	Acid anhydrides
Flour	Insects	Epoxy resins
Fig plants	Silk worm larva	Diisocyanates
Wood dust	Shellfish	Persulphates
Seaweed	Pig or chicken excreta	Para-phenylenediamine
Green coffee beans	Fish feed	Phthalic anhydride
Fungal spores	Animal enzymes	Dimethyl ethanolamine
Tragacanth		Azobisformamide
Castor bean		Azodicarbonamide
Tea		Formaldehyde
Tobacco		Ethylenediamine
Flax		Acrylates
Hemp		Henna
Cotton		
Hops		
Bacterial enzymes		
Colophony		

Metal	Pharmaceutical
Stainless steel	Penicillins
Galvanised steel	Cephalosporins
Aluminium fluoride	Piperazine
Vanadium	Psyllium
Cobalt	Methyldopa
Tungsten carbide (cobalt)	Spiramycin
Platinum salts	Tetracycline
Nickel	Amprolium
Chromium	Cimetidine
	Isoniazid
	Phenylglycine

Table 39. Prescribed causes of occupational asthma in the UK.

Isocyanates

Platinum salts

Fumes or dusts from the use of hardening agents including epoxyresin, curing agents based on phthalic anhydride, tetrachlorophthalic anhydride or trimellitic anhydride

Fumes arising from the use of resin (colophony) as a soldering flux

Proteolytic enzymes

Animals or insects used for the purposes of research or education or in laboratories

Dusts arising from the cultivation, transport, storage and use of barley, oats, rye, wheat or maize or the flour made therefrom

Drugs – antibiotics, cimetidine, ispaghula, ipecacuanha

Castor bean dust

Wood dusts

Azodicarbonamide

Patterns of occupational asthma

The most common pattern is for asthma to progress during the working day, becoming more severe at the end of the working week and, occasionally, continuing into the evening to disturb sleep. After cessation of exposure, recovery may be rapid over a few hours or, as is the case with isocyanate asthma, may be incomplete even after a long absence from work.

617   Challenges with 10 mg ammonium hexachloroplatinate/250 g lactose for 10 minutes

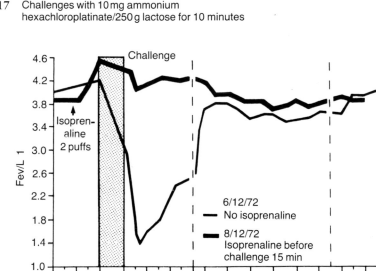

617   Diagnosis of occupational asthma. Immediate bronchoconstriction following inhalational challenge using ammonium hexachlorplatinate dust. Pretreatment with isoprenaline blocks the immediate reaction.

618

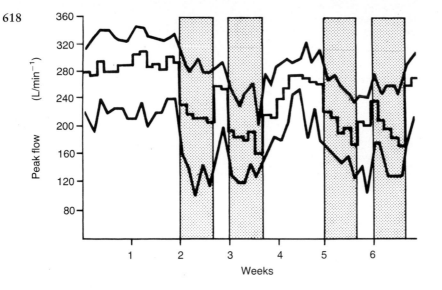

618 Diagnosis of occupational asthma. Serial peak flow recordings made in a platinum refiner. The record shows worsening airway obstruction during the working week, partial recovery during two work-free days at the weekend and complete recovery during a longer period of absence from work. The plot shows the daily maximum (top line), mean (middle line) and minimum peak flow (bottom line). Days at work have a stippled background and days at home a clear background.

22 Interstitial lung disease

The description 'interstitial lung disease' is often used to refer to a wide range of different processes involving the peripheral gas exchanging areas of the lung, which result in functional impairment of gas transfer and a restrictive defect of ventilation. It is implied that the disease process involves the acini and associated supporting tissue.

Acute alveolitis follows in the wake of acinar injury involving type I and type II epithelial cells in the alveolar walls. If the injury persists, the surrounding connective tissue becomes involved, collagenases disrupt collagen, and lung tissue is destroyed. The end-stage histology is of non-specific irreversible pulmonary fibrosis with few helpful diagnostic features. These changes are best described as diffuse pulmonary alveolar or acinar fibrosis. A classification is outlined in **Table 40**.

Table 40. Classification of interstitial lung disease.

Known aetiology	Unknown aetiology

Dusts
    organic (see page 229)
    inorganic (see page 213)
	Necrotising angiitis

	Collagen disorders
	    rheumatoid arthritis
	    progressive systemic sclerosis
	    Sjögren's syndrome

Fumes (see page 228)	
	ankylosing spondylitis (see page 237)
Drugs	
	Inherited disorders

Infections
    Schistosoma mansoni
	tuberous sclerosis
	    neurofibromatosis

Pulmonary oedema	Miscellaneous
	sarcoidosis (see Chapter 23)
Uraemia	Goodpasture's syndrome eosinophilic granuloma

Irradiation	idiopathic haemosiderosis
	    amyloidosis
	    veno-occlusive disease
	    idiopathic pulmonary fibrosis
	    lymphangioleiomyomatosis

Systemic sclerosis

Systemic sclerosis, a multisystem disorder affecting women three times more frequently than men, is characterised by increased production of mature collagen in the skin and involved organs. It is associated with calcinosis, scleroderma (sclerodactyly), Raynaud's phenomenon, oesophageal dysfunction, telangiectasia (collectively known as CREST syndrome), and fibrosis of other organs including kidneys, lungs, heart, lower gastrointestinal tract and skeletal muscle. Antinuclear antibody identification by immunofluorescence shows a speckled pattern and is positive in about 75% of patients.

Pulmonary fibrosis is common, predominantly in the lower zones, resulting in slow progressive deterioration in lung function. Pulmonary hypertension due to widespread obliterative changes in the small arteries and arterioles in the lung develops particularly in the CREST syndrome and tends to be rapidly progressive. Additional problems include recurrent aspiration pneumonia due to oesophageal disease, ventilatory failure with a restrictive pattern of lung function, and an increased incidence of primary lung adenocarcinoma or alveolar cell carcinoma secondary to pulmonary fibrosis.

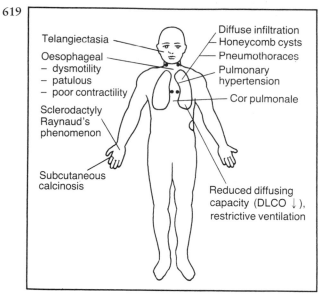

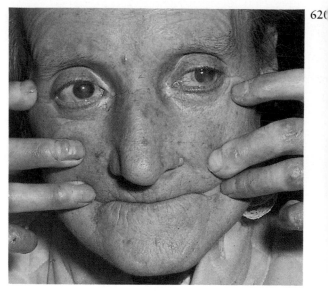

619 Clinical features of systemic sclerosis.

620 **Systemic sclerosis.** Advanced disease. The skin is thickened and contracted around the mouth. Telangiectasia is present on the nose and cheeks. The hands show acrocyanosis.

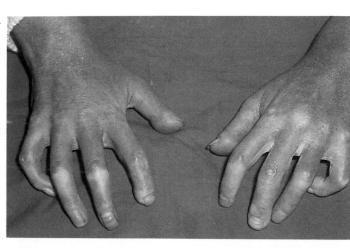

621 **Systemic sclerosis.** Advanced disease. Severe Raynaud's phenomenon, thickening of the skin and gross vascular changes.

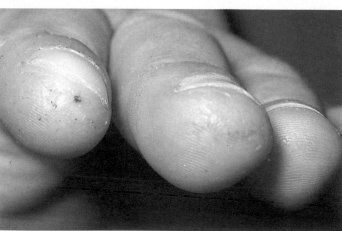

622 **Systemic sclerosis.** Calcinosis of the finger tips.

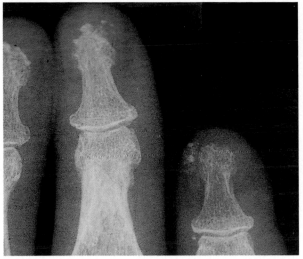

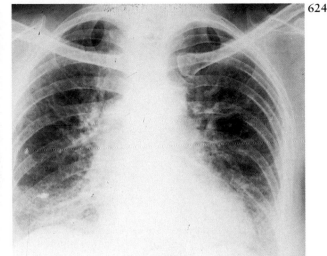

623 Systemic sclerosis. Radiograph of the fingertip showing speckled calcification in the soft tissue.

624 Systemic sclerosis. Chest radiograph showing scleroderma lung with interstitial fibrosis and streaky or honeycomb changes, particularly in the middle and lower zones. These lead to progressive dyspnoea, hypoxaemia and ventilation perfusion imbalance. Measurements of lung volumes show a restrictive defect and gas transfer is reduced. There is an increased risk of adenocarcinoma or alveolar cell carcinoma.

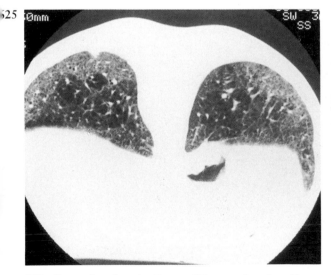

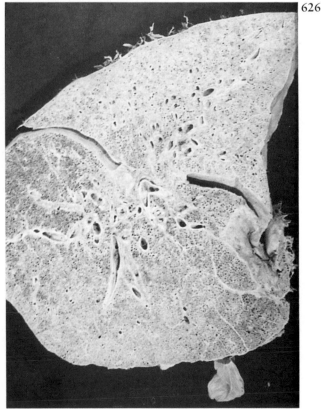

625 Systemic sclerosis. Prone CT scan showing fibrosing alveolitis in scleroderma. The subpleural crescentic distribution of a fine reticulation, together with tiny cysts in the posterior segments of the lower lobes, is typical of the condition. The cupola of the diaphragm and the density of the vertebral column obliterated evidence of the disease on the chest radiograph.

626 Systemic sclerosis. Whole section of scleroderma lung showing diffuse interstitial fibrosis and honeycombing (barium preparation).

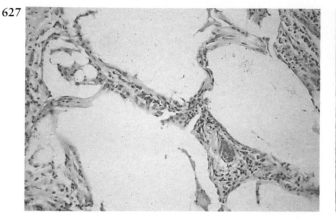

627 Progressive systemic sclerosis. Lung biopsy specimen. Early stage. The prominent alveolar capillaries and thickened cellular alveolar walls are characteristic of the earlier vascular stages. (H & E × 140.)

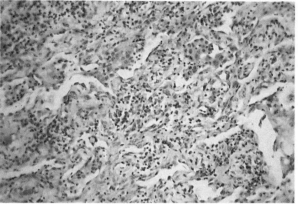

628 Progressive systemic sclerosis. Lung biopsy specimen. Late stage with intra-alveolar and interstitial fibrosis, disruption of alveolar walls and lymphocytic infiltration. (H & E × 140.)

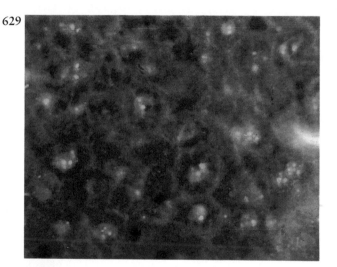

629 Systemic sclerosis. Immunofluorescent preparation showing the common speckled distribution of antinuclear antibody.

Sjögren's syndrome

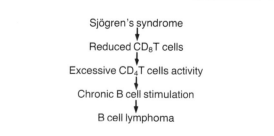

Sjögren's syndrome
↓
Reduced CD_8 T cells
↓
Excessive CD_4 T cells activity
↓
Chronic B cell stimulation
↓
B cell lymphoma

630 Sjögren's syndrome.

This chronic disorder, predominant in menopausal women, is characterised by keratoconjunctivitis sicca, xerostomia and parotid gland enlargement, in association with one of the connective tissue disorders, usually rheumatoid arthritis. It has features of an autoimmune disorder, with circulating autoantibodies, plasma cell infiltration in various tissues and the coexistence of other autoimmune disorders including rheumatoid arthritis. The primary sicca syndrome without arthritis is associated with HLA-DRW3. Rheumatoid arthritis, associated with the secondary sicca syndrome, is HLA-DRW4 associated, indicating the different patterns of the disorder. Circulating immune complexes, a defective clearance rate of the reticuloendothelial system and a high incidence of lymphomas are other features.

Pulmonary abnormalities occur in up to one-third of cases and include pleurisy and pleural effusion, fibrosing alveolitis, lymphoid infiltration of the mucosal bronchial glands, lymphocytic interstitial pneumonia and malignant lymphocytic lymphomas (630). The lack of airways secretions may result in dry cough and a predisposition to pneumonia.

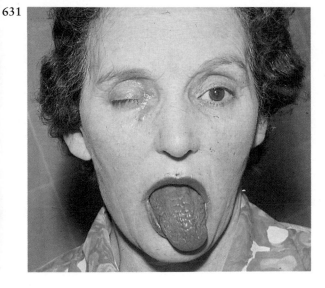

631 Sjögren's syndrome. Dry fissured tongue and keratoconjunctivitis sicca. Because she had very dry eyes, this patient developed corneal ulceration which required tarsorrhaphy.

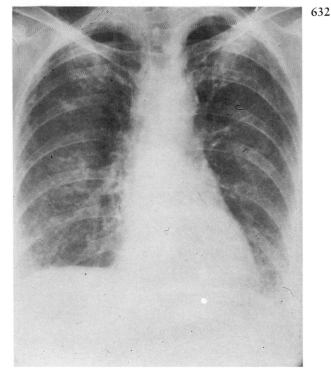

632 Pulmonary fibrosis in Sjögren's syndrome. The alveolar walls are infiltrated by mononuclear cells and become fibrosed. Recurrent pneumonia is common.

Ankylosing spondylitis

Progressive inflammation of spinal joints leads to ankylosis, predominantly in adult males, 90% of whom with this condition are HLA-B27 positive. Extra-articular manifestations include anterior uveitis and proximal aortitis with aortic regurgitation. A restrictive pattern on lung function tests results from increasing fixation of the thoracic cage. Apical lung fibrosis, cavitation and occasional calcification are also described and may be confused with pulmonary tuberculosis. The cavities may be colonised by *Aspergillus* with the formation of a mycetoma.

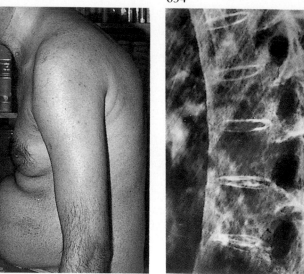

633 Ankylosing spondylitis causes rigidity of the thoracic cage, partly compensated by diaphragmatic movement. The anterior chest is flattened, the back immobile and kyphotic, and the abdomen prominent to allow diaphragmatic breathing.

634 Ankylosing spondylitis. The anterior spinal ligaments of the thoracic spine become calcified ('bamboo' appearance).

Cryptogenic fibrosing alveolitis (CFA)

Synonyms: idiopathic pulmonary fibrosis,
Hamman–Rich syndrome,
Diffuse interstitial pneumonia.

This is a rather uncommon condition in which the lung parenchyma becomes involved in a diffuse fibrotic process, leading to progressive impairment of lung function and dyspnoea. The cause of the condition is not clear.

The disease affects both sexes equally and may occur at any age, but is most common in the fifth and sixth decades.

The presenting symptoms are an insidious onset of exertional dyspnoea and an irritating cough. Finger clubbing is usually present and basal lung crackles are audible on auscultation. Physiological measurements show a restrictive defect of lung function with reduced transfer coefficient (KCo) and hypoxia on exercise.

A number of connective tissue disorders, such as rheumatoid arthritis, systemic lupus erythematosus and systemic sclerosis, are associated with fibrosing alveolitis, with identical histology to that found in lone cryptogenic fibrosing alveolitis. Serum antinuclear antibodies (ANA) are found in one-third of patients with cryptogenic fibrosing alveolitis, and speckled and nucleolar ANA in 6%. Increased Clq

binding levels are observed in 50% of cases and even more frequently when there is also rheumatoid arthritis, the rheumatoid factor and IgG.

Microscopically, the intensity of the pulmonary inflammation varies and tends to be most severe at the periphery of the lung. The two essential features of fibrosing alveolitis are:

1 Cellular thickening of the alveolar wall with a tendency to fibrosis
2 The presence of large mononuclear cells within the alveolar spaces

There is a range of histological appearances. Among these is desquamative interstitial pneumonia (DIP), which is inflammatory, highly cellular and associated with circulating and fixed immune complexes, and with IgG deposition in the alveoli and capillaries. Usual interstitial pneumonia (UIP), is fibrotic, acellular and shows no evidence of immune complex reactivity. Intermediate histology demonstrating cellular and fibrotic changes is common.

The alveolar interstitium becomes disorganised as a result of a breakdown of collagen from a sustained enzymatic attack by collagenase. In the normal lung the ratio between type I and II collagen is 2.5:1, but in cryptogenic fibrosing alveolitis the ratio rises to 5:1. Type I collagen is less yielding; this higher ratio is responsible for the loss of compliance and the restrictive defect. Instead of a regular arrangement of parallel crossbanded fibres of normal Type I collagen, the fibres are randomly twisted and frayed so that alveolar septa are patchily thickened or attenuated.

Treatment is non-specific, mostly unsatisfactory, and relies upon anti-inflammatory corticosteroids and immuno suppression to reduce cellularity and prevent the deposition of firm stable collagen.

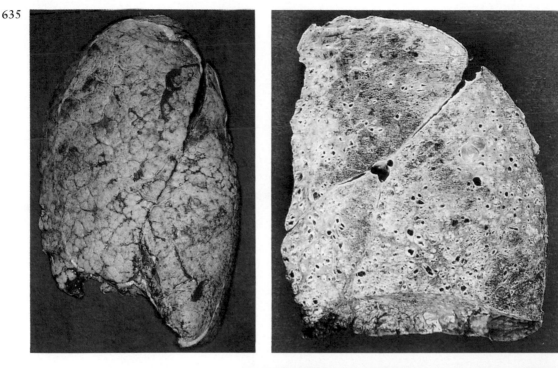

635, 636 Cryptogenic fibrosing alveolitis. Coarse 'cobblestoned' appearance of pleural surface due to underlying lung fibrosis (635). Sagittal section of whole lung showing the peripheral and basal distribution with honeycombing and fibrosis and relative sparing of the more central areas (636).

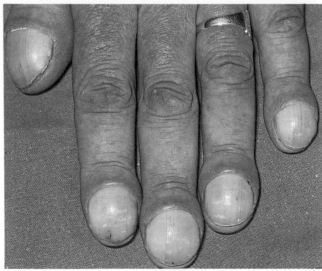

637 Cryptogenic fibrosing alveolitis. Pronounced clubbing of the fingers is characteristic of CFA.

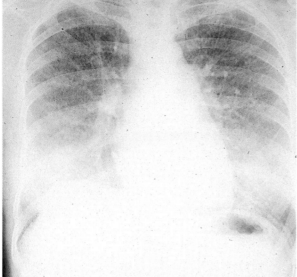

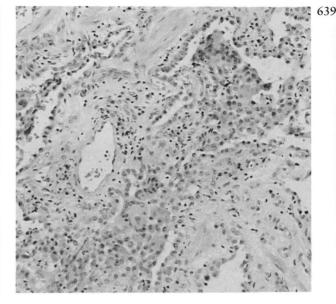

638 Cryptogenic fibrosing alveolitis. Chest radiograph of early progressive disease. Bilateral lower zone pulmonary infiltration with irregular reticulonodular shadows. The predominantly basal distribution differentiates CFA from sarcoidosis and extrinsic allergic alveolitis. Six months earlier, inspiratory crackles were heard on auscultation of the lung bases and lung function showed a moderate restrictive defect.

639 Cryptogenic fibrosing alveolitis. Desquamative interstitial pneumonia (DIP). Cellular pattern with clumps of mononuclear cells filling the intra-alveolar spaces. Lymphocytes and plasma cells are present in the alveolar walls and interstitium. Special stains are required to demonstrate early fibrosis. (H & E × 140.)

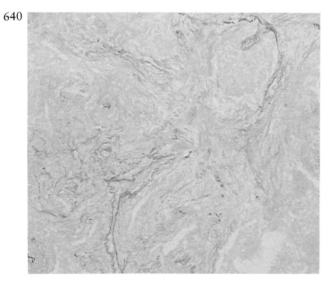

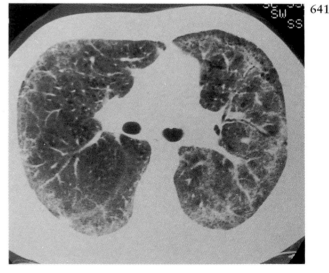

640 Cryptogenic fibrosing alveolitis. Desquamative interstitial pneumonia (DIP), stained to show collagen fibres. Early fibrosis is present, demonstrated as sparse red-staining fibres in the interstitium. (Elastin Van Gieson.)

641 Cryptogenic fibrosing alveolitis. CT scan. Circumferential changes are present in the subpleural region on both sides. Multiple small cysts and nodules are superimposed and an irregular subpleural region of transradiancy is present, especially on the left, a common finding in this condition.

CT scanning is capable of identifying interstitial pulmonary changes before these are evident on a plain radiograph.

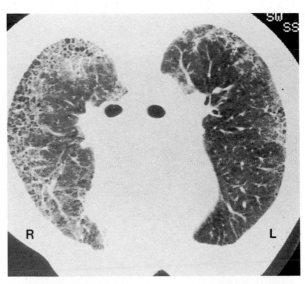

642 Cryptogenic fibrosing alveolitis. CT scan (prone) showing characteristic appearances. The asymmetry of the distribution of the fibrosis is demonstrated. On the right the regimented subpleural cysts are well delineated, whereas on the left the cysts are apparent in one area only. Posteriorly, there is merely air space disease which, on biopsy, showed a mixture of active alveolar wall thickening and interstitial fibrosis.

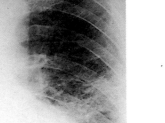

643 Chest radiograph of advanced CFA with extensive destruction and honeycombing of the lung.

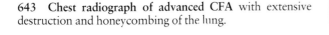

644 Cryptogenic fibrosing alveolitis and emphysema. CT scan. The emphysema has so destroyed and disrupted the lung parenchyma on the right that the underlying pattern of fibrosing alveolitis cannot be identified. On the left the characteristic cystic pattern of the fibrosing alveolitis can still be identified anteriorly (arrowed).

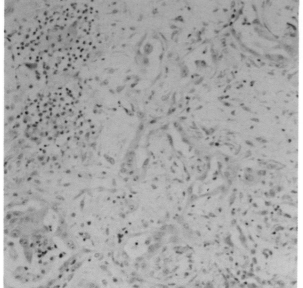

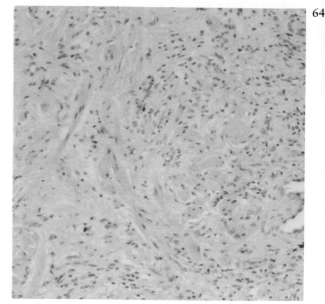

645 Cryptogenic fibrosing alveolitis. Mixed pattern showing patchy cellular infiltration in the fibrotic thickened alveolar walls with attempted air space formation and type 2 pneumocyte hyperplasia. (H & E × 100.)

646 Cryptogenic fibrosing alveolitis. Fibrotic pattern of usual interstitial pneumonia (UIP). The interstitium is thickened with collagen and other connective tissue constituents. The initial acute inflammatory features cannot be identified at this late stage.

647

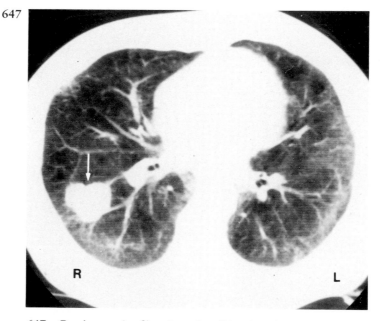

647 Carcinoma in fibrosing alveolitis. Standard (10 mm) CT scan. Because this is not a high resolution scan the pattern detail of the fibrosing alveolitis is not apparent. The mass in the right lower lobe proved to be a bronchogenic carcinoma (arrow). In CFA most patients succumb to respiratory failure and infection, but there is an excess of lung cancer deaths (often adenocarcinoma). CT scanning is very valuable in assessing the presence of neoplastic disease in those conditions where there is a predilection for malignant change, i.e. asbestosis and fibrosing alveolitis.

Cryptogenic organising pneumonitis (bronchiolitis obliterans organising pneumonitis)

This recently described condition is characterised by a rapid onset of cough and dyspnoea, often with fever, malaise and weight loss and, sometimes, with pleuritic chest pain. Lung crackles are frequent, but fingernail clubbing is unusual. The chest radiograph shows patchy infiltration, and lung function testing shows a restrictive defect with reduced gas transfer.

The combination of features is distinctive, but not sufficiently unique to allow diagnosis without histology; confirmation is obtained by lung biopsy. The aetiology of this condition is not clear, but a seasonal environmental agent, infections including HIV, drugs (gold and amiodarone) and collagen vascular disorders may be implicated.

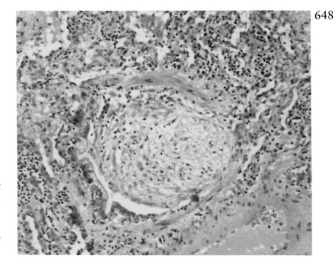

648

648 Cryptogenic organising pneumonitis. Section of lung parenchyma showing a bud of granulation tissue extending out from the wall of an alveolus to occupy the intra-alveolar space, a lymphocyte and plasma cell inflammation of the alveolar walls and a variable amount of interstitial fibrosis. (H & E × 250.)

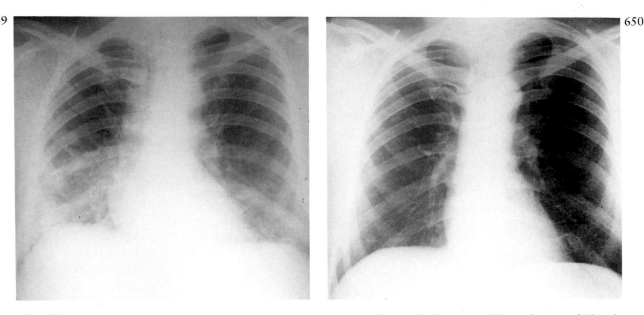

649   650

649, 650 Cryptogenic organising pneumonitis. Presentation chest radiograph showing patchy predominantly basal infiltration (**649**). Following corticosteroid treatment, there was rapid resolution accompanied by dramatic improvement in lung function (**650**). The importance of this condition is the dramatic, occasionally complete, improvement with corticosteroids. If relapse is observed, control is regained by increased doses of corticosteroids.

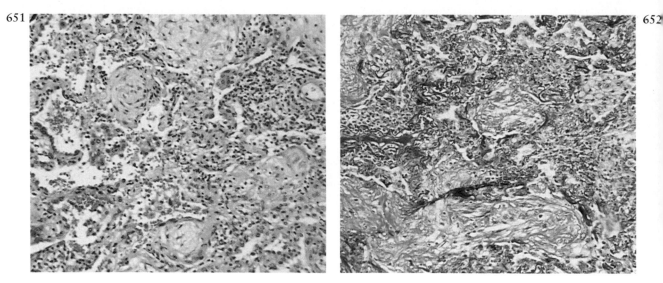

651, 652 **Cryptogenic organising pneumonitis.** Young cellular fibrous tissue filling alveoli and bronchioles. (651, H & E; 652, fibrous tissue green on collagen stain.)

Pulmonary infiltrations

Some rare pulmonary disorders which are not believed to be neoplastic or due to dust exposure may result in diffuse pulmonary radiographic infiltration. These include:

- Histiocytosis X.
- Idiopathic pulmonary haemosiderosis.

- Diffuse pulmonary calcinosis.
- Pulmonary neurofibromatosis.
- Pulmonary tuberous sclerosis.
- Pulmonary alveolar proteinosis.
- Pulmonary amyloidosis.
- Pulmonary lymphangioleiomyomatosis.

Pulmonary histiocytosis X (eosinophilic granuloma)

This describes infiltration of the alveolar septa and bronchial walls by Langerhans'-type histiocytes and eosinophils, leading to diffuse pulmonary fibrosis and, eventually, to multiple cyst formation. Histiocytosis X may affect the lungs alone, but the pulmonary changes are sometimes part of a more generalised disorder (653). Three forms are recognised:

1 Letterer–Siwe disease. A fatal multisystem disorder of infants, with splenomegaly, lymphadenopathy and cystic granulomatous lesions in the lungs.
2 Hand–Schüller–Christian disease. Xanthomatous deposits cause miliary radiographic lung shadows, diabetes insipidus and bone cysts.
3 Eosinophilic granuloma. Bone cysts are common. Pulmonary infiltration leads to fibrosis and bulla formation in around a quarter of patients.

Pulmonary histiocytosis X predominantly affects young adult males. There are five modes of presentation:
1 Abnormal chest radiograph in an asymptomatic patient.
2 Pneumothorax.
3 Cough and dyspnoea.
4 Systemic symptoms, fever, malaise and weight loss.
5 Abnormal chest radiograph associated with multisystem disorder.

In the majority of patients the diagnosis is made by lung biopsy, confirmation depending on the demonstration by electron microscopy of Birbeck granules within the cytoplasm of histiocytic cells.

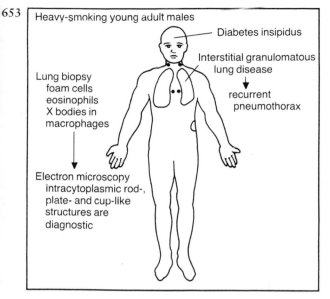

653 Langerhans' cell granulomatosis – clinical features of histiocytosis X.

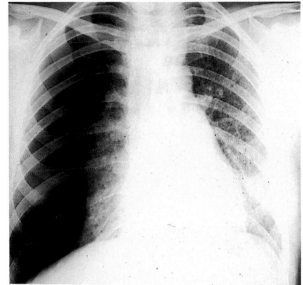

654 **Eosinophilic granuloma** in a young male with diabetes insipidus. The chest radiograph shows miliary mottling involving the left lung. The patient's chest disease was complicated by a right spontaneous pneumothorax.

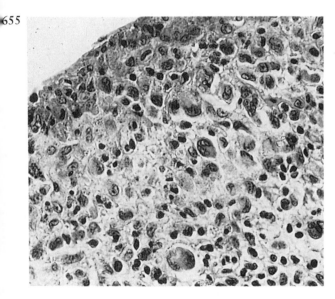

655 **Eosinophilic granuloma.** Bronchial biopsy. Eosinophils, lymphocytes, plasma cells and histiocytic cells (Langerhans' cells) are present; the histiocytic cells are large cells with ample cytoplasm and nuclei with loose chromatin pattern. (H & E × 280.)

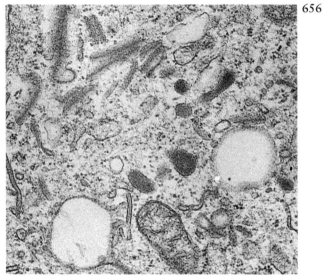

656 **Eosinophilic granuloma.** The presence of the tennis racquet shaped cytoplasmic organelles (Birbeck granules) is diagnostic. (EM × 40,000.)

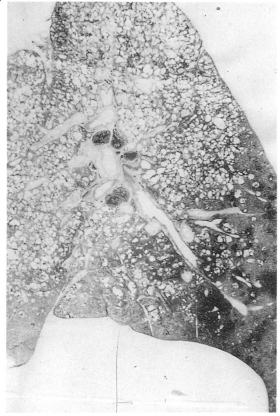

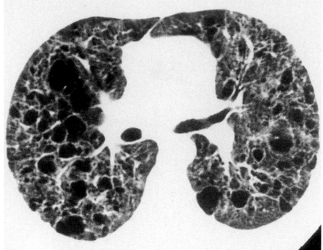

658 Eosinophilic granuloma, late stage. CT scan. Widespread cysts with thickened walls are associated with areas of emphysema and curved and linear fibrosis. There is no volume loss and no significant pleural disease. At this late stage, a similar pattern may be given by cryptogenic fibrosing alveolitis and lymphangioleiomyomatosis (although in this condition the cysts are usually more thinly walled and delicate). At an earlier stage, eosinophilic granuloma usually presents with widespread nodulation in the upper two-thirds of the lung fields.

657 Eosinophilic granuloma. Honeycomb lung with extensive cystic changes, especially in the upper lobes. The bullae ruptured and caused a fatal tension pneumothorax. Premature death is common, mainly from respiratory failure.

Idiopathic pulmonary haemosiderosis (IPH)

This condition is characterised by recurrent intra-pulmonary haemorrhage, producing iron deficiency anaemia, haemoptysis and impairment of lung function. Pulmonary haemorrhage due to cardiac disease, connective tissue disorders and antibody to basal membrane antigen (Goodpasture's syndrome) is excluded.

IPH is most common in children who may develop anaemia in excess of the apparent blood loss from haemoptysis. Repeated attacks may lead to pulmonary hypertension, hepatosplenomegaly and sudden death. In adults the iron deficiency anaemia may be partly due to malabsorption, for in some cases small bowel biopsy shows villus atrophy, suggesting an association between coeliac disease and IPH. Apart from diffuse respiratory crackles on auscultation, fingernail clubbing may also be found. Pulmonary haemosiderosis occurs in chronic passive venous congestion secondary to mitral stenosis and left heart failure and other conditions associated with pulmonary haemorrhage (Goodpasture's vasculitis associated with pulmonary haemorrhage or malignancy).

659

660

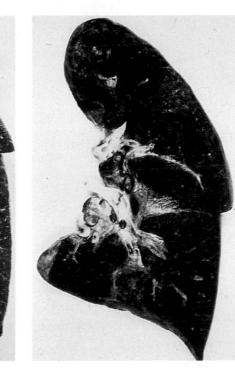

659, 660 Idiopathic pulmonary haemosiderosis. Sagittal section of whole lung. Macroscopically, the lungs and hilar glands show a striking red-brown appearance due to siderosis, with varying degrees of pulmonary fibrosis and honeycombing. The histological appearances are not specific. Iron-laden macrophages pack the alveoli. The prussian blue reaction confirms the presence of haemosiderin (**660**).

661

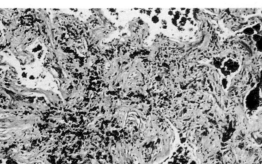

661 Idiopathic pulmonary haemosiderosis. Pigment-containing (iron-laden) macrophages fill the alveolar spaces and there is thickening of the alveolar walls and fibrosis.

662

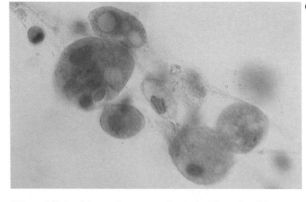

662 Idiopathic pulmonary haemosiderosis. Haemo-siderin-laden macrophages in bronchoalveolar fluid. With the Papanicolaou stain, the macrophages show green (yellowish) granular or globular material containing iron. (PAP×63.)

663

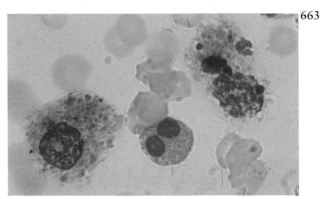

663 Haemosiderin-laden macrophages. There is also some carbon present in the cells. The haemosiderin stains brown with fine granules and the carbon is black with coarse granules of variable size. (May–Grunewald–Giemsa ×63.)

Pulmonary alveolar microlithiasis

This is a rare disorder (sometimes familial) caused by the presence of innumerable minute calcified spherules filling the alveolar spaces, with remarkably little effect on the lung architecture. As a consequence of the alveolar calcium deposition, the lungs are notable for their weight and hardness and they cut with a gritty sensation. Symptoms may be absent in spite of extensive radiograph shadowing, but cough, dyspnoea and respiratory failure eventually supervene.

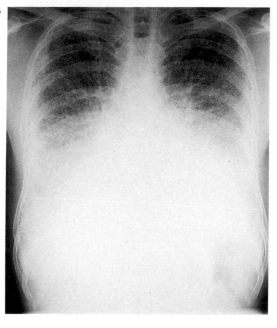

664 Pulmonary alveolar microlithiasis. The radiographic appearance is dense widespread miliary mottling, with a predominance of lower lobe shadowing. The mottling represents extensive intra-alveolar deposits of calcium-containing bodies.

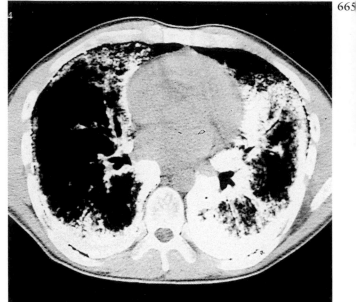

665 Pulmonary alveolar microlithiasis. CT scan, mediastinal setting. The extent of the microlithiasis is shown. It is concentrated mainly in the lower lobes, with the densest infiltration lying in the subpleural tissues.

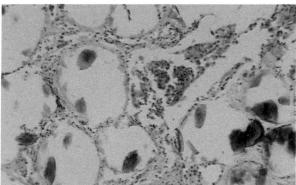

666 Pulmonary alveolar microlithiasis. Scattered calcospherites lying in the predominantly normal alveolar airways. (H & E × 60.)

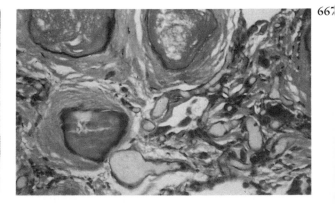

667 Pulmonary alveolar microlithiasis. Multiple intra-alveolar calcospherites with concentric lamination giving rise to an 'onion skin' appearance. The alveolar walls are thickened. (H & E × 250.)

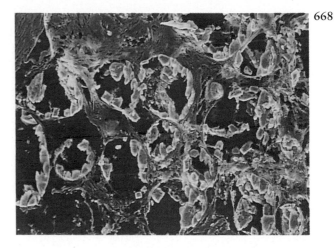

668 Pulmonary alveolar microlithiasis. The calcium salts are seen deposited in the alveolar and bronchiolar basement membranes in this late stage of the disorder. (Photo electron micrograph.)

Neurofibromatosis (Von Recklinghausen's disease)

This is an inherited autosomal dominant disorder, characterised by multiple neurofibromas, which may disfigure the skin, disrupt the nervous system and deform the skeleton. Hyperpigmented skin patches known as 'cafe-au-lait' spots are found and there is a predisposition to meningioma and phaeochromocytoma. In about 5% of cases, neurofibromas undergo sarcomatous change.

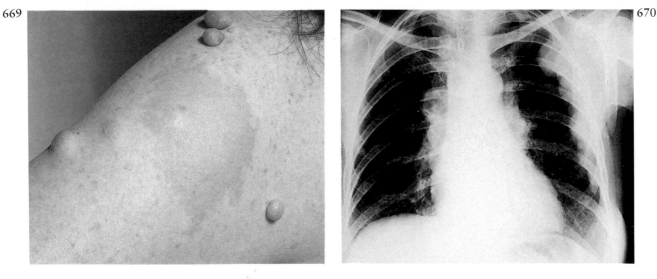

669 Dermal neurofibromatosis together with irregular skin pigmentation, the characteristic 'cafe-au-lait' spots.

670 Neurofibromatosis. Posteroanterior chest x-ray showing multiple thoracic neurofibromas. Two other pulmonary manifestations are described: either honeycomb lung, with non-specific clinical and functional changes; or a fibrosing alveolitis-like picture.

Tuberous sclerosis

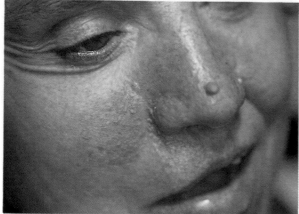

671 Tuberous sclerosis. Malar and nasal adenoma sebaceum in a mentally retarded patient. Similar nodules were present around the fingernails (subungual fibromas). A diffuse non-specific reticulonodular pattern was seen on chest x-ray (not shown).

Originally described in 1880 (Bourneville's disease), this is a rare genetic autosomal dominant disorder, characterised by a classic clinical triad of mental retardation, epileptic seizures and dermal angiofibromas (adenoma sebaceum).

The basic defect is believed to be a disorder of tissue differentiation which leads to multiple hamartomatous proliferative lesions of all germ cell layers, causing parenchymal destructive and diffuse cystic disease generally throughout the body.

Pneumothorax, airflow obstruction with hypoxia and pulmonary cystic disease with focal nodular adenomatoid proliferation are described. Pulmonary function tests show fixed airways obstruction. The most common radiographic abnormality is diffuse bilateral reticular nodular shadowing with honeycomb cystic spaces.

Pulmonary alveolar proteinosis

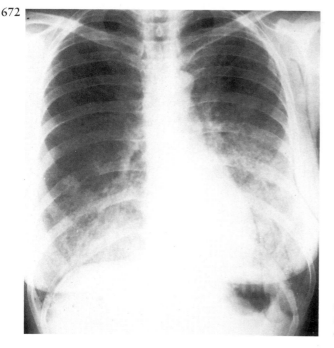

A rare disease of unknown origin, pulmonary alveolar proteinosis is characterised by progressive dyspnoea, febrile episodes, cough which is usually unproductive, weight loss, haemoptysis and chest pain. Physical examination of the chest is normal until the late stages, when bilateral lower-zone crepitations are heard. Finger clubbing occurs in about half of the patients. The condition is believed to be due to a failure of reprocessing of surfactant by type II alveolar cells, which results in an accumulation of phospholipid and glycoprotein-rich material in the alveolar spaces. Opportunistic infections, especially with *Nocardia*, *Aspergillus* and *Cryptococcus*, are common. Exposure to aluminium or silica dust is associated with alveolar proteinosis and the condition can be produced in experimental animals by inhalation of large doses of finely divided mineral dust.

672 Pulmonary alveolar proteinosis. The radiological appearances are often similar to those of pulmonary oedema with a perihilar distribution of opacities.

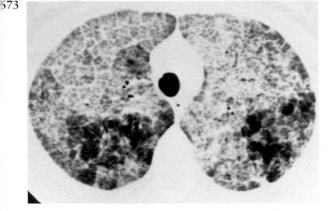

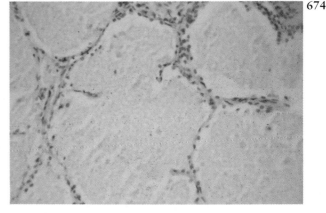

673 Pulmonary alveolar proteinosis. CT scan. A mosaic pattern of uniform density is present throughout the affected area, without deformity of the lung parenchyma. Dense lines surround polygonal areas of lesser density. These lines almost certainly represent septa surrounding lobules. There is no pleural involvement and the pattern is distinctive. It will resolve following successful broncho-alveolar lavage and is a useful monitor in this respect. This characteristic pattern is present in approximately 50% of alveolar proteinosis cases.

674 Pulmonary alveolar proteinosis. The alveoli contain granular eosinophilic exudate which is strongly positive to periodic acid-Schiff (PAS) staining and also stains heavily for lipid. There is no evidence of inflammation in the alveolar spaces of alveoli. Considerable improvement followed bronchial lavage, but deterioration and death as a result of respiratory failure or infection are the usual outcome.

Alveolar macrophages are lipid-rich and stain PAS-positive. They contain lamellar inclusions of whorls of lipoproteinaceous material, filling the cytoplasm of the macrophage. These macrophages provide poor defence against such exotic infections as nocardiasis, to which these patients are peculiarly susceptible. Pulmonary alveolar proteinosis can be diagnosed by broncho-pulmonary lavage, revealing an opaque milky effluent containing few cells but copious large acellular eosino-philic bodies.

Pulmonary amyloidosis

Amyloidosis is a disorder of protein metabolism which is characterised by abnormal extracellular deposition of autologous protein material. It occurs either in local forms, confined to particular organs or tissues, or is systemically distributed throughout the body. Localised amyloid deposition is a very common occurrence in the elderly.

Four macroscopic forms of pulmonary amyloidosis are recognised:

1 Localised bronchial deposits, usually found in lobar or segmental bronchi as large sessile smooth grey/white tumours. They may protrude into the lumen, causing bronchial obstruction.
2 Diffuse multiple submucosal bronchial deposits, which may extend into the peribronchial connective tissue.
3 Nodular pulmonary amyloid.
4 Diffuse parenchymal amyloid, usually associated with generalised amyloidosis.

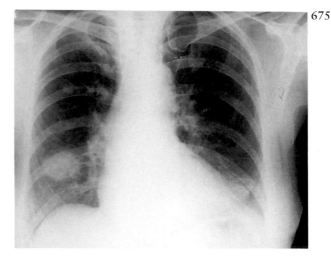

675 Nodular pulmonary amyloidosis chest x-ray. Opacity of the right lower lobe due to a localised amyloid deposit. Amyloid deposits may be single or multiple, may vary in size up to 8 cm and can be confused with primary or secondary tumours.

The diagnosis is usually made either at bronchoscopy, where the amyloid deposits appear as multiple plaques, or at lung biopsy.

With extensive nodular or diffuse disease, a restrictive pattern of lung function with reduced gas transfer may be seen. Tracheobronchial involvement can result in proximal airways obstruction.

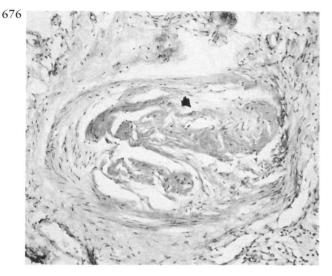

676 Nodular pulmonary amyloidosis. Periarterial and alveolar capillary obliterations and alveolar thickening. (Congo red×140.)

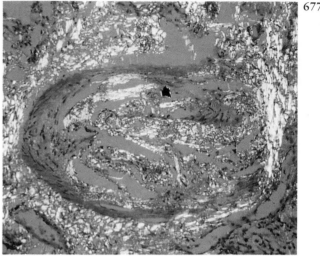

677 Nodular pulmonary amyloidosis. Birefringent amyloid fibres seen under polarised light.

Pulmonary lymphangioleiomyomatosis

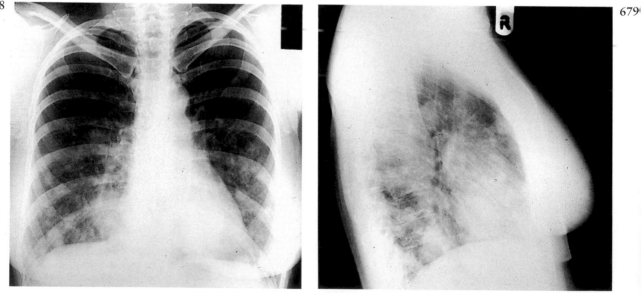

678, 679 Pulmonary lymphangioleiomyomatosis. Progressive fine reticulonodular infiltrates are characteristic of early disease, with progression to a honeycomb appearance due to multiple cyst formation. Most patients die from respiratory failure within 10 years of diagnosis.

There is a proliferation of smooth muscle cells in the lungs, lymphatics and lymph nodes in women of reproductive age presenting with interstitial lung disease progressing to destructive cystic disease, emphysematous changes, spontaneous pneumothorax and chylous effusions. Extrapulmonary manifestations include leiomyomas of kidneys, uterus and adnexae, or retroperitoneal tissues.

The presenting symptoms are haemoptysis, dyspnoea and pleural pain due to recurrent pneumothoraces.

 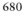

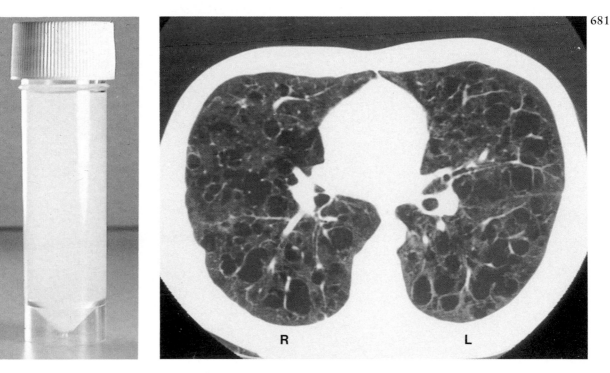

680 Pulmonary lymphangioleiomyomatosis. Chylous effusion is a diagnostic clue.

681 Pulmonary lymphangioleiomyomatosis. CT scan. Multiple thin-walled cysts are present throughout both lung fields, associated with large volume lungs. This appearance has been said to be characteristic of the condition, but it may also be seen in the late stages of fibrosing alveolitis and histiocytosis X.

Drug and radiation induced lung disease

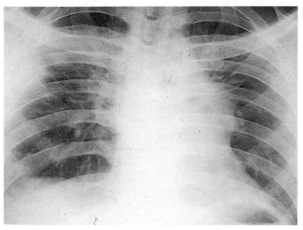

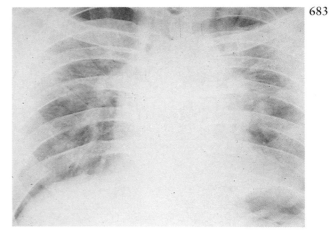

682 Cyclophosphamide lung. This diffuse pneumonitis developed in a 17-year-old boy who received the drug for 3 years as treatment for glomerulonephritis.

683 Cyclophosphamide lung. Widespread and progressive fibrosis with severe restriction in lung volumes 3 years after the drug was discontinued.

Drugs may cause a variety of adverse effects on the lung parenchyma, the airways or the pulmonary vasculature. The rapidly expanding pharmacopoeia has generated many additional problems, with a wide spectrum of iatrogenic lung diseases. Some examples are listed in **Table 41**.

Table 41. Drug-induced lung disease.

Bronchial hyper-reactivity	Cholinergic agents	Pilocarpine
	B sympathomimetic antagonist	B-blocking drugs
	Histamine release	Curare, opiates
	ACE inhibitors	
	Anaphylaxis	Penicillin
	Analgesic drugs	Aspirin and derivatives
Non-cardiogenic pulmonary oedema	Opiates	
	Aspirin	
Diffuse alveolitis/fibrosis	Cytotoxic drugs	Busulphan, cyclophosphamide
	Cardiac drugs	Amiodarone
	Antibiotics	Nitrofurantoin
	Paraquat	
Eosinophilia	Cytotoxic drugs	Methotrexate
		Bleomycin
	Antibiotics	Nitrofurantoin
		Sulphonamides
		Penicillin
	Antirheumatics	Gold
		Penicillamine
	Anticonvulsants	Phenytoin
		Carbamazepine
Lung haemorrhage	Penicillamine	
	Amphotericin B	
Pleurisy/SLE reaction	Procainamide	
	Hydralazine	
	Isoniazid	

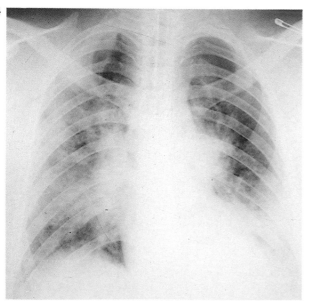

684 Non-cardiogenic pulmonary oedema. Severe pulmonary oedema as a result of heroin abuse. Assisted ventilation was required.

685 Bleomycin lung. In this prone scan, nodular and linear densities are superimposed to form crescentic subpleural zones of high attenuation posteriorly in the lower lobes. The changes are not diagnostic and are usually associated with irregular areas of confluent density, coarse reticulation and nodulation scattered across the lung field. On occasion, the pattern may simulate fibrosing alveolitis and may involve the anterior segments of the upper lobes, but changes elsewhere in the lung fields invariably exclude a diagnosis of interstitial fibrosis.

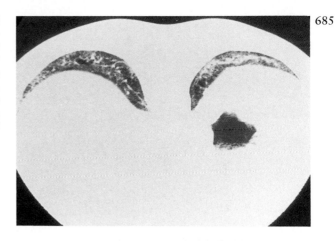

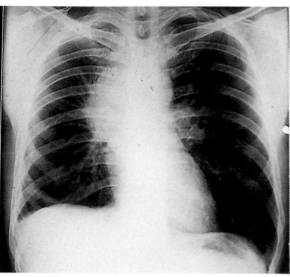

686 Radiation changes in the lung. Posteroanterior film showing a right paratracheal mass caused by a proximal bronchial carcinoma. The patient presented with haemoptysis.

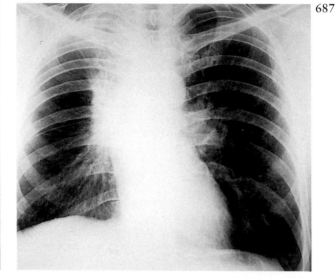

687 Radiation changes in the lung. Twelve months after radiotherapy. Fibrosis gradually develops after a latent period. The right upper zone is avascular with streaky fibrosis and there is radiation mediastinal and lung fibrosis.

Inflammatory bowel disease and lung involvement

A number of pulmonary disorders may be loosely associated with ulcerative colitis and Crohn's disease, due either to an inflammatory reaction affecting the airways or to the well-known association of alveolitis with sulphasalazine treatment (**Table 42**). Biopsy shows basement membrane thickening and submucosal inflammatory cell infiltrates reminiscent of the colonic mucosal disease. Several reports show an increase in progressive bronchitis and bronchiectasis after proctocolectomy.

Table 42. Lung associations of inflammatory bowel disease.

Bronchitis in non-smokers
Bronchiectasis
Asthma
Lung fibrosis
Fibrosing alveolitis
Pulmonary eosinophilia (sulphasalazine)

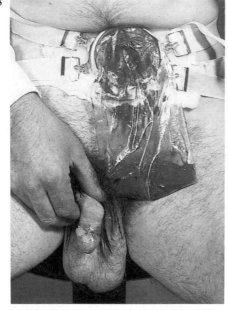

688

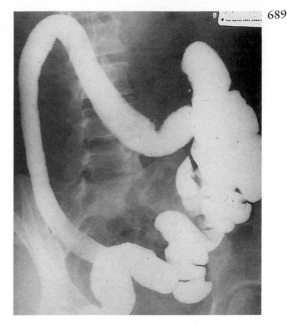

689

688 Crohn's disease. Colectomy for severe colitis. The disease is still active with mucocutaneous ulceration, especially florid on the glans penis. Bronchoalveolar lavage disclosed pulmonary lymphocytic alveolitis.

689 Ulcerative colitis. Barium enema showing featureless colon due to long-standing inflammatory bowel disease.

Coeliac disease

Definite associations between lung and coeliac disease include previous pulmonary tuberculosis, eczema and asthma, as well as interstitial lung fibrosis, sometimes associated with sarcoidosis and extrinsic allergic alveolitis.

690

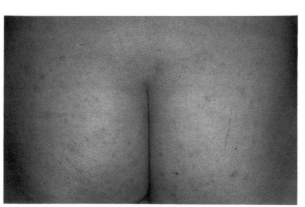

691

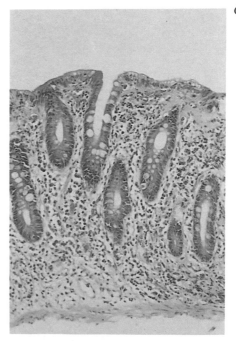

690 Coeliac disease. Dermatitis herpetiformis, a skin manifestation of coeliac disease, in a 35-year-old asthmatic patient who presented with an intensely itchy discrete vesicular and papular rash over extensor surfaces. Biopsy showed characteristic granular deposition of IgA in the dermis.

691 Coeliac disease. Small bowel biopsy showing subtotal villous atrophy and abundant inflammatory cells between the crypts. There is an increased incidence of small bowel lymphoma and oesophageal carcinoma in coeliac disease.

23 Sarcoidosis

Sarcoidosis, a multisystem disorder (**Table 43**) of unknown aetiology, is one of a number of granulomatous disorders in which the common feature is the presence of epithelioid cell granulomata.

Sarcoidosis most commonly affects adults, with a peak incidence in the third and fourth decades. The diagnosis is established by histological evidence of widespread non-caseating epithelioid cell granulomata in more than one organ and/or a positive Kveim–Siltzbach skin test. This skin test also reflects the activity of the disease. Immunological features are depression of delayed type hypersensitivity, indicating T cell anergy, and raised serum immunoglobulins, indicating B cell overactivity (**692**). There may also be hypercalciuria, with or without hypercalcaemia. The course and prognosis correlate with the mode of onset: an acute onset usually heralds a self-limiting course with spontaneous resolution, while an insidious onset may be followed by relentless progressive fibrosis (**Table 44**).

Corticosteroids relieve symptoms and suppress inflammation and granuloma formation. Serum angiotensin converting enzyme (SACE) is elevated in most patients and is a biochemical marker of activity. It falls towards normal with corticosteroid therapy and has proved a useful monitor of progress.

Although sarcoidosis is found worldwide, population studies reveal a variable prevalence. In England the overall incidence is about 20 per 100,000; Irish women in London demonstrate an incidence of 200 per 100,000. Sarcoidosis is more common in black patients than in white in the USA.

Table 43. Features of 818 patients with sarcoidosis.

Features	Number of patients	Percentage
Total	818	100
Women	500	61
Presentation under 40 years of age	604	74
Intrathoracic	716	88
Peripheral lymph adenopathy	225	27
Splenomegaly	101	12
Erythema nodosum	215	31
Other skin lesions	147	21
Ocular lesions	224	27
Nervous system	77	9
Parotid	52	6
Lacrimal	22	3
Bone	31	3
Heart	27	3
Kidney	10	1
Positive Kveim	430/658	65
Negative tuberculin	488/702	70
Hyperglobulinaemia	161/526	31
Hypercalcaemia	99/547	18
Corticosteroid therapy	344	42
Mortality caused by		
sarcoidosis	25	3
other causes	23	3

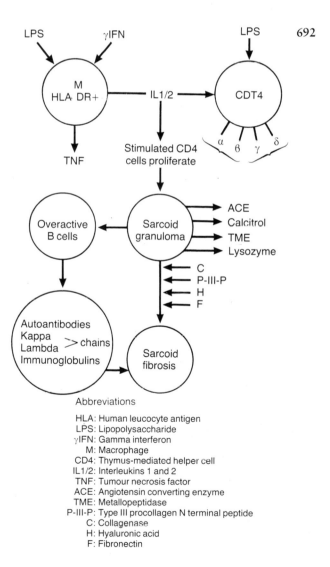

Abbreviations

HLA: Human leucocyte antigen
LPS: Lipopolysaccharide
γIFN: Gamma interferon
M: Macrophage
CD4: Thymus-mediated helper cell
IL1/2: Interleukins 1 and 2
TNF: Tumour necrosis factor
ACE: Angiotensin converting enzyme
TME: Metallopeptidase
P-III-P: Type III procollagen N terminal peptide
C: Collagenase
H: Hyaluronic acid
F: Fibronectin

692 Sarcoid granuloma. Interplay between macrophages, T and B lymphocytes and cytokines.

Table 44. A comparison of acute and chronic sarcoidosis.

Features	Acute transient	Chronic persistent
Age (years)	<30	>40
Onset	Abrupt	Insidious
Skin lesions	Erythema nodosum Maculopapular rashes Vesicles	Lupus pernio Plaques Scars Keloids Skin ulcers
Eyes	Acute iritis Conjunctivitis Conjunctival nodules	Chronic uveitis Glaucoma Cataracts Keraconjunctivitis sicca
Parotids Lymphadenopathy Splenomegaly Facial palsy	Usually transient	Rarely persistent
Bone cysts	No	Yes
Chest x-ray	Hilar adenopathy	Pulmonary infiltration fibrosis
Heart	Arrhythmias	Cor pulmonale
Histology	Epithelioid and giant cells	Hyaline fibrosis
Calcium metabolism	Hypercalcaemia Hypercalciuria	Nephrocalcinosis
Hydroxyprolinuria	Increased	Normal
Kveim test	Positive	May be negative
Gallium	+	±
Lymphocytic alveolitis	+	−
Serum angiotensin converting enzyme (SACE)	Elevated	Normal
Spontaneous remission	Frequent	Rare
Steroid therapy	Abortive effect	Symptomatic relief
Recurrence after steroid	Rare	Frequent
Prognosis	Good	Fair

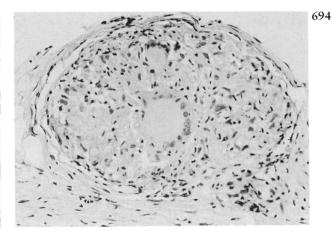

693 **Sarcoid granuloma lung.** Early stage of development. The centre is occupied by a collection of pale-staining histiocytic cells (epithelioid cells), all at the same stage of development. At the periphery is a ring of lymphocytes. (H&E×100.)

694 **Sarcoid granuloma lung.** A later stage of development than that shown in 693. The histiocyte cells have fused to form well-defined multinucleate giant cells. These may measure 300 μm in diameter and contain as many as 30 peripherally arranged nuclei. Necrosis, if it occurs, is minimal and in consequence the reticulin between the histiocytes and around the nodules remains intact. Acid-fast organisms are almost invariably absent.

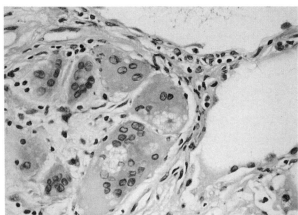

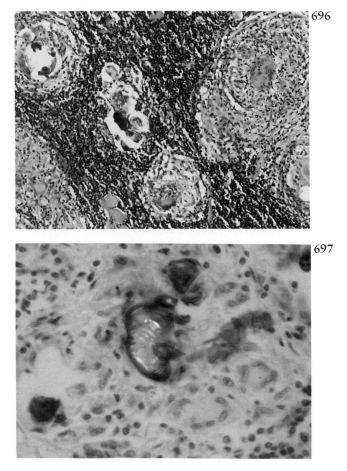

695–697 **Inclusion bodies in sarcoid granuloma lung.** The giant cells in the granulomata are metabolically active and as a consequence may contain a variety of intracytoplasmic inclusions. These are not unique to sarcoidosis. Three types are described:

1 Asteroid bodies (**695**) are found within the multinucleate giant cells and consist of a central core with radiating spinous projections. They measure 5–20 μm in diameter. (H&E×200.)
2 Residual bodies are doubly refractile and are composed of calcium carbonate and iron.
3 Schaumann bodies. These are round or oval, vary in size and are composed of calcium carbonate, iron and impregnated lipomucoglycoproteins with central birefringent, possibly calcite, crystals. (**696**, H&E×200; **697**, H&E×200, polarised light.)

698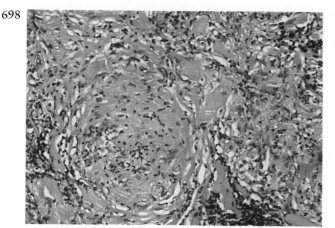

698 Sarcoid granuloma lung. Chronic sarcoidosis with fibrosis. The granulomata are mostly replaced with featureless hyalinised collagen. (H & E × 120.)

699 Clinical features of sarcoidosis.

699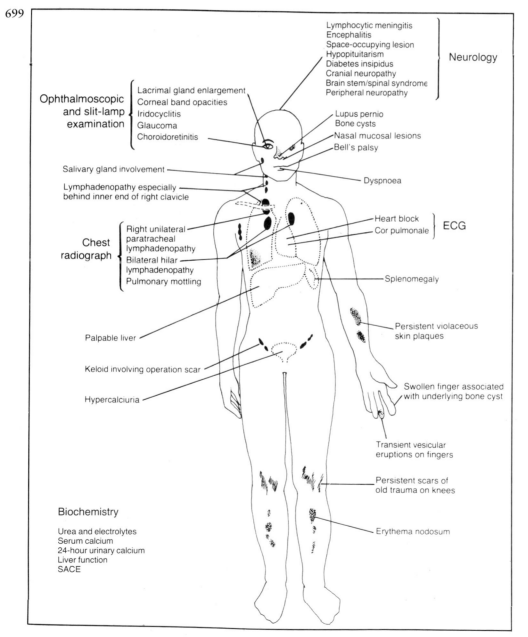

Neurology
Lymphocytic meningitis
Encephalitis
Space-occupying lesion
Hypopituitarism
Diabetes insipidus
Cranial neuropathy
Brain stem/spinal syndrome
Peripheral neuropathy

Ophthalmoscopic and slit-lamp examination
Lacrimal gland enlargement
Corneal band opacities
Iridocyclitis
Glaucoma
Choroidoretinitis

Lupus pernio
Bone cysts
Nasal mucosal lesions
Bell's palsy

Salivary gland involvement

Lymphadenopathy especially behind inner end of right clavicle

Dyspnoea

Chest radiograph
Right unilateral paratracheal lymphadenopathy
Bilateral hilar lymphadenopathy
Pulmonary mottling

Heart block
Cor pulmonale
} ECG

Splenomegaly

Persistent violaceous skin plaques

Palpable liver

Keloid involving operation scar

Hypercalciuria

Swollen finger associated with underlying bone cyst

Transient vesicular eruptions on fingers

Persistent scars of old trauma on knees

Erythema nodosum

Biochemistry

Urea and electrolytes
Serum calcium
24-hour urinary calcium
Liver function
SACE

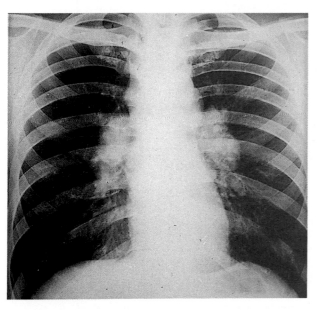

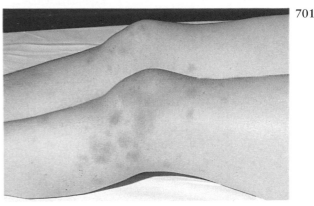

701 **Erythema nodosum and arthralgia** are features of abrupt onset sarcoidosis.

700 **Bilateral hilar lymphadenopathy (BHL).** The combination of erythema nodosum and hilar lymphadenopathy (Lofgren's syndrome), often with anterior uveitis, indicates acute exudative sarcoidosis. This acute onset syndrome has a favourable outcome. Bilateral hilar lymphadenopathy is frequently a chance radiographic finding in a symptom-free patient. It may be expected to subside eventually in 60% of patients.

In sarcoidosis the diversity of possible clinical manifestations is such that patients may present to almost any branch of medicine. The more abrupt the onset, the better the prognosis. Lofgren's syndrome, with bilateral hilar lymphadenopathy and erythema nodosum, is a typical acute presentation.

Erythema nodosum is a non-specific hypersensitivity reaction provoked by many antigens (see **Table 21**). The classic account of erythema nodosum by Robert Willan (1808) is as apt today as when he described it.

In erythema nodosum many of the red patches are large and rounded. The central parts of them are very gradually elevated and on the sixth or seventh day form hard and painful protuberances. From the seventh to the tenth day they constantly soften and subside without ulceration. On the eighth or ninth day the red colour changes to bluish or livid, and the affected limb appears as if it had been severely bruised. This appearance remains for a week or 10 days, when the cuticle begins to separate in scurf. Erythema nodosum usually affects the fore parts of the legs. I have only seen it in females, most of whom were servants. It is preceded by irregular shiverings, nausea, headaches and fretfulness with a quick unequal pulse and a whitish fur on the tongue. These symptoms continue for a week or more but they usually abate on the appearance of the erythema.

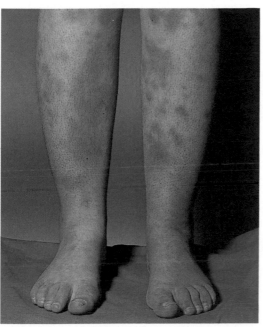

702 **Erythema nodosum.** As the condition subsides, there is a play of colours from bright red to a brownish yellow discoloration resembling a bruise.

261

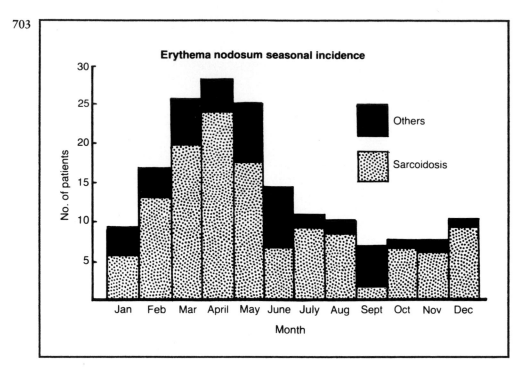

703 **Erythema nodosum** occurs most commonly in the spring. It arises most frequently in women of child-bearing age who are predominantly HLA–B8:A1.

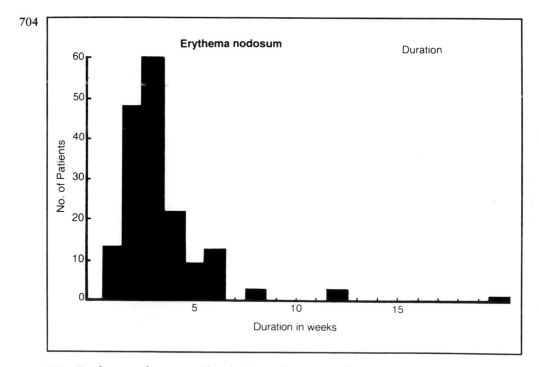

704 **Erythema nodosum** usually subsides within one month.

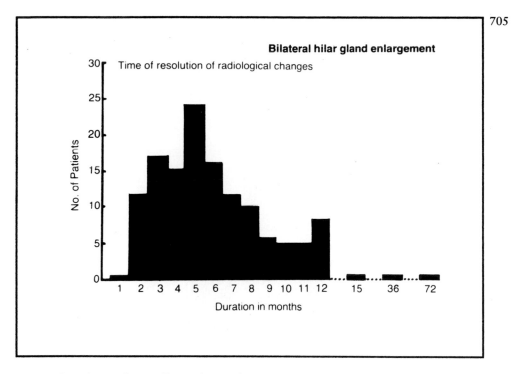

Bilateral hilar gland enlargement

Time of resolution of radiological changes

(y-axis) No. of Patients

(x-axis) Duration in months

705 **Hilar adenopathy** usually resolves within one year.

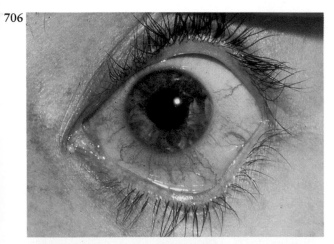

706 **Acute anterior uveitis.** Because sarcoidosis is a multisystem disorder, clinical examination must be thorough and should include slit-lamp examination of the eyes. Uveitis occurs in around a quarter of patients.

707, 708 **Acute anterior uveitis in sarcoidosis.** The eyes are red, with circumcorneal ciliary congestion, papillary irregularity and fine keratitic precipitates floating in the anterior chamber. Keratitic precipitates are best demonstrated by slit-lamp examination of the eyes (**708**).

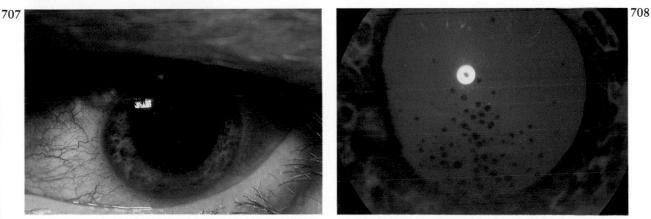

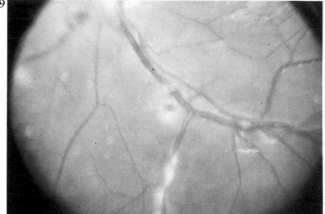

709 **Sarcoidosis.** Acute choroidoretinitis, exudates and retinal haemorrhages.

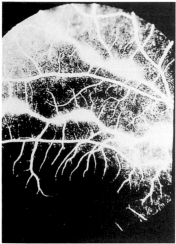 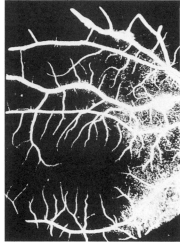

710 711

710, 711 **Acute choroidoretinitis.** Fluorescein angiography shows a fluffy appearance of the vessels which are the site of a vasculitis. Intravenous fluorescein leaks through diseased retinal vessels. There is considerable improvement after only three weeks of treatment with prednisolone (**711**).

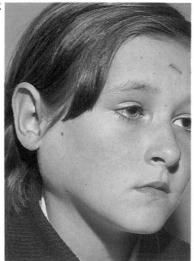

712

712 **Parotid gland enlargement** may be associated with the Heerfordt–Waldenström syndrome ('uveoparotid fever'). This uncommon condition presents acutely, running a chronic course with parotid gland enlargement, uveitis, fever and cranial nerve palsies. The facial nerves especially are involved. Other components include bizarre neurological manifestations, lethargy, meningism and cerebrospinal fluid pleocytosis.

713 **Left Bell's palsy.** Lower motor neurone paralysis of the facial nerve is usually unilateral and may be associated with uveitis and parotitis.

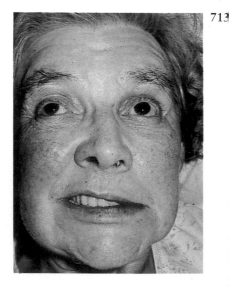

713

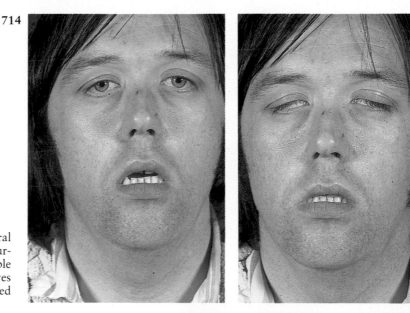

714, 715 Sarcoidosis. Bilateral facial nerve palsy is rare, but occurred in this patient who was unable to close his lips or eyelids. (Eyes open **714**, eyes and mouth closed **715**.)

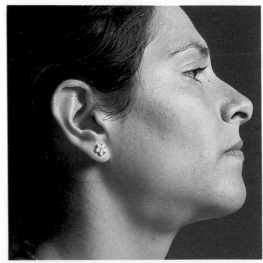

716 Submandibular lymphadenopathy. Enlargement of the superficial lymph nodes is a frequent finding during the course of sarcoidosis. The cervical lymph nodes are most commonly involved. Enlargement is seldom sufficient to attract the patient's attention. In this instance, considerable enlargement of the submandibular glands is evident.

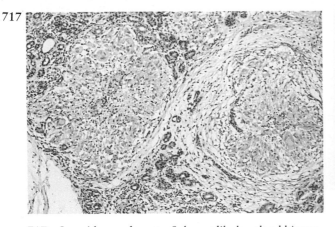

717 Sarcoid granulomata. Submandibular gland biopsy, performed because lymphoma was suspected, showing two classic sarcoid granulomata. (Same patient as shown in **716**.)

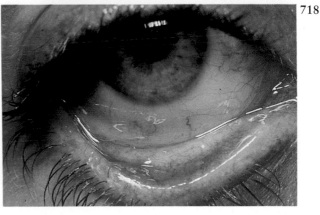

718 Conjunctival follicles in sarcoidosis. Biopsy revealed typical granuloma.

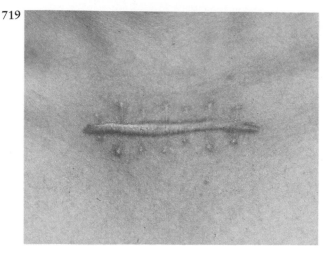

719 **The scar after mediastinoscopy** may develop into a keloid or become infiltrated with sarcoid tissue. Surgical scars become red and livid with exacerbations or activity of sarcoidosis, as in this case.

Chronic sarcoidosis

The hallmarks of chronicity of sarcoidosis are chronic skin lesions and bone cysts. Their insidious onset suggests to the chest physician that the lung changes are also chronic, fibrotic and irreversible. The more insidious the onset, the more protracted is the course of the disease.

Chronic cutaneous sarcoidosis

Lupus pernio of the face is a most disfiguring form of chronic fibrotic sarcoidosis, ranging from a few small nasal nodules to exuberant plaques covering the nose and spreading across both cheeks. It occurs predominantly in women in the fourth and fifth decades, presenting with nasal congestion or obstruction and followed by a purple macular eruption. It always involves nasal mucosa.

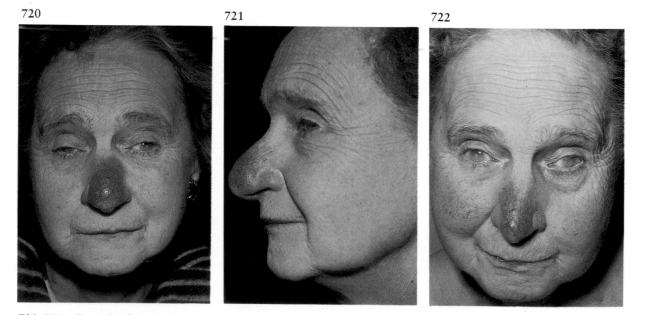

720–722 **Extensive lupus pernio.** As this patient developed the condition in pre-cortisone days, her bilateral uveitis progressed to blindness (**722**).

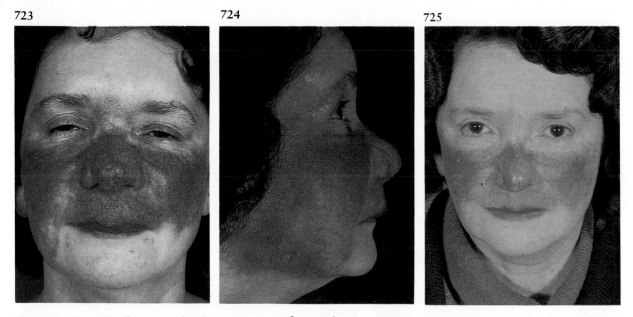

723–725 Extensive lupus pernio. Cosmetic camouflage and corticosteroids helped this patient, but the condition persisted as shown in **725**, taken 10 years later.

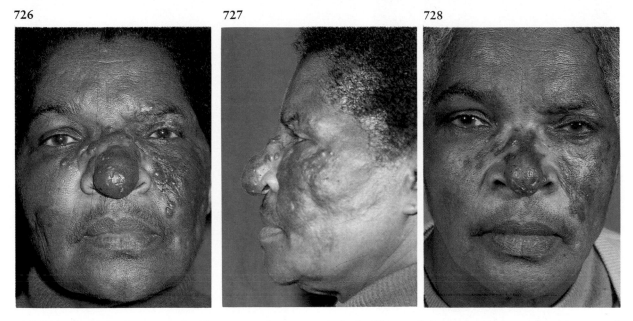

726–728 Extensive lupus pernio. Plaques on the nose and cheek. The condition was quiescent after 15 years of corticosteroid treatment, leaving disfigured depigmented skin, a complication which sometimes worries the patients as much as the disease.

267

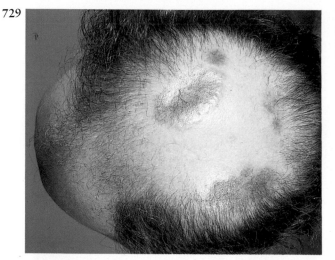

729   **Plaques on the scalp.** These were associated with progressive pulmonary fibrosis. A sarcoid skin plaque is generally rounded or oval and has a nodular slightly raised rim of pinkish brown encircling a clearer atrophic central area.

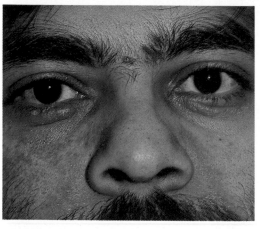

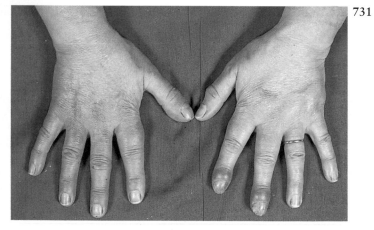

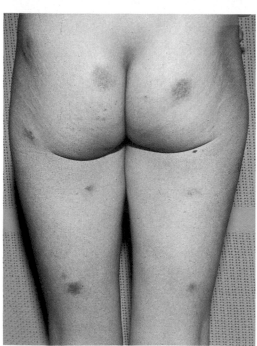

730   **Sarcoidosis.** Nodular lesions on the face.

731   **Lupus pernio of the extremities.** Smooth chilblain-like swellings are present on the fingers. The underlying phalange is usually involved and the nail is often dystrophic.

732   **Sarcoidosis.** Skin plaques on the trunk.

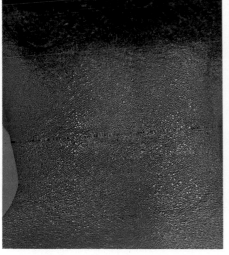

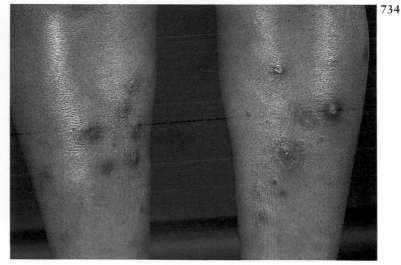

733 Skin plaques caused by sarcoidosis on the nape of the neck often look like grains of salt.

734 Sarcoidosis. Nodular infiltration on both legs.

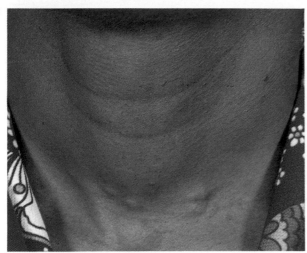

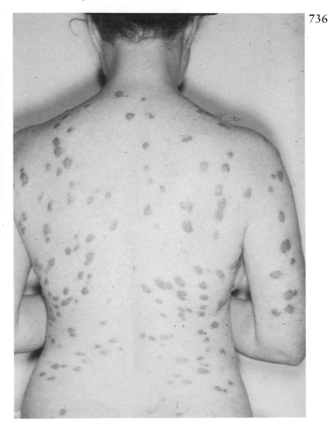

735 Sarcoidosis. Subcutaneous nodules may be palpable in the neck, trunk and limbs.

736 Small nodular infiltrations are commonly multiple, affecting the arms and trunk. Skin plaques, like the accompanying lung lesions, persist indefinitely. It is little wonder that sarcoidosis has occasionally been subtitled 'European leprosy'.

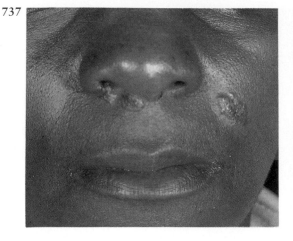

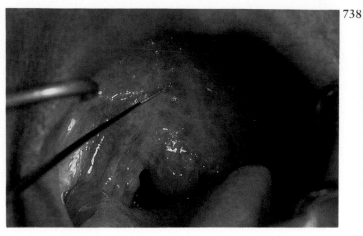

737 **Skin plaques on the face and right nostril.** Plaques at the nostril are frequently associated with upper respiratory tract sarcoidosis.

738 **Extensive granulomatous lesions in the larynx and pharynx.** The sarcoid granulomata have a cobblestone appearance. This patient presented with a sore throat and hoarseness.

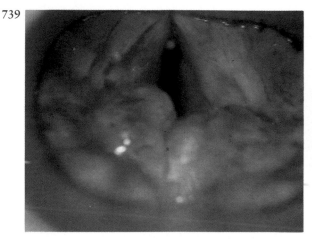

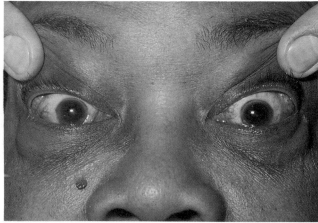

739 **Sarcoid granulomata of the larynx.**

740 **Sarcoidosis.** Lacrimal gland involvement is more frequent in black than in white persons. It may cause dry gritty eyes and swelling of the lateral portion of the upper eyelids.

Infiltration of old scars may occur without other evidence of skin sarcoidosis. Its course follows that of the lung changes, the scar reverting to its normal flat pale state as the sarcoidosis activity wanes.

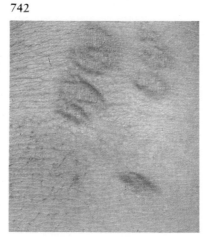

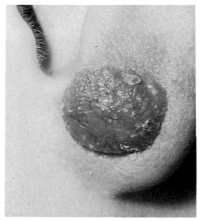

741 Stab wound infiltrated by sarcoid tissue.

742 Sarcoidosis nodules at venesection sites in the antecubital fossa.

743 Sarcoid nodules at the site of earlobe piercing.

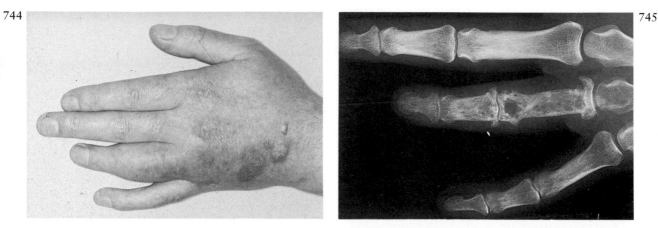

744, 745 Chronic skin plaques and bone cysts. These bone changes rarely heal completely. There is residual shortening of the fourth digit, with a bone cyst involving the medulla of the middle phalanx.

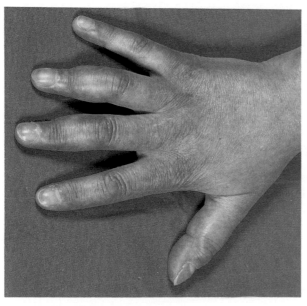

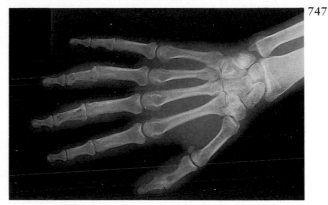

746 Phalangeal bone cysts causing sausage-shaped swelling of the fingers in this patient with chronic pulmonary sarcoidosis.

747 Phalangeal bone cysts. Lytic, reticular permeative and deforming lesions are shown on the x-ray. (Same patient as shown in **746**.)

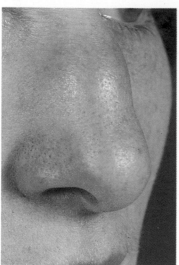 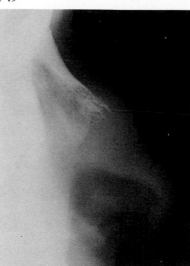

748 Sarcoidosis of the upper respiratory tract is closely associated with lupus pernio. This patient with chronic sarcoidosis complained of nasal obstruction and a broadening of the bridge of the nose.

749 Sarcoidosis of the upper respiratory tract. This lateral radiograph shows osteoporotic changes in the nasal bones, together with a soft tissue swelling. The nasal symptoms responded to steroid therapy, but there was no improvement in the disfiguring bone changes.

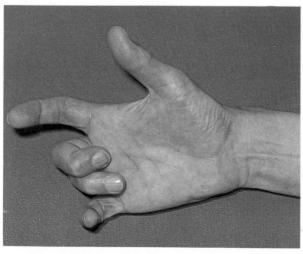

750 Sarcoidosis of skeletal muscle. Contraction of the third, fourth and fifth fingers developed, with a fixed flexion deformity at the wrist. Biopsy of the muscles of the forearm and biceps showed sarcoid granulomata. In chronic sarcoidosis, muscle wasting, weakness, contracture and tender palpable nodules may occur.

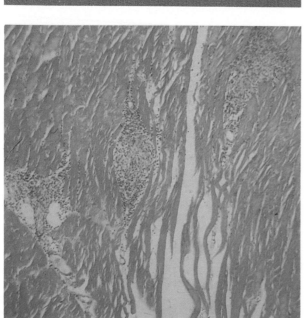

751 Sarcoidosis. Quadriceps muscle biopsy showing granuloma in striated muscle. (H & E × 40.)

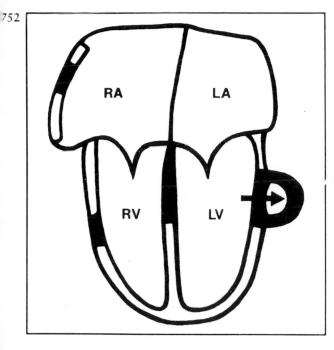

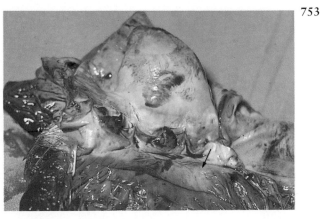

753 Myocardial sarcoidosis. Fibrosis involving the bundle of His in a fatal case (arrow).

752 Involvement of the heart in sarcoidosis. The interventricular septum, bundle of His and the free ventricular wall of both ventricles are most frequently involved. Less commonly, the right atrium may be affected. Cardiac involvement may be silent or present with arrhythmias, conduction block or cardiac failure due to cardiac fibrosis and ventricular hypokinesia. The high incidence of sudden death reflects the very real risk of conduction system involvement.

754 Myocardial sarcoidosis. Numerous granulomata with extensive fibrosis of the ventricular wall. (H& E×50.)

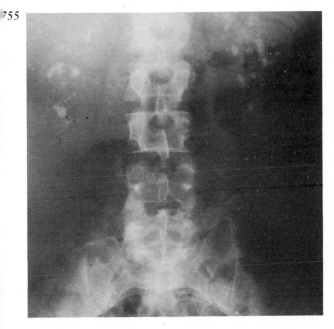

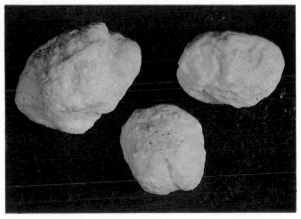

756 Renal calculi. The calcium stones caused acute renal colic. Renal calculi and nephrocalcinosis are complications of persistent hypercalciuria and reflect abnormal calcium metabolism, which occurs in about 20% of patients.

755 Nephrocalcinosis. A plain film of the abdomen. Renal involvement is unusual and nephrocalcinosis is present in only 1% of cases of sarcoidosis. It may lead to pyelonephritis and chronic renal failure.

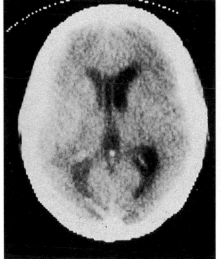

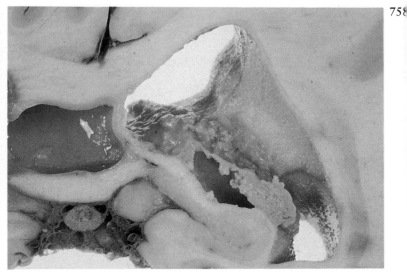

757 Cerebral sarcoidosis – internal hydrocephalus. CT scan of the brain showing a dilated left ventricle in a patient who complained of severe unrelieved headaches. Chronic sarcoidosis may be associated with granulomatous changes in the brain, spinal cord and meninges.

758 Cerebral sarcoidosis. Necropsy specimen. Grape-like clusters of granulomata on the lateral ventricle, and also widely scattered elsewhere, were revealed on necropsy (same patient as shown in **757**). The presence of internal hydrocephalus carries a gloomy prognosis.

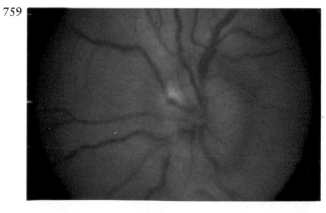

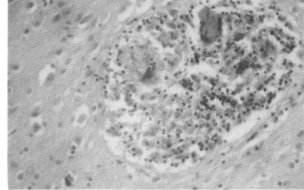

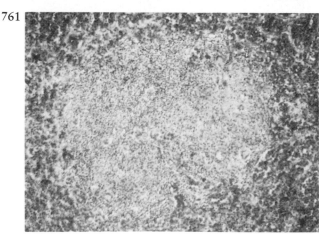

759 Cerebral sarcoidosis. Papilloedema in a patient presenting with a space-occupying nodular cerebral lesion.

760 Cerebral sarcoidosis granulomata in brain tissue. These are most abundant over the base of the brain, with involvement of both veins and arteries.

761 Cerebral sarcoidosis granuloma in posterior pituitary gland. Diabetes insipidus is a rare complication of pulmonary sarcoidosis. The differential diagnosis is histiocytosis X. Granulomata in the posterior pituitary or hypothalamus may result in diabetes insipidus, hypothalamic hypothyroidism, or hypopituitarism and somnolence with hypercapnia.

Radiographic features

It is customary to stage intrathoracic sarcoidosis in the following way:

Stage 0 Clear chest radiograph.
Stage 1 Hilar lymphadenopathy.
Stage 2 Hilar lymphadenopathy and pulmonary infiltration.
Stage 3 Pulmonary infiltration.
Stage 4 Irreversible pulmonary fibrosis.

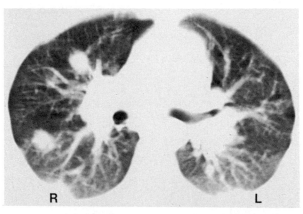

762 Pulmonary sarcoidosis. Stage 1: florid bilateral hilar and right paratracheal gland lymphadenopathy. This may be expected to subside in 60% of patients. Sarcoidosis was diagnosed histologically by mediastinoscopy.

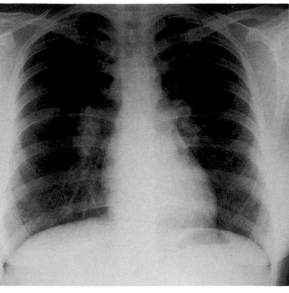

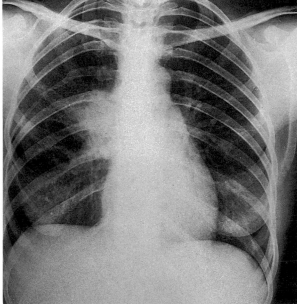

763, 764 Pulmonary sarcoidosis. Stage 1: discrete bilateral hilar gland enlargement. The lung fields are radiographically clear on the posteroanterior film. The CT scan (**764**) confirms the bilateral hilar adenopathy and also demonstrates unsuspected nodular shadows in both the right and the left lung fields.

765 Unilateral hilar adenopathy due to sarcoidosis is only one-tenth as frequent as its bilateral counterpart. The differential diagnosis includes tuberculosis, reticulosis or bronchogenic carcinoma.

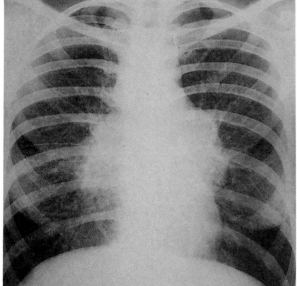

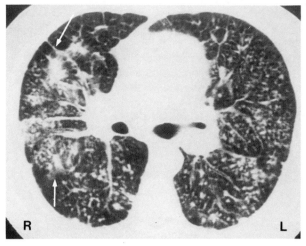

766 Pulmonary sarcoidosis. Stage 2: bilateral hilar lymphadenopathy with pulmonary infiltration. This subsides in 40% of patients.

767 Pulmonary sarcoidosis (active and healing). CT scan. Widespread nodules of varied size and shape are present throughout the lung fields. The nodules in sarcoidosis may be well defined, angular or irregular and are usually less than 5 mm in diameter. They are most often deployed along the bronchovascular bundles, lymphatics and interlobular septa, and may be subpleural in location. The widespread nodules are more discrete on the left. On the right, areas of irregular fibrosis and thickened bronchovascular bundles are beginning to pull, stretch and deform the lung parenchyma (arrowed). This characteristic appearance is quite unlike the pattern found in fibrosing alveolitis and other diffuse fibrosing diseases.

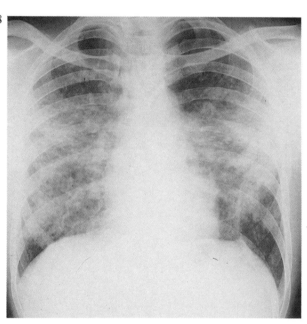

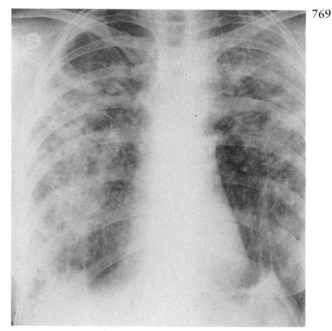

768 Pulmonary sarcoidosis. Stage 3: diffuse symmetrical infiltration showing the characteristic preponderance of shadowing in the mid-zone.

769 Pulmonary sarcoidosis. Stage 4: upper zone fibrosis with loss of volume in the upper zones elevating the hilar shadows. The lower zones are hypertransradiant, suggesting 'compensatory' lower lobe emphysema.

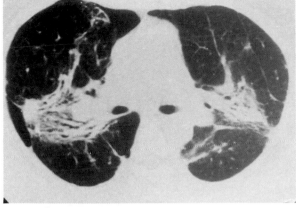

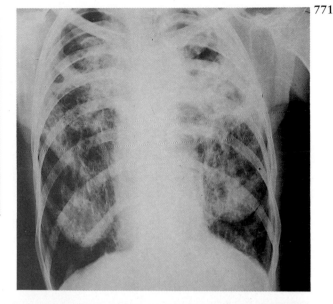

770 Pulmonary sarcoidosis – CT scan. Stage 4: there is severe fibrosis in both mid-zones. Dilated bronchi are present within fibrotic masses surrounded by emphysematous lung.

771 Pulmonary sarcoidosis. Stage 4: irreversible lung fibrosis with formation of upper zone bullae.

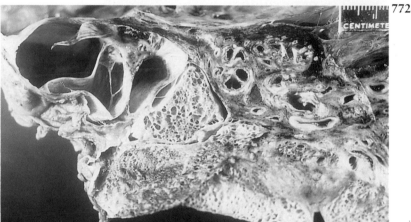

772 Pulmonary fibrosis and bulla formation. Large bullae are unusual and may be colonised by mycetoma.

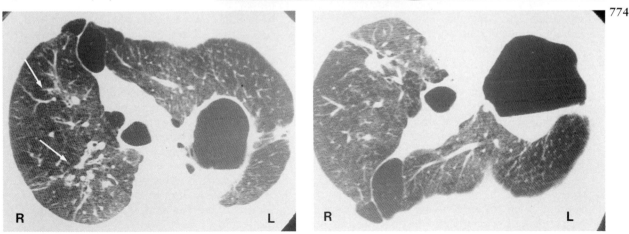

773, 774 Chronic sarcoidosis (CT scan) has caused thickened bronchial walls and bronchiectasis in the right upper lobe (arrowed), with volume loss and mediastinal deviation (supine CT). On the left a large cavity contains fluid which obscures the posterior wall of the cavity. In the prone position (774) the fluid in the cavity now lies anteriorly and the cavity wall is seen to be smooth posteriorly. CT scanning carried out in the prone position frequently resolves diagnostic difficulties where overlying densities are due to dependent factors, e.g. hypervascularity, fluid, mycetomas.

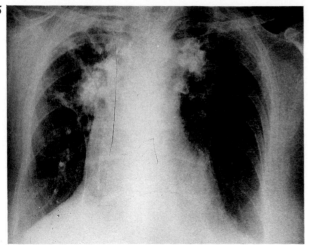

775 Pulmonary sarcoidosis. Stage 4: chronic fibrosis with bilateral upper lobe shrinkage. The hilar glands are densely calcified, a legacy of previous hypercalcaemia. This patient also developed nephrocalcinosis and renal impairment.

Diagnosis of sarcoidosis

When sarcoidosis is suspected, histological confirmation of the clinical and radiographic findings should be followed by an assessment of activity of the disease.

Diagnosis is inferred from the clinical features at presentation, in combination with the radiographic, biochemical and immunological findings. Some clinical presentations are so highly characteristic, for instance the erythema nodosum arthropathy–bilateral hilar lymphadenopathy syndrome, that histological confirmation may not be required, provided that there are no discordant features. With less characteristic clinical presentations, the diagnosis may only be accepted after positive biopsies have been obtained from a number of sites.

Clinical investigation of suspected sarcoidosis
This should include the following in most cases:

1 Full history including enquiry about BCG vaccination, and detailed clinical examination including ophthalmoscopy.
2 Slit-lamp examination of the eyes.
3 Chest x-ray is essential irrespective of the presenting symptoms. If equivocal, it can be helpful to locate any previous films.
4 Routine haematological and biochemical tests including serum calcium and a 24-hour urine collection for calcium excretion.
5 Tuberculin test series up to a concentration of 1:100. This is negative in two-thirds of patients with sarcoidosis. Strongly positive reactions are unusual.
6 Sputum, if any, or bronchoalveolar lavage should be examined to exclude acid-fast bacilli.
7 Histological confirmation by specific organ biopsy, bronchial or transbronchial biopsy, or by Kveim–Siltzbach skin test.
8 Assessment of activity in confirmed cases. This will routinely include serial chest x-rays and respiratory function tests. Serial measurements of serum angiotensin converting enzyme (SACE) can be useful. Bronchoalveolar lavage (BAL) and Gallium-67 scanning are both sensitive and specific methods for assessing the intensity of the alveolitis in sarcoidosis, valuable in research but of unproven value in routine clinical practice.

These investigations enable the clinician to classify the disease as acute or chronic and aid in the assessment of activity and need for treatment with corticosteroids.

Tissue diagnosis

The preferred site for biopsy is influenced both by the availability of facilities and by the mode of presentation. The general requirement is to confirm the diagnosis without undue discomfort or hazard.

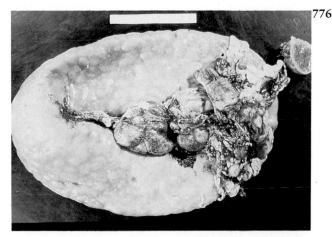

776 Human sarcoid spleen. The spleen is enlarged and infiltrated by sarcoid granulomata, which have produced the surface's nodularity. The Kveim–Siltzbach test material is a finely particulate saline suspension of human sarcoid spleen which is phenolised, pasteurised at 58°C and irradiated.

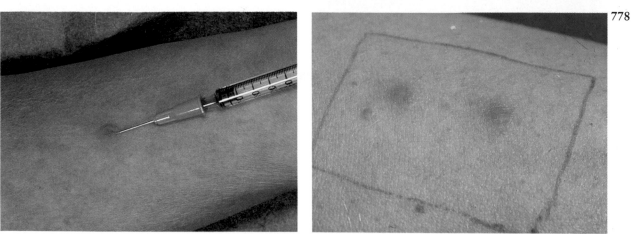

777, 778 Kveim–Siltzbach test. The test dose (0.15 ml) is injected intracutaneously (777). In most reactive individuals a palpable papule is present at the injection site after 4–6 weeks (778).

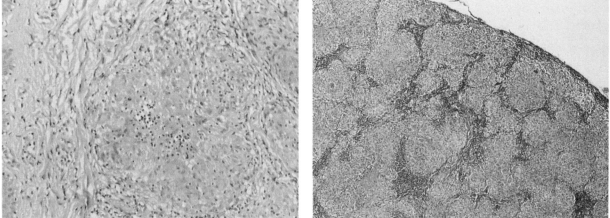

779 Histology from a positive Kveim–Siltzbach test showing subdermal granulomata. The test is positive in about two-thirds of sarcoidosis patients. (H & E×25.)

780 Sarcoidosis. Scalene node biopsy specimen infiltrated with numerous granulomata. Lymph node tissue may be readily obtained at mediastinoscopy.

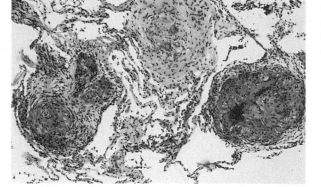

781 Sarcoidosis. Bronchoscopic transbronchial lung biopsy will show granulomata in two-thirds of patients with active sarcoidosis. The small specimens may cause difficulty in pathological interpretation. This specimen shows a number of classic non-caseating sarcoid granulomata. (H & E × 25.)

782, 783 Sarcoidosis. Hepatic biopsy specimens showing active sarcoid granuloma (782) and healing with hyaline fibrosis (783). Hepatic granulomata are usually isolated, randomly distributed (often within portal tracts) and seldom give rise to symptoms.

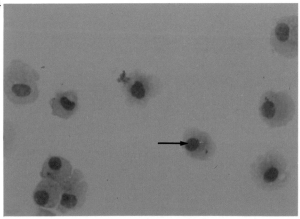

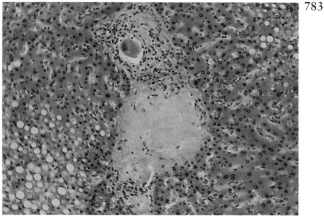

Bronchial lavage

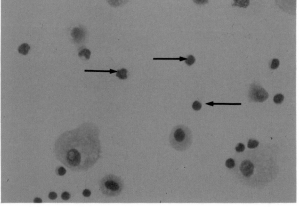

784 Bronchial lavage from normal lung. The differential cell count from lavage of a normal non-smoking adult reveals 93% macrophages, 6% lymphocytes and only 1% neutrophils. The average total cell count is from 5 to 10 cells per 100 ml of lavage. A larger number of cells is obtained from smokers' lungs containing 'activated macrophages' and an excess of neutrophils. (Arrow indicates macrophage.)

785 Bronchial lavage from active stage 2 sarcoidosis. This differential count showed 55% lymphocytes, 39% macrophages and 6% neutrophils. The unexpected finding of an elevated lymphocyte ratio suggests a granulomatous disorder.

In sarcoidosis the lymphocytes are predominantly CDT_4 but in hypersensitivity pneumonitis are CDT_8. (Arrows indicate lymphocytes.)

Table 45. Bronchoalveolar lavage findings.	
CDT4 helper	Sarcoidosis
	Beryllium
	Asthma
CDT8 suppressor	Hypersensitivity pneumonitis
	Talc
	Asthma
Neutrophils	Smokers
	Fibrosing alveolitis
	ARDS
	AIDS
	Mineral dusts
	Collagen
Eosinophils	Drugs
	Asthma
	Pneumonia
Mast cell	Sarcoidosis
	Asthma
Malignant	Lymphangitic carcinoma
	Hodgkin's
Plasma cell	Myeloma
Multinucleate giant cells	Cobalt

Cells and protein may be harvested from the lower respiratory tract by instilling sodium chloride 0.9% solution through a fibreoptic bronchoscope or catheter and immediately suctioning the fluid back into a container.

Bronchial lavage recovers cells and proteins present on the epithelial surface of the lower respiratory tract, which compare closely with the cellular and protein constituents obtained by open lung biopsy.

In interstitial lung disease the differential count allows disorders to be separated broadly into those with high lymphocyte ratios and those with elevated neutrophil ratios. High lymphocyte ratios are found in extrinsic allergic alveolitis (hypersensitivity pneumonitis) or sarcoidosis, and high neutrophil ratios in idiopathic pulmonary fibrosis and asbestosis (Table 45).

Biochemical markers in sarcoidosis

Serum angiotensin converting enzyme (SACE), transcobalamin II, B2 microglobulin, calcium and lysozyme activity are all elevated in patients with active sarcoidosis. Measurement provides supporting, but not specific, diagnostic information.

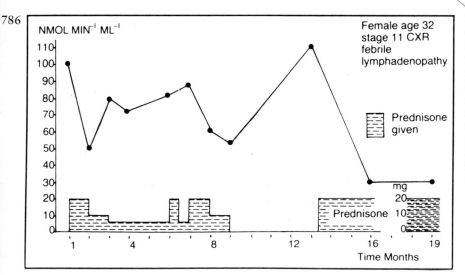

786

786 Serum angiotensin converting enzyme (SACE). Changes in SACE activity with steroid therapy are shown in a 32-year-old Afro-Caribbean woman with histologically proven pulmonary sarcoidosis. SACE is a monitor of progress, since it falls towards normal when steroid therapy suppresses activity of the granulomata. It also heralds relapses in the patient who is no longer receiving steroid therapy.

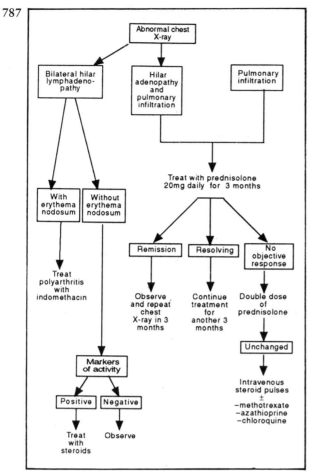

787 Treatment schedule for pulmonary sarcoidosis.

Table 46. Differences between sarcoidosis and tuberculosis.

Features	Tuberculosis	Sarcoidosis
Ethnic grouping	Pakistani/Indian/ Bangladeshi	West Indian/ Irish
Age (year)	Over 50	20–50
Fever	Common	Rare
Erythema nodosum	Uncommon	Common
Uveitis Skin involvement Enlarged parotids Bone cysts	Very rare	Common
Ulceration and sinuses	Common	No
Involvement of: Pleura Peritoneum Pericardium Meninges Small intestine	Common	Very rare
Caseation	Maximal	Minimal
Acid-fast bacilli	Present	Absent
Tuberculin test	Positive in most	Negative in 65%
Kveim–Siltzbach test	Negative	Positive in 80%
Hypercalcaemia	No	Yes
Hypercalciuria	No	Yes
Serum angiotensin converting enzyme	Elevated in up to 10%	Elevated in 60%
Calcification	Yes	Rare
Hilar lymphadenopathy	Unilateral	Bilateral
Pulmonary cavities	Common, early	Rare, late
Ghon focus	Yes	No
Corticosteroids	Harmful alone	Helpful
Antituberculous drugs	Treatment of choice	Unhelpful

24 Chronic obstructive pulmonary disease (COPD)

The terminology used to describe those disorders characterised by airways obstruction is imperfect. The designation 'chronic obstructive pulmonary disease' is widely used to describe airflow limitation, often irreversible, associated with bronchitis and emphysema.

Chronic bronchitis is defined clinically as chronic or recurrent excessive mucous secretion in the bronchial tree. It is diagnosed by the presence of cough and expectoration, not attributable to other lung diseases, on most days for at least three months in two consecutive years.

Chronic bronchitis may be subdivided into:

- Simple chronic bronchitis with mucoid expectoration.
- Chronic or recurrent mucopurulent bronchitis.
- Chronic obstructive bronchitis with persistent widespread narrowing of the intrapulmonary airways.

Emphysema is defined anatomically as an increase beyond normal in the size of air spaces distal to the terminal bronchiole, accompanied by destruction of their walls and without obvious fibrosis. This anatomical description can be confirmed only by histological examination of lung tissue.

Airways obstruction, which may be severe, is a feature of both conditions.

The definitions are not exclusive since bronchitis and emphysema may co-exist; the boundary between COPD and asthma is undefined. Individuals suffering from chronic obstructive bronchitis may show significant improvement in airways obstruction when treated with bronchodilating drugs.

Numerous studies have related the presence of bronchitis and emphysema to increasing age, the cumulative effects of cigarette smoking, atmospheric pollution, certain occupations in which there is inhalation of inorganic or organic dusts and fumes, recurrent childhood respiratory tract infections and genetic factors, especially those concerned with antiprotease activity.

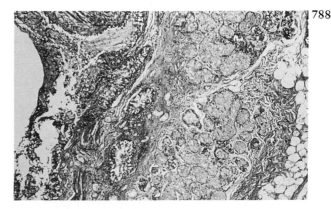

788

788 Chronic bronchitis. Mucous gland hyperplasia and chronic inflammation. The mucous glands in the submucosa usually make up less than 40% of the total wall thickness. In this example there is mucous gland hypertrophy (blue staining). *Haemophilus influenzae* and *Streptococcus pneumoniae* are the common infective organisms found in the mucopurulent sputum of the bronchitic. (Alcian blue×100.)

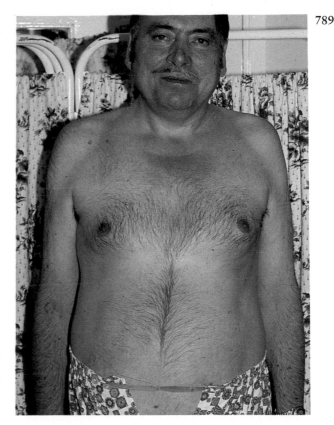

789

789 Chronic obstructive pulmonary disease. Cyanosed polycythaemic obese patient who was receiving treatment for central congestive cardiac failure. 'Blue and bloated' aptly describes these patients' appearance. This patient did not complain of breathlessness in spite of hypoxic–hypercapnoic respiratory failure.

283

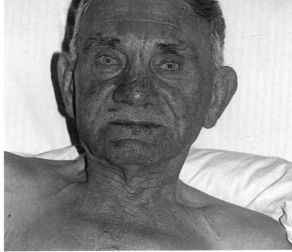

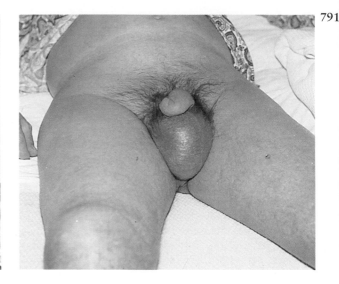

790 Chronic obstructive pulmonary disease. Central cyanosis and engorged neck veins caused by secondary right heart failure – cor pulmonale. The herpes skin rash on the lip points to a recent infective exacerbation.

791 Chronic obstructive pulmonary disease. Cardio-respiratory failure, with ascites and gross oedema including the genitalia. Breathlessness was not severe in spite of severe hypoxia and elevation of the arterial carbon dioxide tension.

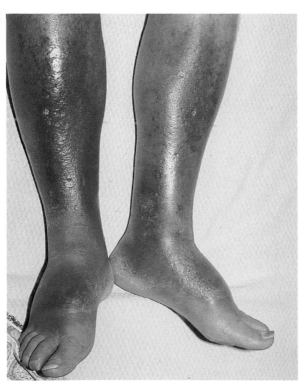

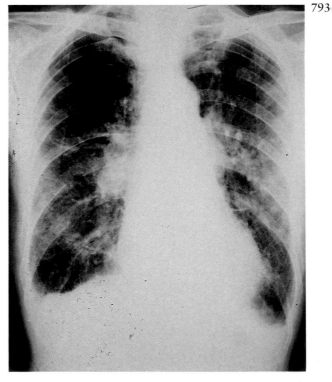

792 Chronic obstructive pulmonary disease. Gross peripheral oedema secondary to hypoxic right heart failure.

793 Chronic obstructive pulmonary disease. Chest radiograph showing typical appearances of cor pulmonale, with cardiomegaly, dilatation of the proximal pulmonary vessels and small bilateral pleural effusions. Same patient as shown in **791** and **792**.

794 Chronic obstructive pulmonary disease. Cor pulmonale. Treatment with diuretics, venesection for polycythaemia, controlled oxygen therapy and antibiotics for infection produced considerable improvement. The pleural effusions have cleared and the dilated heart is smaller. Same patient as shown in **791–793** after four weeks in hospital.

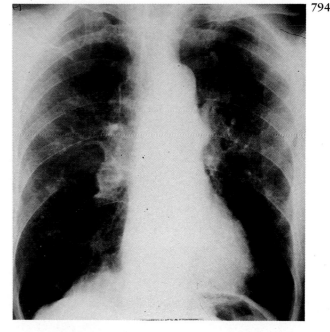

Two patterns of disturbance may be discerned during the progress of advanced COPD, which mainly differ in the extent to which ventilatory drive is maintained.

Type B or blue bloater (789–792)

The picture of poor respiratory drive. Individuals tend to show the following features:

- Relatively mild dyspnoea.
- Obese and plethoric.
- Oedema, congestive heart failure.
- Large volume sputum.
- Hypoxia and hypercapnia.
- Polycythemia.
- Nocturnal hypoxaemia (sleep apnoea).
- Unexpectedly well preserved lung function.
- No radiological emphysema.
- Poor prognosis, 70% five year mortality.

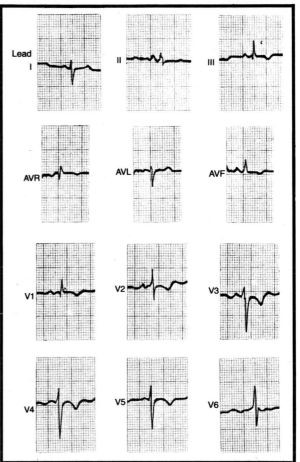

795 Chronic obstructive pulmonary disease. Right ventricular hypertrophy. Electrocardiogram of patient shown in **791–794**. The criteria for right ventricular hypertrophy are an R wave of 7mm or more in V1, a combined voltage of R wave in V1 and S wave in V6 of 10mm or more, an R wave taller than the S wave in V6 and right axis deviation. Right atrial enlargement associated with P. pulmonale causing a tall peaked P wave in standard lead II is a frequent finding, but not apparent in this example.

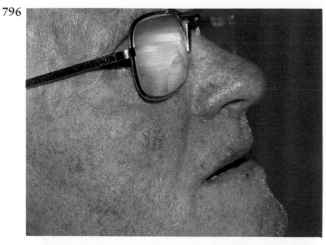

796

Table 47. Signs and symptoms of hypercapnia.

Warm peripheries	Enlarged retinal veins
Bounding full pulse	Papilloedema
Flapping tremor	Depressed tendon reflexes
Headache	Extensor plantar response
Confusion/drowsiness	Coma
Small pupils	

796 **Pursed lip expiration** is a common feature in severe airflow obstruction. In an attempt to prevent premature airways collapse and air trapping, the patient maintains an elevated intrathoracic presure by exhaling slowly against a raised intralaryngeal or oral pressure. The lips are cyanosed.

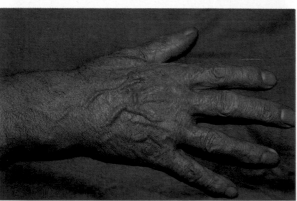

797

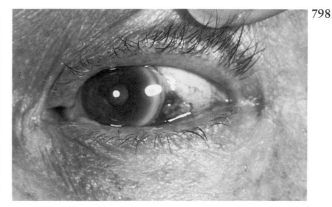

798

797 **Peripheral signs of carbon dioxide retention** include dilated veins, a bounding pulse and flapping tremor of the dorsiflexed outstretched hands that is similar to that seen in hepatic encephalopathy. Peripheral cyanosis always accompanies central cyanosis and may be seen in the nail vascular beds.

798 **Subconjunctival flame-shaped haemorrhage** indicates transient elevation of the venous pressure during a bout of coughing. Cough syncope, in which the patient faints during a bout of coughing, also indicates raised venous and intrathoracic pressure with transient reduction in cardiac output, causing cerebral hypoxia and transient loss of consciousness.

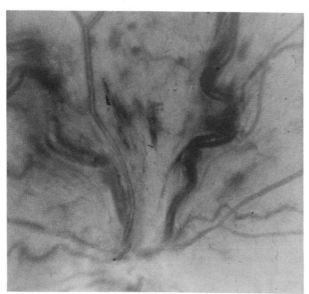

799

799 **Chronic obstructive pulmonary disease.** The cerebral vessels dilate in response to hypercapnia and the patient may complain of headache, drowsiness and confusion. Fundal examination may show the dilated vessels, sometimes accompanied by papilloedema.

Pathological classification of emphysema

Four main types of emphysema are recognised. They are classified according to the distribution of the abnormally large air spaces within the acinar unit.

- Panacinar emphysema. Abnormally large air spaces evenly distributed throughout the acinar unit.
- Centriacinar or centrilobular emphysema. Abnormal air spaces found within the respiratory bronchioles.
- Periacinar or paraseptal emphysema. Abnormal air spaces at the edge of the acinar unit.
- Irregular emphysema found adjacent to lung scars.

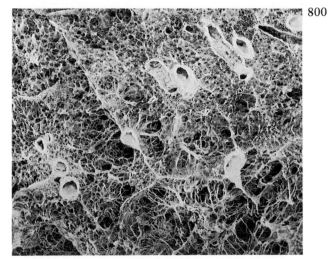

800

800 **Panacinar emphysema (panlobular).** The air spaces beyond the terminal bronchioles are destroyed in a relatively uniform manner throughout the affected lobule. Compare the extensively destroyed alveolar walls in the lower portions of the photograph with the more normal appearance above. (Barium sulphate lung slice impregnation specimen ×15.)

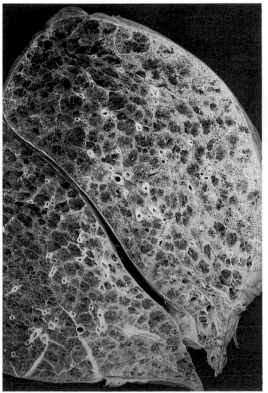

801

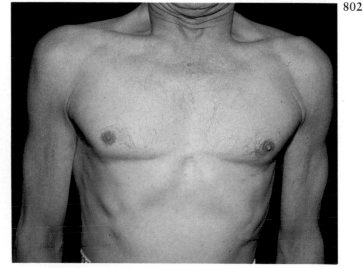

802

802 **Barrel-shaped chest in emphysema** is a sign of hyperinflation and air trapping. The horizontal position of the ribs, prominent sternal angle and increased anteroposterior diameter of the chest are characteristic of hyperinflation due to emphysema.

801 **Centrilobular emphysema** (centriacinar). Sagittal lung section. This form of emphysema involves air spaces in the centre of lobules. This whole left lung section shows patchy centrilobular emphysema.

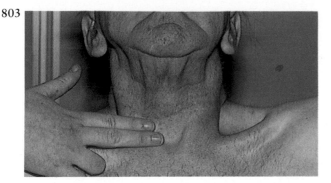

803 **Tracheal tug.** Inspiratory shortening of the distance between the thyroid cartilage and the suprasternal notch is attributed to contraction of a low flat diaphragm. The distance between the cricothyroid cartilage and the suprasternal notch measures the length of the trachea outside the thorax and is normally at least three finger widths in vertical distance.

Type A or pink puffer (802–805)
The picture of preserved respiratory drive. Individuals tend to show the following features:

- Severe dyspnoea with purse-lip breathing.
- Thin and often elderly.
- Heart failure uncommon.
- Near normal blood gases.
- Very severe airways obstruction.
- Reduced transfer factor.
- Raised total lung capacity.
- Radiological evidence of emphysema.

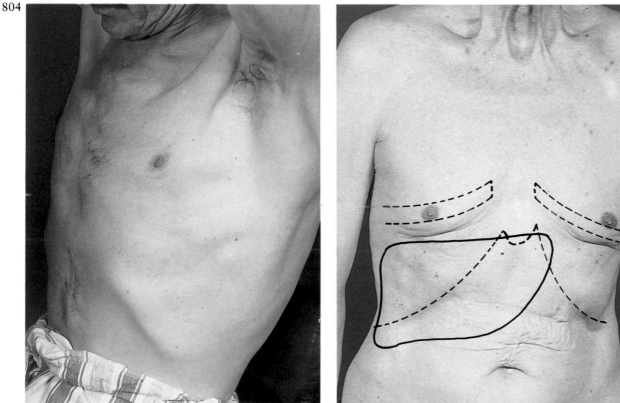

804 **Indrawing of the intercostal spaces** is another sign of hyperinflation of the chest.

805 **Emphysema.** The liver is displaced downwards so that the lower edge is palpable. The upper border of the liver is normally at the level of the fifth rib.

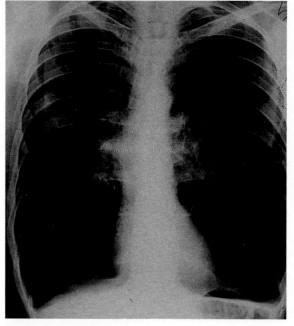 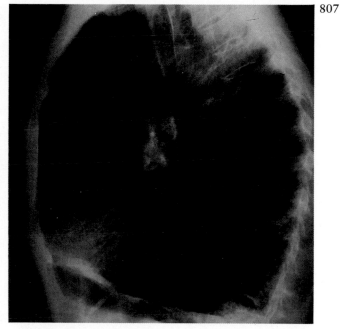

806 Emphysema. The posteroanterior radiograph shows hyperinflation, with low flat diaphragms at the level of the eleventh rib and oligaemia caused by loss of the pulmonary vessels.

807 Emphysema. The lateral radiograph shows an increased retrosternal air space and deep postero-anterior diameter. The heart is of normal size.

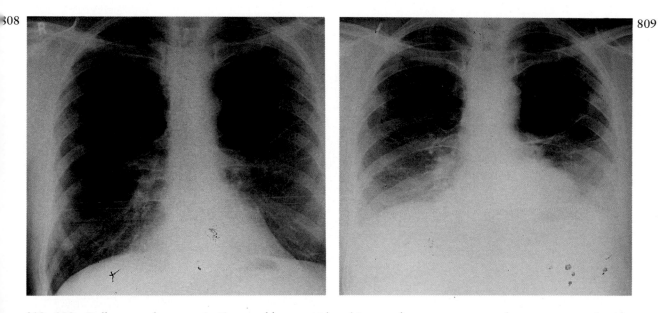

808, 809 Bullous emphysema. A 48-year-old man with a history of recurrent pneumothoraces presented with moderately severe exertional dyspnoea. Posteroanterior chest radiographs on inspiration (808) and expiration (809) show hypertransradiant upper zones with bilateral large bullae.

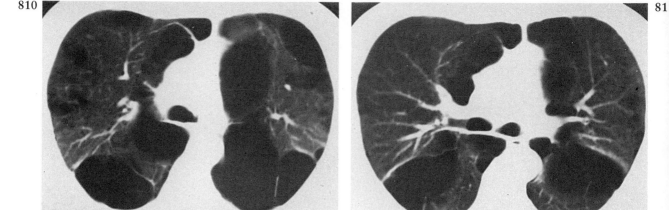

810, 811   Bullous emphysema, same patient as shown in 808, 809. CT scans remove the overlap of the superimposed walls of bullae seen on standard chest radiographs to give a clear picture of the number, position and size of the bullae (**810** at level of mid trachea, **811** at level of carina).

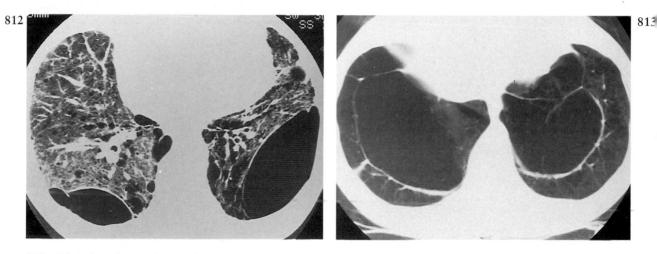

812 Chronic obstructive pulmonary disease. CT scanning accurately demonstrated the ovoid bullae lying posteriorly. These were not visible on the posteroanterior radiograph, although they could be seen on the lateral film. Small paramediastinal bullae are present. These cannot be identified on the standard chest radiograph and are a common finding on CT.

813 Bullous emphysema. By removing the overlap of the superimposed walls of bullae, which results in inaccurate interpretation from the radiograph, CT scanning gives a clear picture of the number, position and size of the bullae. This may be of importance where operative removal is contemplated.

Alpha 1 protease inhibitor deficiency (Alpha 1 P1) (Alpha 1 antitrypsin deficiency)

This inherited metabolic deficit is associated with basal pulmonary emphysema in adults, and with neonatal hepatitis and cirrhosis in children. Alpha 1 P1, a polymorphic glycoprotein synthesised in the liver, is responsible for most antiprotease activity in the serum and is the principal antiprotease inhibiting neutrophil elastase in the lung.

The inheritance is autosomal codominant and the major alleles are designated M, S and Z. The rare homozygous ZZ state is associated with severe emphysema in early middle life (**Table 48, 815**).

The Z gene occurs more frequently in Scandinavia than in Southern Europe and is absent from Black and Asian populations. The incidence is about 1 in 1,000 in Sweden and 1 in 3,000 in the UK. Replacement therapy for alpha 1 P1 deficiency is potentially available, either with frequent normal plasma transfusions or a recently developed genetic recombinant DNA form of alpha 1 protease. Treatment of established emphysema is limited. Lung transplantation may be life saving.

Table 48. Alpha 1 phenotypes.

Phenotype	MM	MS	MZ	SZ	ZZ
P1 activity (%)	100	85	60	45	<20
Frequency (%)	85	9.0	3.0	0.2	0.1

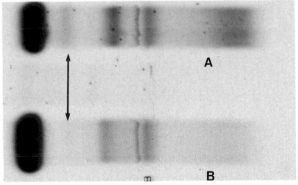

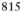

814 Alpha 1 P1 deficiency. Serum protein electrophoretic strip abnormality in the alpha 1 globulin region due to alpha 1 P1 deficiency (arrowed). The basic defect is a failure of cellular transport from the hepatocyte to the blood. (A = normal, B = alpha 1 P1 deficiency.)

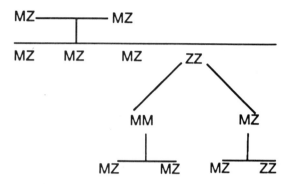

815 Alpha 1 P1 inheritance from union of two MZ carriers.

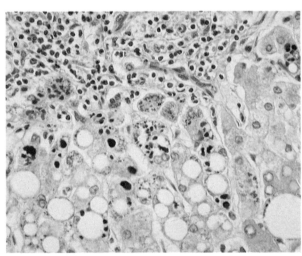

816 Alpha 1 antiprotease deficiency. A liver biopsy of a patient with alpha 1 P1 deficiency (homozygous type ZZ) shows brightly staining diastase-resistant inclusions concentrated around the portal tracts. Release into the circulation is defective and the red granular inclusions represent accumulated alpha 1 antiprotease in the liver. (Stained with periodic acid-Schiff after diastase digestion.)

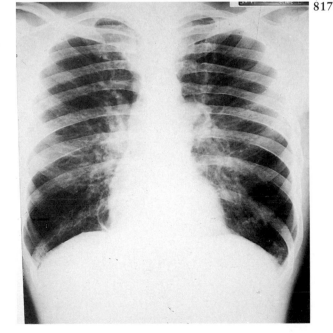

817 Alpha 1 antiprotease deficiency. Chest x-ray showing severe, predominantly basal, emphysema and enlarged pulmonary arteries in a 37-year-old man. Death from cor pulmonale occurred soon afterwards. Homozygous type ZZ alpha 1 P1 deficiency is associated with early death from emphysema, especially in cigarette smokers.

25 Pulmonary vascular disease

Pulmonary thromboembolic disease

The term 'thromboembolism' implies clinically significant obstruction of a part or the whole of the pulmonary arterial system. This is usually a result of a thrombus that becomes detached from its extra-pulmonary site of formation in the venous system to be swept into the pulmonary circulation. Thrombo-embolism often follows deep vein thrombosis of the thigh and leg veins or of the pelvic veins. Less commonly, thrombi may embolise from axillary and arm veins or from the right heart cavities.

Pulmonary embolism is preceded by venous thrombosis; the factors predisposing to both conditions are similar and fit Virchow's triad of venous stasis, injury to the vessel walls and enhanced coagulability of the blood. The contributing factors include: bedrest and immobility; surgery, trauma and burns; previous venous thrombosis and cardiac disease; obesity and paralytic disorders; malignant disease, treatment with the contraceptive pill and antithrombin III deficiency. The single most important diagnostic factor is the awareness of the possibility of embolism in these high risk groups (**Table 49**) as the various tests tend to be non-specific (**Table 50**).

Uncommon non-thrombotic embolism may be caused by air, fat, malignant cells, amniotic fluid, parasites and foreign material.

Table 49. Clinical features of pulmonary thromboembolism.

Type	Symptoms	Signs	Remarks
Silent	Asymptomatic		Probably more frequent than is realised
Acute minor (without infarction)	Dyspnoea Anxiety	Tachycardia Hypoxia	Usually transient
Acute minor (with infarction)	Dyspnoea Anxiety Pleurisy Haemoptysis	Tachycardia Hypoxia Pleural friction rub Fever Bronchospasm Consolidation Effusion	If you wait for these features you will miss perhaps 60% of patients with embolism
Acute massive (haemodynamic impairment)	Syncope Angina Pleurisy Severe dyspnoea	Tachycardia (sinus) Gallop rhythm Cyanosis Raised venous pressure Hypotension/low cardiac output Loud split P2 Consolidation Effusion Pleural friction rub	This means obstruction of 50% or more of pulmonary vascular bed

Table 50. Value of tests for thromboembolism.

Test	Abnormal features	Remarks
Chest x-ray	Elevated diaphragm Wedge-shaped peripheral opacity Oligaemia (Westermarks' sign) Atelectasis Dilated azygous vein Serosanguineous pleural effusions	It may be normal after acute minor embolism or immediately following massive pulmonary embolism
Electrocardiogram	Sinus tachycardia S1, Q3, T3, P. pulmonale Right axis deviation Incomplete RBBB T wave inversion Arrhythmias	Chest x-ray and electrocardiogram should be routine ECG changes common but seldom specific
Ventilation/perfusion V/Q scintography	Abnormal lung perfusion 'Hot' and 'cold' spots	Unfortunately non-specific. A normal perfusion scan with a normal chest x-ray rules out pulmonary embolism. False positives with tumours, consolidation and COPD. Don't do it if chest x-ray abnormal.
Echocardiography	Thrombus right atrium Dilated right ventricle	Non-invasive. Limited usefulness.
Pulmonary arteriogram	Intravascular filling defect or vessel 'cut-off'	Reliable but unfortunately an invasive technique associated with definite mortality
Leucocyte count	Under 15,000	If over 15,000 consider bacterial sepsis
Isoenzyme pattern	Normal	Only helpful in distinguishing embolism from myocardial infarction
Arterial oxygen tension	Decreased	Non-specific
Alveolar–arterial oxygen tension difference	Increased difference	Even more sensitive but still non-specific

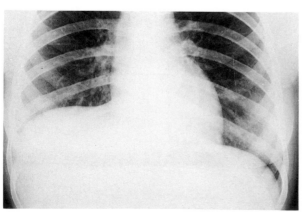

818 **Acute minor pulmonary embolism** in a 23-year-old woman using the contraceptive pill. The abrupt onset of right-sided pleuritic chest pain and severe dyspnoea led to an x-ray showing slight elevation of the right diaphragm, with a small pleural reaction. Three recent episodes of breathlessness and hyperventilation had been incorrectly attributed to anxiety when chest x-rays had appeared normal. The radiographic evolution is shown in **821** and **822**.

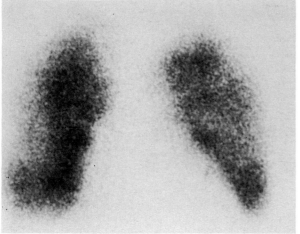

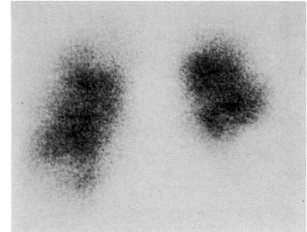

819 Acute minor pulmonary embolism. Technetium 99m (^{99}Tc) labelled albumen microsphere perfusion scan. A wedge-shaped perfusion defect is evident in the right lower lobe and there are extensive perfusion defects in the radiographically normal left lower lobe.

820 Acute minor pulmonary embolism. Krypton 81m ventilation scan. The radioactive emission is evenly distributed throughout both lung fields. The perfusion scan defects do not match with the ventilation scan and are typical of multiple pulmonary embolism.

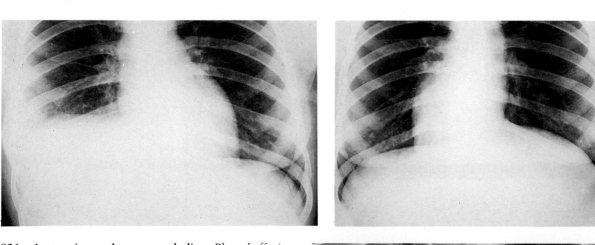

821 Acute minor pulmonary embolism. Pleural effusion formed by the sixth day. Pulmonary infarction is common when minor pulmonary arteries are occluded. Such an event is not associated with a significant circulatory disturbance.

822 Acute minor pulmonary embolism. The x-ray (822) and isotope perfusion scan (Technetium 99m) were normal after six weeks' therapy with anticoagulants.

823 Acute massive pulmonary embolism. The pulmonary angiogram shows multiple bilateral filling defects due to a recent embolism. There is good filling of the right upper and left lower lobe vessels only. The remaining vessels show varying degrees of embolic occlusion. A repeat angiogram two months later showed normal perfusion.

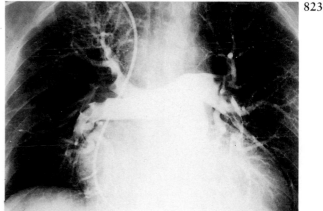

824

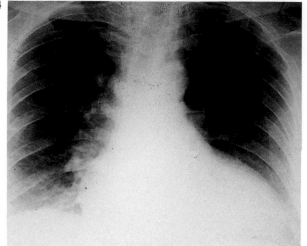

824 Acute massive pulmonary embolism. Chest x-ray. The heart is large and the lung fields, especially in the left mid and upper zones, are oligaemic.

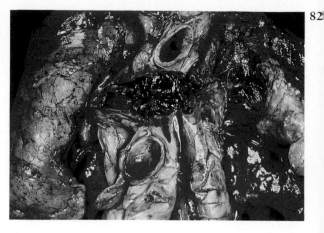

825 Acute massive pulmonary embolism. Postmortem demonstration of a fatal pulmonary embolism straddling the main pulmonary artery and occluding its major branches eight days after hysterectomy. Necropsy shows a granular laminated antemortem clot which had arisen from the pelvic veins. A smooth shiny postmortem clot is present. The coiled thrombi, extracted at necropsy from the pulmonary artery, corresponded in calibre to the leg veins from which they arose.

826

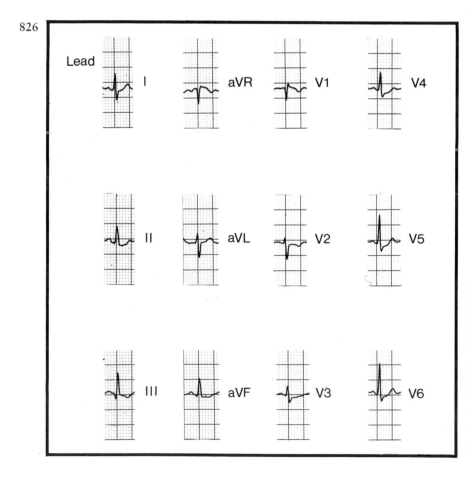

826 Acute massive pulmonary embolism. The classic changes are tachycardia, right axis shift, the appearance of an S wave in lead I and Q wave in lead III, T wave inversion in lead III and over the right ventricle and incomplete right bundle branch block. This case shows classic features with tachycardia, T wave changes in lead III and the precordial leads and a deep S wave in lead I. ECG changes are not invariable and are often non-specific.

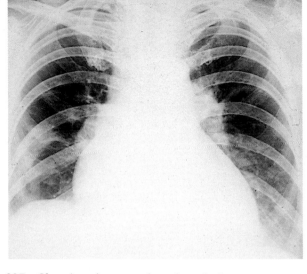

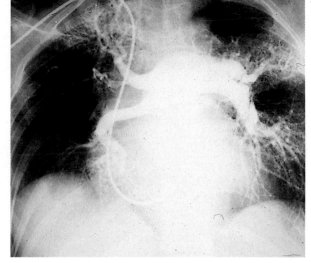

827 Chronic pulmonary thromboembolism. Prominent pulmonary arteries, patchy reduction in mid-lung and peripheral vessels and huge cardiac silhouette due to pulmonary hypertension. This 45-year-old man, a chronic respiratory invalid, had experienced an insidious onset of dyspnoea attributed to recurrent pulmonary emboli. Right heart catheter studies showed a right ventricular pressure of 88/6 and pulmonary artery pressure of 88/30.

828 Chronic pulmonary thromboembolism. Pulmonary angiogram. Perfusion to the right middle and lower lobes and left upper lobes is obstructed. The left proximal pulmonary artery is dilated secondary to pulmonary hypertension.

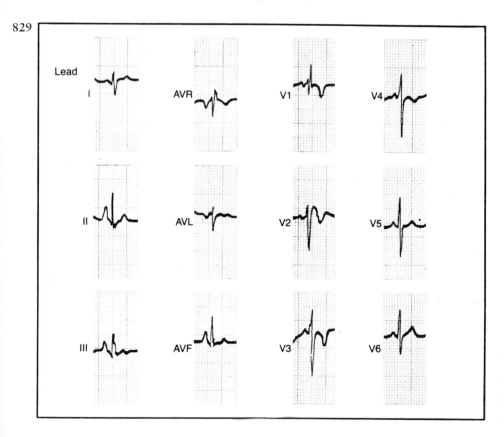

829 Pulmonary hypertension. The electrocardiogram of the patient in 827 shows a right axis shift, the appearance of an S wave in lead I, and changes due to right ventricular strain with ST depression and T wave inversion in V1–V4. P. pulmonale is also present.

Pulmonary hypertension

Pulmonary hypertension is a common sequel to a number of cardiopulmonary diseases (**Table 51**). The clinical features reflect both the underlying cause and the physiological changes in the pulmonary circulation, which result in a low cardiac output or an inability to increase cardiac output during exercise. Breathlessness on exercise is invariable. Other symptoms include syncope, angina, cough and haemoptysis. Commonly observed physical signs include a loud pulmonary component to the second heart sound (P2), a parasternal heave from right ventricular hypertrophy and an abnormal jugular venous pulse with prominent presystolic 'a' wave due to the increased force of right atrial contraction, or 'v' wave in the presence of tricuspid incompetence. The physical signs are due to a progression from pulmonary hypertension to right ventricular hypertrophy, leading eventually to right heart failure.

Table 51. Causes of pulmonary hypertension.

Increased vascular resistance	*Hypoxic*
	Chronic airflow obstruction
	Restrictive lung disease
	High altitude (Monge's disease)
	Hypoventilation syndrome
	Obstructive
	Primary pulmonary hypertension
	Drugs
	Collagen vascular disorders
	Thromboembolism
	Tumour emboli
	Parasites, schistosomiasis
	Veno-occlusive disease
Increased left atrial pressure	Mitral valve disease
	Left ventricular failure
Increased pulmonary flow	Atrial/ventricular septal defect
	Patent ductus arteriosus

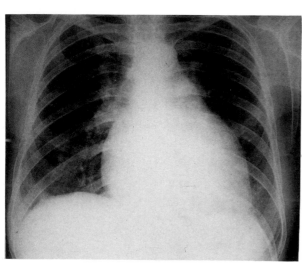

830 **Chronic hypoxic pulmonary hypertension.** Chest x-ray of a 67-year-old man with long-standing severe COPD. There was massive cardiomegaly, dilatation of proximal pulmonary vessels and reduction in vascularity in the left lung.

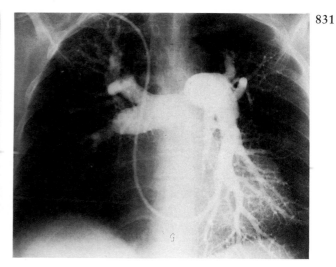

831 **Chronic hypoxic pulmonary hypertension.** Pulmonary angiogram showing proximal pulmonary artery enlargement. There are no discrete filling defects, but most of the vessels taper quickly and the peripheral vessels are attenuated, except those in the left lower lobe. The condition was due to severe COPD and previous thromboembolism.

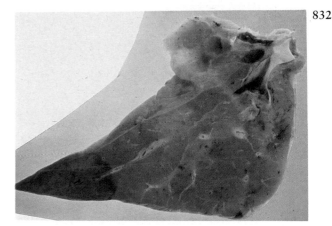

832 Peripheral pulmonary infarction. Postmortem specimen with peripheral wedge-shaped pulmonary infarct and thromboembolism occluding the feeding pulmonary artery. The symptoms included severe pleuritic pain that impeded breathing. Minor pulmonary embolism does not compromise the right ventricle.

Non-thrombotic pulmonary embolism

A wide variety of substances can embolise to the lungs, some of which produce a characteristic clinical picture.

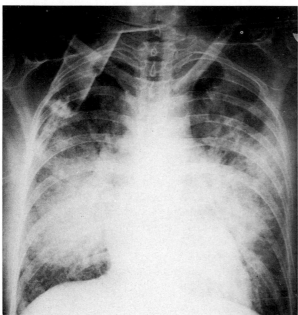

833 Fat embolism. Major trauma, usually to the long bones of the legs and pelvis, may force fat and marrow tissue into the blood. Most of the embolic material impacts in the pulmonary circulation, but the fat droplets may pass through the lungs to embolise systemically. This woman fractured the neck of her femur in a road traffic accident; 48 hours later she was confused, cyanosed and had developed a petechial skin rash. The x-ray shows a pattern simulating pulmonary oedema. Fat droplets were present in the sputum and urine. This condition may also result from a jockey's riding injury.

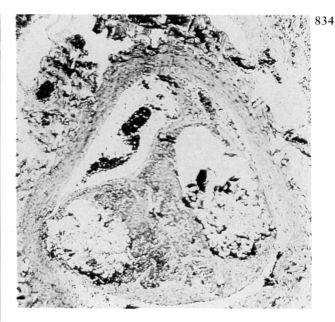

834 Cotton fibre emboli lying in a small pulmonary artery. A granulomatous foreign body reaction is stimulated, resulting in damage to the vessel wall and the ultimate extension of the lesion into the perivascular tissues. Schistosome eggs are similarly extruded through pulmonary vessel walls.

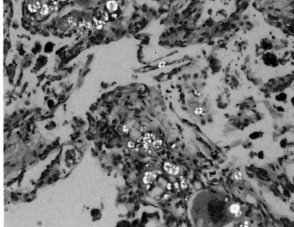

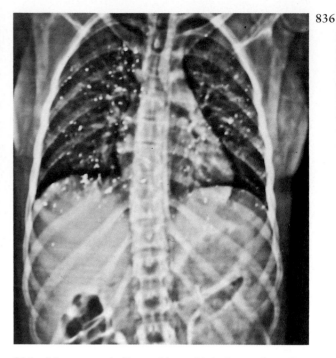

835 Talc emboli in a drug addict's lung. Lung biopsy showing a foreign body granuloma and birefringent particles under polarising light. The high price and scarcity of illicit drugs leads to their adulteration with inert 'fillers' of starch, lactulose or talc, which can cause a granulomatous reaction and pulmonary hypertension. An incidental finding was emphysema due to alpha 1 P1 deficiency. (Polarised light, H & E × 140.)

836 Mercury embolism with multiple intensely radio-opaque opacities shown in preliminary CT scan. This disturbed patient presented with a factitious fever and during a hospital admission self-administered mercury obtained from three thermometers by injecting it through an indwelling venous cannula.

Pulmonary arteriovenous malformations (AVM)

Pulmonary arteriovenous fistula
This abnormality is caused by the persistence of foetal capillary anastomosis between the pulmonary arteries and veins. In about one-fifth of cases the lesions are multiple and similar lesions may develop in other organs. About half are associated with hereditary haemorrhagic telangiectasia (Rendu–Osler–Weber syndrome). Not all patients experience symptoms, but in those that do, dyspnoea, cyanosis, polycythaemia, facial telangiectasia, gastrointestinal or pulmonary bleeding and finger clubbing are features. Major right-to-left shunts of deoxygenated blood may occur. Occasionally, other complications common to any right-to-left shunt develop; these include paradoxical embolism and an increased risk of cerebral abscesses.

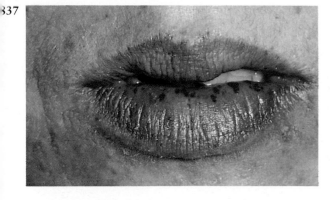

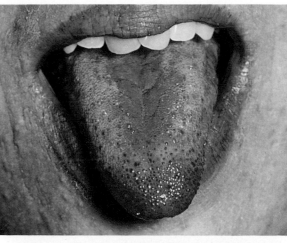

837–839 Pulmonary arteriovenous fistula. Telangiectasia of the lips, tongue and fingers is a helpful clue. A florid example of hereditary haemorrhagic telangiectasia (Rendu–Osler–Weber disease).

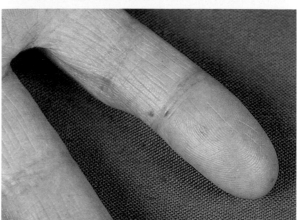

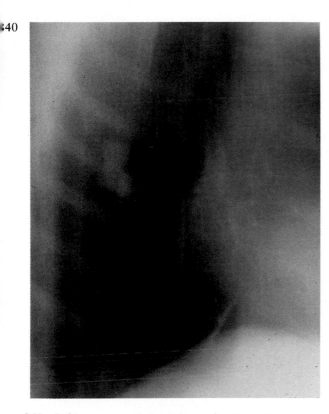

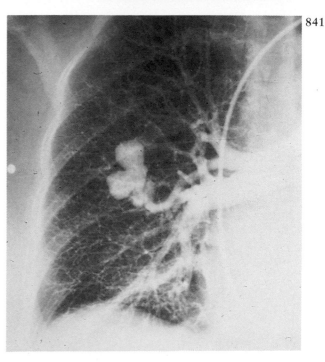

840 Pulmonary arteriovenous fistula. Tomogram showing a lobulated opacity in a patient presenting with haemoptysis.

841 Pulmonary artery angiogram showing an AVM in a patient with hereditary haemorrhagic telangiectasia. The vascular abnormalities are often multiple and most likely to occur in the lower lobes.

Anomalous pulmonary venous drainage (scimitar syndrome)
This congenital abnormality of the right lung's pulmonary venous system may be partial or total, with direct venous drainage to the superior or inferior vena cava, hepatic vein or the right atrium.

A common form is a large vein running vertically in the right lung, gathering tributaries and passing downwards through the diaphragm at the right cardiophrenic angle to the inferior vena cava. Because of its shape it is known as the scimitar syndrome and is frequently associated with hypoplasia of the right lung.

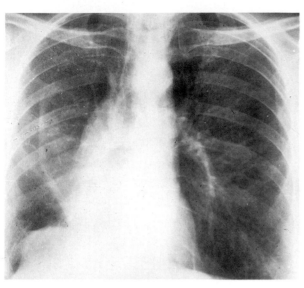 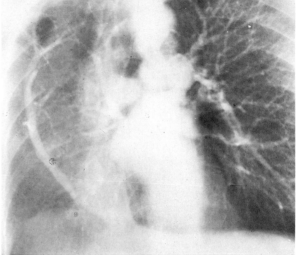

842 **The anomalous vein** is seen as a 'scimitar-like' shadow adjacent to the heart border. Hypoplasia of the right lung is also present.

843 **Angiogram showing drainage into the vena cava.** A significant left-to-right shunt may occur.

Pulmonary atresia

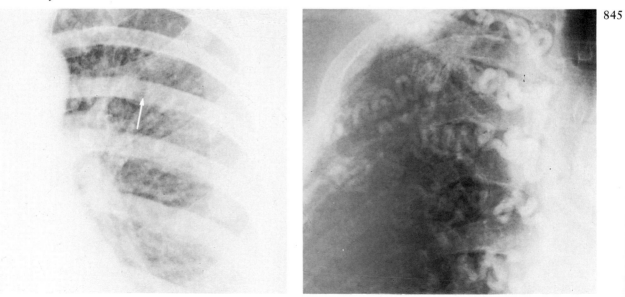

844, 845 **Pulmonary atresia.** The posteroanterior film shows notching of the ribs (arrowed) (**844**). The aortic angiogram shows tortuous and dilated intercostal arteries (**845**). Rib notching can also occur in coarctation of the aorta.

Pulmonary sequestration

Sequestration is the term used to describe developmental pulmonary abnormalities that result in malformations of the lung and pulmonary vasculature. Various defects are described, but the common feature is a disconnection or abnormal communication with a bronchopulmonary mass, accompanied by normal or anomalous arterial supply and venous drainage.

Sequestrations may be intrapulmonary and lie within the boundary formed by the visceral pleura, or extrapulmonary and lie outside the visceral pleura.

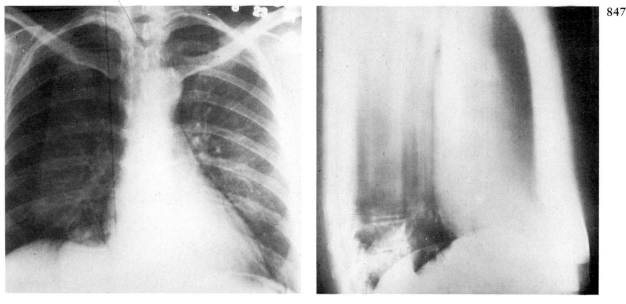

846   **847**

846, 847 Intrapulmonary sequestration commonly lies in the posterior segment of the lower lobes (60%) and accounts for 90% of sequestrations. The aberrant systemic arterial blood supply arises from the lower thoracic or upper abdominal aorta in most cases. Communication with normal proximal airways is usually absent, but air and infection may enter through pores of Kohn. Symptoms include cough, chronic suppuration and haemoptysis.

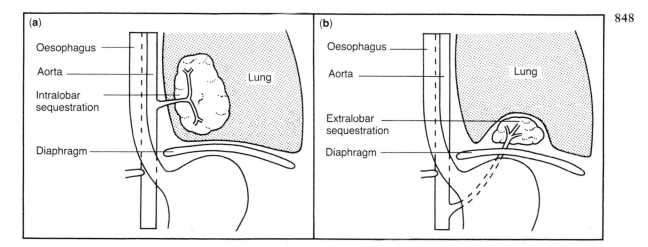

848

848   Diagrams of (a) intrapulmonary and (b) extrapulmonary sequestration.

303

849

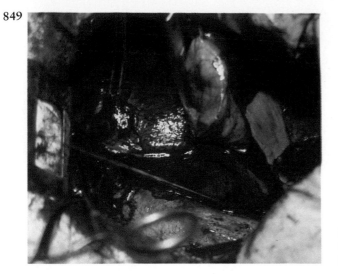

849 Resected pulmonary sequestration. The large feeding vessels arose directly from the thoracic aorta and were the source of a significant arteriovenous shunt.

26 Respiratory failure and adult respiratory distress syndrome

Oxygen is needed continuously for metabolic function of the mitochrondria and its delivery depends upon alveolar ventilation, alveolar perfusion and the oxygen-carrying ability of the circulation. Respiratory failure is a defect in pulmonary gas exchange, leading to hypoxaemia with or without hypercapnia.

The arbitrary limits defining this failure are an arterial oxygen tension (PaO_2) of less than 60 mmHg (8 kPa) and an arterial carbon dioxide tension ($PaCO_2$) of more than 50 mmHg (6.7 kPa), the patient being at rest and breathing air at sea level. This level of PaO_2 lies at the critical point on the oxygen dissociation curve, below which small reductions in PaO_2 are associated with large falls in blood oxygen content and percentage haemoglobin saturation (SaO_2).

Respiratory failure may result from chemoreceptor or medullary respiratory centre depression, mechanical disorders limiting ribcage movement, physiological shunting with mismatch of ventilation and perfusion, or anatomical shunting of blood through congenital cardiac defects. As in heart failure, respiratory failure often commences with exertional dyspnoea, followed later by dyspnoea at rest. The onset may be acute as, for example, in opiate overdose, or chronic with permanent blood gas disturbance, as in severe COPD. Failure, both acute and chronic, can be divided into two main groups according to the arterial $PaCO_2$ level:

Type I Hypoxaemia without hypercapnia
>   Cardiogenic pulmonary oedema
>   Adult respiratory distress syndrome
>   Acute pneumonia
>   Pulmonary thromboembolism
>   Severe bronchial asthma
>   R–L shunts in congenital cardiac disease
>   R–L shunts in pulmonary arteriovenous malformation

Type II Hypoxaemia with hypercapnia
>   Primary alveolar hypoventilation
>   Chronic airflow obstruction
>   Respiratory sedative drugs
>   Ribcage trauma
>   Cerebrovascular disease – stroke, space-occupying lesion
>   High spinal cord lesion or polyneuritis
>   Myopathies

O₂ dissociation curve

O_2 forms an easily reversible combination with haemoglobin (Hb). The saturation of arterial blood with a PaO_2 of 100 mmHg is about 97.5%, whereas that of mixed venous blood with a PaO_2 of 40 mmHg is about 75%. Cyanosis is clinically apparent with a saturation of less than 85%.

The curved shape of the O_2 dissociation curve is advantageous (**850**). The flat top end of the curve tends to stabilise the quantity of oxygen in the arterial blood, while the steep middle part of the curve ensures that a large proportion of the oxygen that is carried by the blood is delivered to the tissues at a relatively high tension. The position of the O_2 dissociation curve is influenced by pH, $PaCO_2$ and temperature; acidosis and fever increase the oxygen uptake in the tissues.

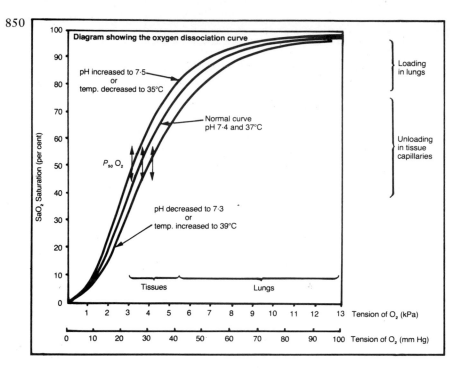

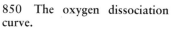

850 The oxygen dissociation curve.

Adult respiratory distress syndrome

The adult respiratory distress syndrome (ARDS) is caused by acute lung injury and is an important form of acute respiratory failure. There are many causes (**Table 52**), all of which result in increased permeability of the alveolar capillary membrane.

The syndrome is best recognised in patients who have suffered an acute, often multisystem, illness. Characteristically, there is a short latent period of 12–24 hours between the primary event and the onset of dyspnoea, tachypnoea and a low arterial oxygen tension (PaO_2 <50mmHg) in spite of high inspired oxygen concentrations (FiO_2 >60%). The chest x-ray shows diffuse patchy shadows, with sparing of the lung bases.

The diagnostic criteria include refractory hypoxaemia, bilateral pulmonary infiltrates suggestive of oedema and normal capillary wedge, and plasma oncotic pressures. In defining ARDS it is important to exclude primary left ventricular failure and most forms of chronic lung disease.

Regardless of the mechanism of lung injury, noncardiogenic pulmonary oedema develops secondary to an increase in the permeability of the alveolar capillary endothelium. Pneumocytes are damaged and surfactant synthesis reduced. The total respiratory compliance falls and the inspiratory pressures required to inflate the stiff lungs are high. There are many similarities between ARDS and hyaline membrane disease of the newborn.

The average mortality among patients with ARDS is 50–60%. Those who recover seldom suffer significant impairment of lung function, although up to 20% may show a mild restrictive defect.

Table 52. Clinical conditions associated with the adult respiratory distress syndrome.

Respiratory	Non-respiratory
Pneumonia – viral – bacterial – fungal – *Pneumocystis carinii*	Massive haemorrhage or multiple transfusions
	Disseminated intravascular coagulation
Aspiration – gastric contents – drowning	Major trauma/burns
	Pre-eclampsia
Inhalation of toxic fumes	Amniotic fluid embolism
	Sepsis from any cause – Gram-negative – staphylococcal
Trauma – lung contusion – fat emboli	
	Drug overdose
Oxygen toxicity	
Drug-induced – Bleomycin/paraquat	

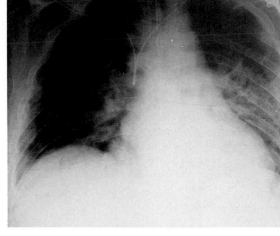

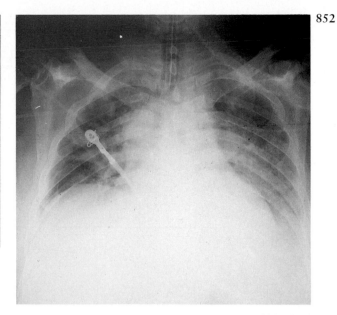

851   Adult respiratory distress syndrome – first day. Acute cyanosis and dyspnoea 12 hours after aspiration of gastric contents during grand mal epileptic convulsion. Before ventilation the arterial PO_2 was 3.9 kPa. An endobronchial tube, misplaced subclavian line and dense left alveolar infiltrate are present.

852   Adult respiratory distress syndrome – fifth day. Same patient as shown in **851**. More extensive and bilateral alveolar infiltrate. Inspired O_2 tension of 60% (FiO_2) was necessary to maintain an arterial PO_2 of 9 kPa. Death finally resulted from infection.

Abnormal breathing during sleep (sleep apnoea syndrome)

Irregularity of breathing and occasional short episodes of apnoea occur in normal subjects, particularly during rapid eye movement (REM) sleep.

Abnormal breathing during sleep is common, may affect 3–10% of the population and can lead to periods of profound oxygen desaturation. Sleep apnoea is a cessation of breathing during sleep, which is usually repetitive and lasts for more than 10 seconds. The sleep apnoea or sleep hyperpnoea syndromes are characterised by night-time restlessness, snoring and nocturnal choking attacks, fatigue and headache on awakening and daytime somnolence. In time, this may cause daytime hypoxaemia, leading eventually to respiratory failure, polycythaemia and pulmonary hypertension (**853**).

There are essentially two types of disorder:
1   Obstructive sleep apnoea. Cessation of airflow in spite of continued respiratory effort (**Table 53**).
2   Central (non-obstructive) sleep apnoea. Cessation of airflow and respiratory effort.

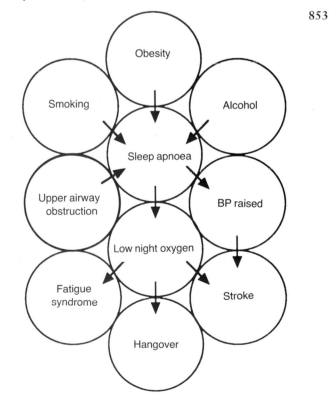

853   Factors associated with obstructive sleep apnoea.

Table 53. Factors predisposing to obstructive sleep apnoea.

Upper airway obstruction	Large tonsils
	Obesity
	Acromegaly
	Micrognathia
	Superior vena cava (SVC) obstruction
	Upper airway/pharyngeal tumour
	Hypothyroidism
Nasal airway obstruction	Nasal trauma
	Septal deviation
	Polyps/adenoids
Decreased upper airway muscle tone	Alcohol
	Night sedation

854

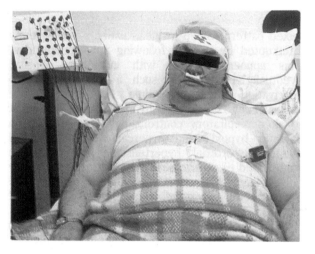

855

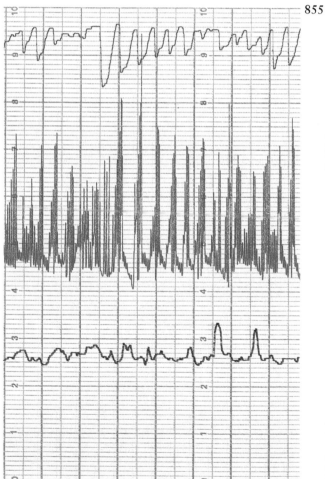

854 Sleep apnoea syndrome. Polysomnography study in patient suffering from sleep apnoea syndrome due to morbid centripetal obesity. This sleep study showed profound nocturnal hypoxaemia with frequent obstructive episodes. Sleep apnoea is conventionally defined as episodes of complete cessation of airflow for at least 10 seconds, with at least 40 episodes in a night of 7 hours sleep.

855 Sleep apnoea syndrome. Polysomnography trace with continuous measurement of oxygen saturation (SiO_2) (red line), chest and abdominal wall movement by impedance plethysmography (blue line) and heart rate (black line). The EEG trace (not shown) identifies periods of REM (rapid eye movement) sleep, and thermistors measure airflow at the mouth and nose. Note the repeated falls in SiO_2 accompanied by increased heart rate and chest wall movement.

Treatment depends upon the severity and type of sleep apnoea. Weight loss, avoidance of drugs that depress central ventilatory drive and protryptiline to alter REM sleep may help in mild cases. Continuous nasal positive airway pressure (CPAP), surgery to the nasopharynx or even tracheostomy may be considered for those more severely affected.

Lung function tests

Routine lung function testing is carried out to assess, in a simple and relatively non-invasive way, the performance of the lungs. The features measured are:

- The size of the lungs and compartments.
- The calibre of the airway.
- Diffusing capacity.
- Arterial blood gas tensions.

The most useful clinical information is obtained from the most easily performed tests, especially forced expiratory volumes and arterial blood gas tensions. Measurement of airway resistance and static lung volumes may complete this picture if more detail is required.

Simple bedside lung function tests

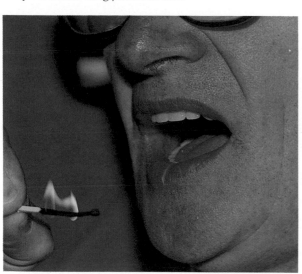

856 Bedside lung function tested with a lighted match. Airflow obstruction prevents the patient exhaling rapidly enough through the open mouth to extinguish the flame.

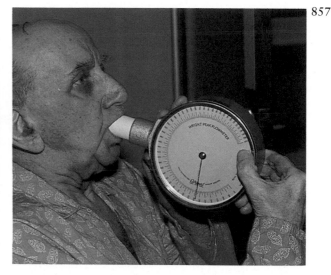

857 Bedside lung function measurement of peak expiratory flow (PEF). This is a convenient test for routine assessment. Flow is averaged over a 10 ms period coinciding with the peak maximum expiratory flow volume. In normal subjects the reading is effort dependent and reflects expiratory muscle force, the calibre of the airways and lung volume. The PEF is directly related to height and inversely to age. It is greater in men than in women.

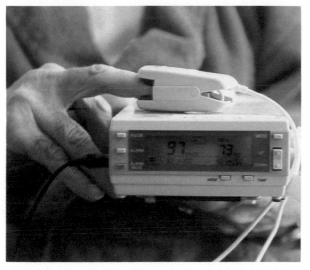

858 Pulse oximeter measuring oxygen saturation (SiO_2) using a finger sensing probe in a patient with COPD. Chronic hypoxaemia was corrected with oxygen at 2 litres per minute, delivered by nasal cannulae from an oxygen concentrator. This technique provides a simple non-invasive serial assessment of SiO_2.

Results for maximum expiratory flow–volume curves (MEFV)

These tests are based on a forced expiration from total lung capacity (TLC) to residual volume (RV). The MEFV curve is a graphic plot of flow rates achieved during inspiration and expiration, usually using maximum effort. The curve defines the maximum at any lung volume, and declines almost linearly as lung volume falls from TLC to RV.

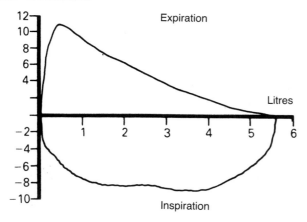

859 Litres/second

859 Maximum expiratory flow–volume curve in a normal subject. The curve peaks at the maximum expiratory flow rate and is then followed by the effort – independent part of the curve. The inspiratory curve is effort dependent.

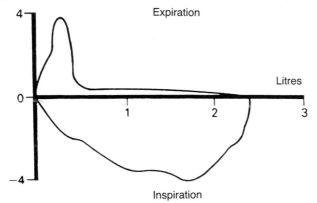

860 Litres/second

860 Maximum expiratory flow–volume curve in severe emphysema. A severe obstructive ventilatory defect with pressure-dependent airflow limitation. Inspiration is relatively easy and deep, but expiration is limited abruptly as soon as the pleural pressure rises. The early stages of airflow obstruction are characterised by preservation of the peak of the curve, but with a decrease in maximum flow at lower lung volumes giving a concave appearance to the curve. In more severe airflow obstruction this concavity is more marked.

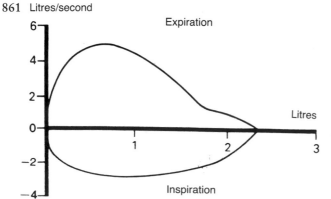

861 Litres/second

861 Flow volume curve showing a restrictive defect in fibrosing alveolitis. The lungs are stiff and less compliant, and airway patency is maintained during expiration. Thus, breathing out is easy and breathing in is difficult. In diffuse pulmonary fibrosis the normal shape of the curve is preserved but with reduced vital capacity and flow rates.

Results from the timed expiratory volume–time tests
The simple measurement of forced expiratory volume in one second (FEV_1) and forced vital capacity (FVC) gives valuable information. A forced delivery of air from maximum inspiration to maximum expiration (FVC) is mandatory and therefore patient cooperation is essential.

The results of spirometry can be compared with tabulated predicted values dependent upon age, sex and height.

Three broad categories of result may be obtained.

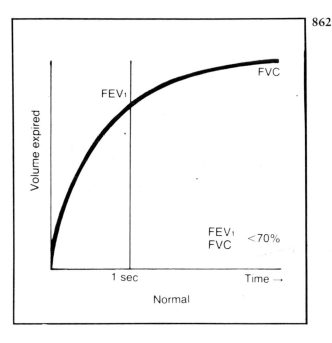

862 Normal spirogram. Values of FEV_1 and FVC at predicted level and FEV_1/FVC ratio 70%.

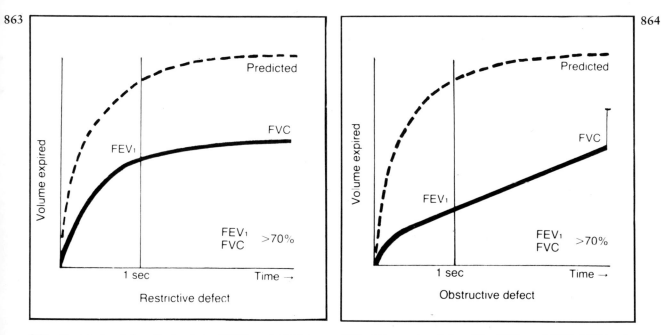

863 Restrictive defect. Reduction of FEV_1 and FVC, but preservation of a normal FEV_1/FVC ratio. Restrictive lung diseases may be divided into two groups: extrapulmonary restriction caused by chest wall rigidity, respiratory muscle weakness or pleural thickening; and intrapulmonary restriction caused by lung fibrosis.

864 Obstructive defect. The FEV_1 and FEV_1/FVC ratio are considerably reduced. The forced expiratory time required to reach FVC is prolonged. This picture is seen in chronic airflow limitation and bronchospasm.

27 Tumours of the lung

A wide range of tumours may arise in the lung. The commonly used term 'lung cancer' is used to describe a heterogeneous group of malignant epithelial tumours of the airways, which form about 95% of all types of lung tumour.

Table 54. World Health Organisation classification of epithelial tumours of the lung (1981).

A Benign

1 *Papillomas*
   Squamous cell papilloma
   'Traditional' papilloma

2 *Adenomas*
   Pleomorphic adenoma ('mixed tumour')
   Monomorphic adenoma
   Others

B Dysplasia/carcinoma *in situ*

C Malignant

1 *Squamous cell carcinoma*
      (epidermoid carcinoma) variant
   Spindle cell (squamoid) carcinoma

2 *Small cell carcinoma*
   Oat-cell carcinoma
   Intermediate cell type
   Combined oat-cell carcinoma

3 *Adenocarcinoma*
   Acinar adenocarcinoma
   Papillary adenocarcinoma
   Bronchio-alveolar carcinoma
   Solid carcinoma with mucus formation

4 *Large cell carcinoma variants*
   Giant cell carcinoma
   Clear cell carcinoma

5 *Adenosquamous carcinoma*

6 *Carcinoid tumour*

7 *Bronchial gland carcinomas*
   Adenoid cystic carcinomas
   Mucoepidermoid carcinoma
   Others

8 Others

865 Distribution of histological types of bronchial carcinoma.

Lung cancer

Lung cancer is the most common malignant disease in the Western world, accounting for 200,000 deaths per year in the USA and 35,000 deaths per year in Britain. The mortality rate from bronchial carcinoma has risen dramatically during the past 50 years: it is now the cause of death in 1 in 11 British males and is responsible for 40% of male cancer deaths. Men are affected more frequently than women, but the ratio of male to female lung cancer deaths has narrowed (2.5:1 in Britain in 1982) as more women have used tobacco. The average age of presentation is 70–74 years for men and 65 years for women.

Lung cancer can present with a variety of symptoms (**Table 55**); most patients who develop it have a history of heavy cigarette consumption and thus chronic bronchitic symptoms are common. Lung cancer symptoms may be classified as follows:
- Intrathoracic symptoms caused by the primary tumour.
- Intrathoracic symptoms caused by local metastases.
- Extrathoracic symptoms.
- Symptoms from non-metastatic (paramalignant) manifestations of lung cancer.

Table 55. Common symptoms associated with lung cancer.

Intrathoracic symptoms

Cough	Haemoptysis
Dyspnoea	Unilateral wheeze
Persistent chest infections	Chest pain
Hoarseness	Dysphagia

Extrathoracic symptoms

Pain (ribs, spine, pelvis)	Neurological lesions
Weight loss and malaise	(Cerebral metastases)
Abdominal discomfort	

Paramalignant symptoms

Ectopic hormone production	Hypercalcaemia
Peripheral neuropathy	Proximal myopathy
Clubbing of fingernails	Confusion
Hypertrophic pulmonary osteoarthropathy	

Aetiological factors in lung cancer

1 Tobacco

The single most important factor in the causation of lung cancer is cigarette consumption, the risk increasing with the duration of consumption and the number of cigarettes smoked. The risk of lung cancer in relation to cigarette smoking is summarised in **866**. Smokers of over 25 cigarettes per day show a risk of carcinoma of the bronchus over 25 times that of non-smokers.

If smokers of less than 20 cigarettes per day stop, the incidence of lung cancer declines, reaching the level of non-smokers after 13 years.

In smokers of more than 20 cigarettes per day there always appears to be a small increase in risk.

In non-smokers the predominant cell type is adenocarcinoma.

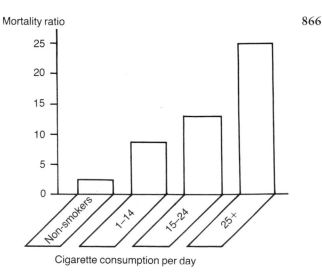

866 Relative risk of developing lung cancer for male smokers according to cigarette consumption.

Cigarette smokers occupationally exposed to asbestos show a dramatic 40-fold increased risk of lung cancer.

Passive smokers – those who involuntarily inhale side-stream smoke that is emitted into the environment while an active smoker pursues his or her habit – also have an increased risk of developing lung cancer.

2 Occupational
Certain occupations are associated with a higher than expected incidence of lung cancer (**Table 56**).

3 Air pollution
The reduction in air pollution due to smoke from domestic fires is claimed to have contributed to the decline in lung cancer deaths among younger people.

4 Diet
There is some evidence to support the hypothesis that the risk for certain cancers, including lung cancer, varies inversely with the consumption of vitamin A.

5 Genetics
The possibility for a genetic role in the development of lung cancer seems likely, but the mechanism remains uncertain.

Table 56. Known causes of occupational lung cancer.

Substance	Occupation
Asbestos	Mining, processing, usage
Arsenic (arsenic trioxide, arsenates, arsenites)	Copper, zinc, lead smelting Insecticides Chemical industry
Nickel dust/fumes	Refining ore
Chromium salts	Refining Chemical industry
Chloroethers (chloromethyl methyl ether, bis-chloromethyl ether)	Organic chemical industry
Coal carbonisation volatiles	Coking plants, gas workers, carbonisation of steel
Radioactivity (radon gas)	Metal ore mining (uranium, fluorspar)

Lung cancer – the growth of tumours
It is unusual to visualise a bronchial neoplasm that is less than 1 cm in size. The growth rate of individual tumours varies considerably, but it is possible to estimate broadly the rate of cell division or doubling (see **867**). If growth was exponential, a single malignant cell would become a 1 mm tumour mass after its volume had doubled 20 times and a 1 cm tumour mass after 30 doublings. If death were to occur when the primary tumour mass was 5 cm in diameter, the duration of life from the onset of growth would be 3.2 years for oat-cell carcinoma, 9.6 years for squamous cell carcinomas and more than 17 years for adenocarcinomas (**867**).

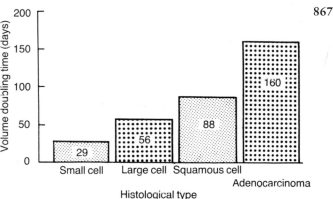

867

867 Lung cancer volume doubling times.

868 869 870 871

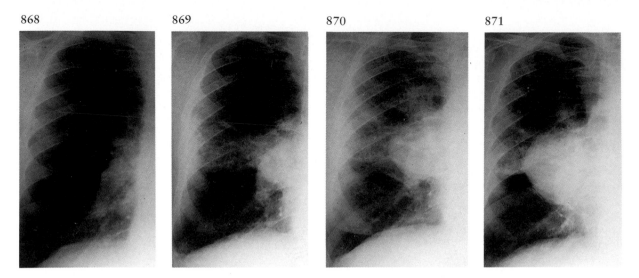

868–871 Growth of small cell carcinoma. A 55-year-old smoker with severe COAD had a routine chest x-ray (**868**) and six months later presented with haemoptysis and dyspnoea at rest. The second chest x-ray (**869**) showed a right hilar mass, and bronchial biopsy revealed small cell carcinoma. All treatment was declined. Repeat chest radiographs taken six (**870**) and ten weeks (**871**) after **869** show a rapidly enlarging mass at the right hilum.

872

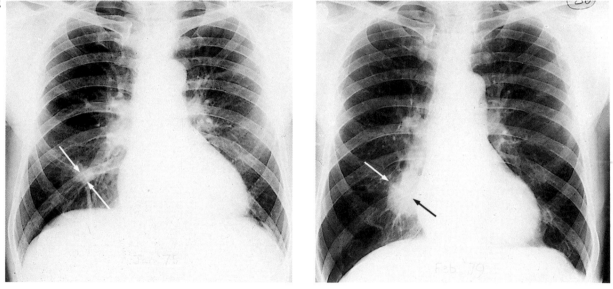

873

872, 873 Growth of squamous cell carcinoma. This elderly bronchitic was found to have dense circular opacity in the right lower lobe. Numerous sputum specimens revealed squamous cell carcinoma. Regular follow-up films demonstrated slow tumour growth, with an increase in diameter of only 2 cm between 1973 (**872**) and 1979 (**873**). Fatal cerebral metastases finally developed.

Lung cancer – clinical features and presentation

There are no early or specific symptoms of bronchial carcinoma, but cough, dyspnoea, haemoptysis, weight loss and chest pain are common presenting symptoms.

Intrathoracic symptoms caused by the primary tumour

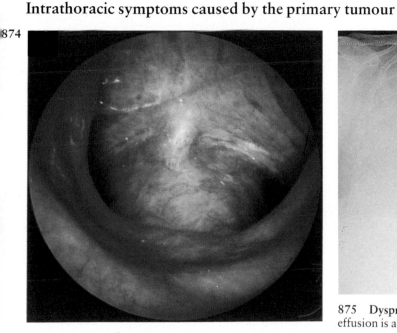

874 **Dyspnoea.** Bronchoscopy shows widened carina caused by enlarged mediastinal glands. Dyspnoea occurs in about 60% of patients. Occlusion of a major airway by a carcinoma causes a rapid onset of breathlessness, often accompanied by wheezing or stridor.

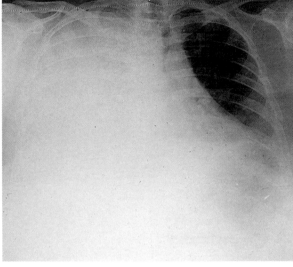

875 **Dyspnoea.** The development of a large pleural effusion is another cause of breathlessness.

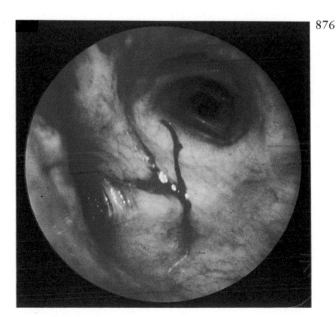

876 **Haemoptysis** is a presenting symptom in up to 50% of cases, due to ulceration of bronchial mucosa. Blood streaking of the sputum for several days in succession is common. Haemoptysis is seldom severe and massive haemoptysis at presentation is very rare. At fibreoptic bronchoscopy, blood is seen lying proximally in a large bronchus. Cough and shortness of breath may be attributed to smokers' bronchitis and ignored, but haemoptysis and chest pain are seldom neglected.

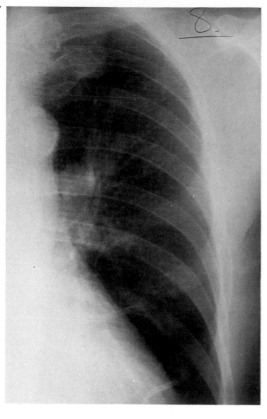

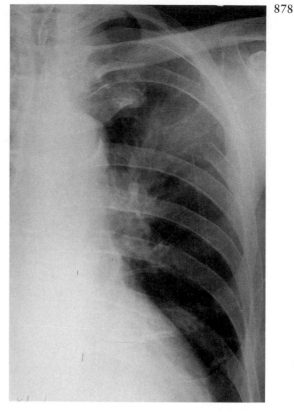

877 **Chest pain** is a presenting feature in one-third of patients and is frequently mild and poorly localised. This man presented with left pleuritic pain, but his initial x-ray was considered normal.

878 **Chest pain** (same patient as shown in 877). Four months later the left hilum is more prominent. The fourth left rib is eroded. The histology was squamous cell carcinoma.

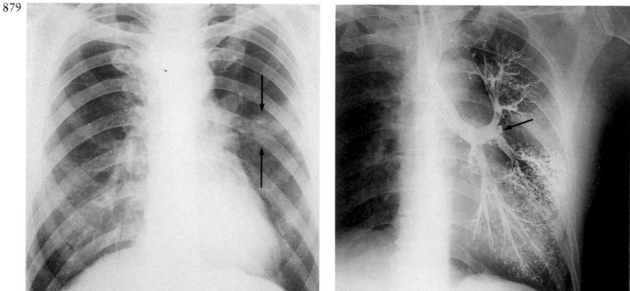

879 **Recurrent chest infections.** Patchy infiltration in the left mid-zone. The patient's symptoms were of left pleurisy and recurrent infections.

880 **Bronchogram** reveals a block corresponding with this shadow due to a bronchial neoplasm.

Intrathoracic metastatic manifestations

Spread of lung cancer to the hilar and mediastinal nodes may be followed by specific clinical features due to malignant invasion of adjacent intrathoracic structures.

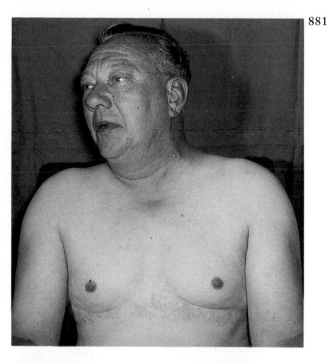

881 Superior vena cava obstruction (SVCO) in a 53-year-old man who presented with headaches, distended jugular veins, bloated face, swollen arms and dilated veins over the lower chest. The x-ray shows a large proximal tumour and bronchial biopsy confirmed squamous cell carcinoma.

SVCO may be caused by malignant glands compressing the superior vena cava (SVC) or by thrombosis when a tumour directly invades and damages the luminal surface of the SVC. It is almost always associated with metastatic spread into the right paratracheal lymph node chain and occurs in 4% of all presentations and 10% of small cell carcinomas. The patient may complain of dyspnoea, dysphagia, stridor caused by vocal cord oedema, blackouts and severe headache on coughing. The circulation is maintained by a well-developed collateral circulation with dilated veins across the lower chest. Periorbital oedema, facial and upper limb swelling may occur.

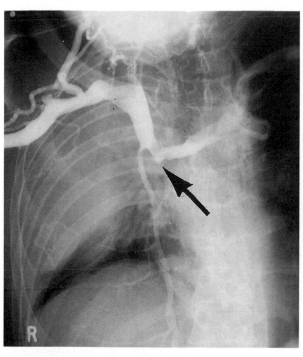

882 Superior vena cavogram. The early phase of this bilateral vena cavogram shows occlusion below the origin of the patent azygos vein (arrowed). Same patient as shown in **881**.

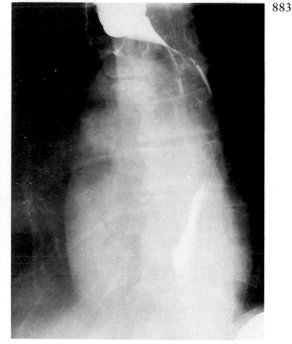

883 Dysphagia. Metastatic mediastinal lymph nodes may compress the oesophagus. This barium swallow shows considerable deviation of the oesophagus, caused by enlarged mediastinal glands. Dysphagia may result from extrinsic pressure upon the oesophagus from enlarged glands, or from stenosis by direct infiltration of tumour into the oesophagus.

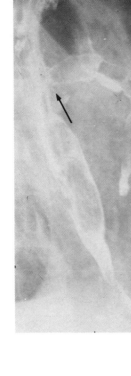

884 Tracheo-oesophageal fistula. This oat-cell carcinoma invaded the oesophagus which then perforated during a course of palliative radiotherapy. (75% of bronchial carcinomas arise centrally so they are often inoperable.) Note the fistula (arrowed) and the right main bronchus outlined by barium.

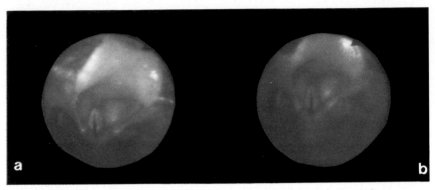

885 Dysphonia. Hoarseness secondary to entrapment of the left recurrent laryngeal nerve as it loops under the arch of the aorta is a presenting symptom in up to 18% of patients. It causes a weak 'bovine' cough and predisposes to aspiration pneumonia. This example shows bilateral cord paralysis due to mediastinal and thoracic inlet malignant disease infiltrating both recurrent laryngeal nerves (a – inspiration, b – expiration).

Extrathoracic metastatic manifestations

About one-third of patients present with symptoms due to metastases.

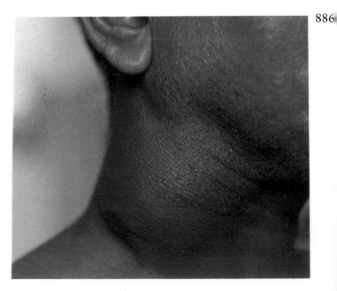

886 Lymphadenopathy. Large cervical lymph nodes. Supraclavicular and cervical lymph nodes are involved in 5% of presentations and occur in 15–20% of cases in the course of the disease.

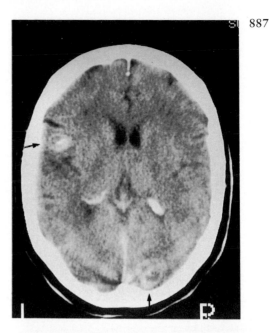

887 Neurological lesions. CT scan of the brain after intravenous contrast injection. This shows two circular opacities within the cerebral cortex (arrowed) due to metastases from a primary bronchogenic carcinoma. Intracranial deposits account for 10% of all metastatic presentations and metastatic lung cancer is the most common cerebral tumour in adults (50% coming to necropsy). Spinal metastatic deposits are less common and usually occur in patients with cerebral metastases.

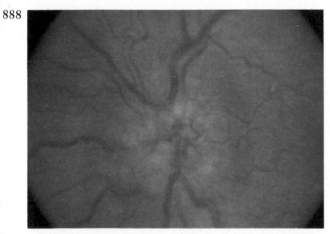

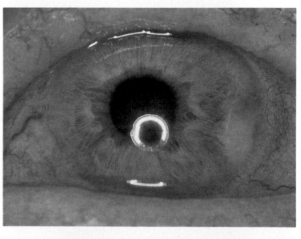

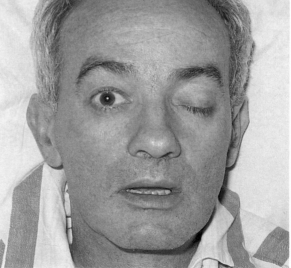

888 Neurological lesion. Papilloedema secondary to cerebral metastases. Intracranial deposits may present with headache and papilloedema.

889 Secondary deposit in the iris from squamous bronchial carcinoma is comparatively rare.

890 Brainstem lesion resulting in third nerve palsy. The eye is completely closed, the pupil widely dilated and, as all but the superior oblique and lateral rectus muscles are paralysed, the eye points downwards and laterally. This contrasts with partial ptosis, which follows interruption of the sympathetic nerve supply.

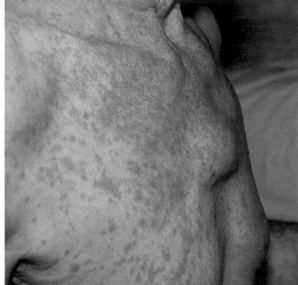

891 Bone metastases in the sternum. The skin rash is caused by ampicillin sensitivity which developed during treatment for recurrent pneumonia. Bone pain is reported in 20% of cases. Bone metastases are particularly common in small cell lung cancer; in all cell types, metastases predominate in the ribs, vertebrae, humeri and femora.

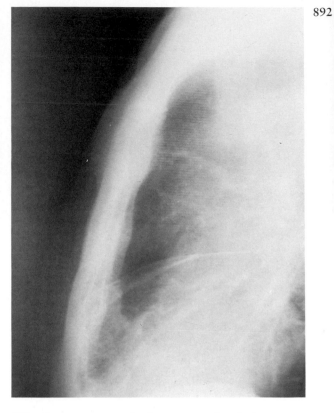

892 Bone metastases in the sternum. A soft tissue mass is visible over the sternum (same patient as shown in **891**).

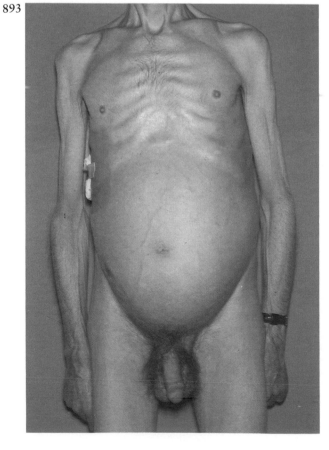

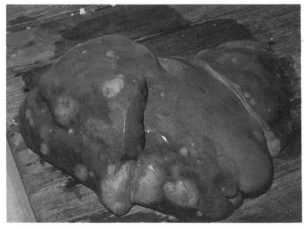

893 Hepatic metastases. Weight loss, malaise and ascites. Hepatic metastases tend to be a late feature of lung cancer. Liver function is disturbed only when the metastases are numerous, jaundice being unusual. An irregular firm liver may be palpable in about one-fifth of cases at diagnosis of small cell carcinoma; the incidence of hepatic metastases is much lower in other cell types.

894 Multiple hepatic metastases (necroscopy specimen) from oat-cell carcinoma.

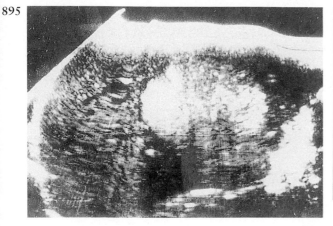

895 Large solitary hepatic metastasis. Parasagittal abdominal ultrasound scan picture.

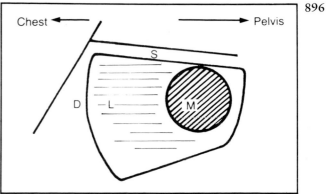

896 Diagrammatic representation of 895. Parasagittal abdominal ultrasound scan – 7 cm right of the midline showing skin (S), diaphragm (D), normal liver (L) and metastases (M).

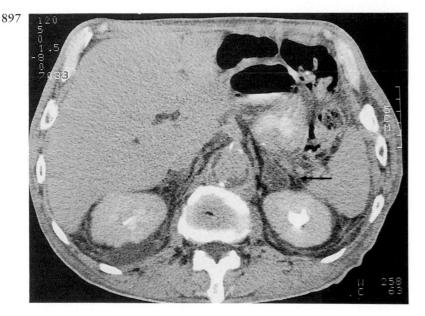

897 Adrenal metastases. Abdominal CT scan. A low attenuation mass is present in the left adrenal gland (arrowed). It was a solitary and clinically silent metastasis from a bronchogenic carcinoma. Adrenal and para-aortic lymph node metastases are visualised by abdominal CT scanning and occur in 8% of small cell tumours at presentation.

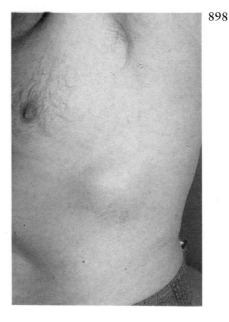

898 Large firm skin metastases tethered to the rib cage at a site of previous pleural biopsy. The underlying diagnosis was adenocarcinoma.

Superior sulcus tumours (Pancoast)

Tumours situated at the extreme apex of the lung produce a characteristic clinical picture of severe unremitting pain in the lower part of the shoulder and inner aspect of the arm (C8, T1 and T2 distribution), accompanied by sensory loss in the same distribution and by wasting and weakness of the small muscles of the hand and of the medial forearm, wrist and finger flexors. Pain is caused by erosion of the upper ribs and involvement of the brachial plexus nerve roots (C8, T1, T2).

A further neurological component is involvement of the sympathetic chain at or above the T1 (stellate ganglion) level to produce Horner's syndrome (ipsilateral partial ptosis, enophthalmos, a small pupil and hypohydrosis).

Dysphonia with hoarseness may develop should the tumour invade the adjacent recurrent laryngeal nerves.

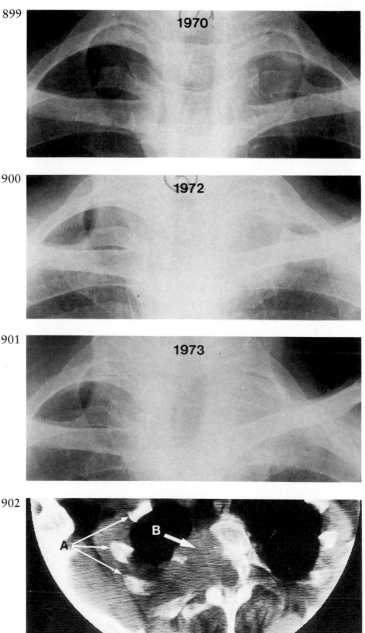

899–901 **Superior sulcus tumour.** Progressive tumour presenting with shoulder pain attributed to arthritis (**899**). Two years later weakness and pain were experienced in the left hand (**900**) and after three years rib erosion occurred (**901**).

902 **Superior sulcus tumour.** The plane of the CT scan is at apical level. The obliquity of the ribs causes them to be seen as short white opacities and they are normal (arrow A). On the right, there is a soft tissue mass in the paravertebral gutter, which has eroded deeply into the vertebral body and extends into the spinal canal (arrow B). The extent of the vertebral body erosion could not be appreciated from the radiograph, but is always clearly demonstrated by CT scanning (bone erosion is also well demonstrated by magnetic resonance imaging).

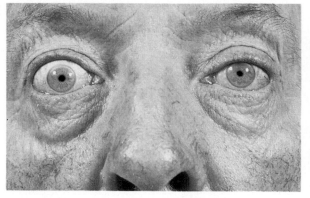

903 **Superior sulcus tumour (Horner's syndrome).** Left ptosis and a constricted pupil, caused by involvement of the inferior cervical sympathetic ganglia. The patient said he did not sweat on the affected side of the face.

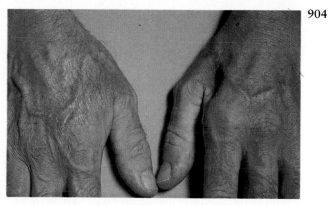

904 **Superior sulcus tumour (brachial plexus involvement).** The small muscles of the hand and thenar eminence show gross wasting. This is caused by infiltration of the left C8 T1 nerve roots and by disuse atrophy.

Table 57. Non-metastatic paramalignant manifestations.

SIADH
Hypercalcaemia
Gynaecomastia
Hyperthyroidism
Neuromyopathies
   peripheral neuropathy
   autonomic neuropathy
   cerebellar ataxia
   myasthenic syndrome (Eaton–Lambert)
Dermatomyositis

Hypertrophic pulmonary osteoarthropathy (HPOA)

This condition is uncommon and painful and characterised by warm painful swelling of the wrists and ankles, usually accompanied by fingernail clubbing. The mechanism by which lung cancer produces HPOA remains unknown. Although its major association is with primary lung cancer, it was originally described with chronic pleuro-pulmonary sepsis. In lung cancer it occurs most commonly with squamous tumours and, occasionally, with adenocarcinomas and large cell un-differentiated tumours. It does not occur in small cell lung cancer. In severe cases walking becomes impossible because of pain and swelling; the facial features can become thickened and gynaecomastia is present in a few cases.

Table 58. Some associations of HPOA.

Thymic carcinoma
Chronic myeloid leukaemia
Thyroid carcinoma
Hodgkin's disease
Adenocarcinoma of the oesophagus
Bronchial carcinoid
Lymphosarcoma
Cyanotic congenital heart disease
Pleural fibroma
Graves' disease
Oesophageal achalasia
Portal cirrhosis
Inflammatory bowel disease
Leiomyoma of the oesophagus
Cystic fibrosis

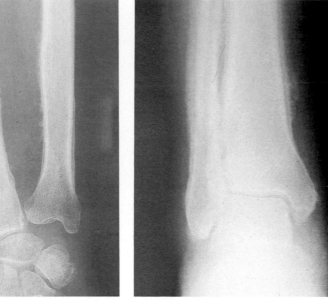

905 HPOA. Subperiosteal new bone formation at the wrist.

906 HPOA. Subperiosteal new bone formation at the ankle. The 1–2 mm wide line-shadows parallel to the cortex indicate where new bone has been deposited. Effective relief of symptoms, with resolution of the radiograph changes, frequently follows prostaglandin inhibitor drug therapy. Successful resection of the tumour is curative.

Fingernail clubbing

The earliest sign is loss of the angle between the nail and the dorsum of the terminal phalanx, caused by hypertrophy of the nail bed tissue. There is a 10–30% incidence with lung cancer, predominantly associated with squamous cell carcinoma and, occasionally, adenocarcinoma. Its mechanism is unknown; it may disappear after resection of the tumour.

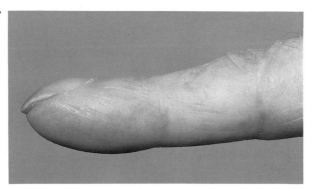

907   Fingernail clubbing.

Table 59. Causes of fingernail clubbing.

Respiratory
Bronchial neoplasms, especially squamous cell
Pleural tumours
Bronchiectasis, lung abscess and empyema
Lung fibrosis, especially asbestosis and cryptogenic
   fibrosing alveolitis

Cardiovascular
Bacterial endocarditis
Cyanotic congenital lesions with right-to-left shunts
Pulmonary arteriovenous fistula
Aortic aneurysm

Gastrointestinal
Cirrhosis
Chronic diarrhoea
   coeliac disease
   ulcerative colitis
   Crohn's disease

Familial clubbing

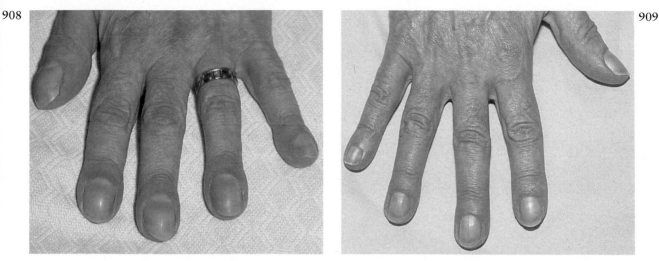

908, 909 Pre-operative fingernail clubbing (908) promptly regressed after successful resection of a bronchial squamous cell carcinoma (909).

Skin changes in bronchial malignancy

The cutaneous manifestations of malignant tumours, in addition to metastatic lesions, include changes ranging from non-specific rashes and pigmentation to the following characteristic markers, which may precede the underlying cancer by several years.

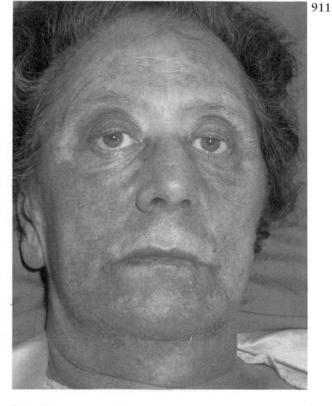

910

911

910 Purpura caused by thrombocytopenia. The bone marrow was extensively infiltrated by oat-cell carcinoma.

911 Dermatomyositis appears as patchy heliotrope markings on the face, eyelids and extremities.

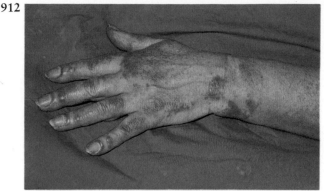

912 **Dermatomyositis.** Heliotrope markings are present over the finger joints (Gottron's sign). In up to 50% of cases the onset of dermatomyositis in middle-aged adults is associated with a variety of internal neoplasms including carcinoma of the breast, prostate, intestinal tract and lungs.

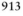

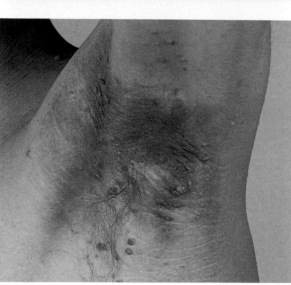

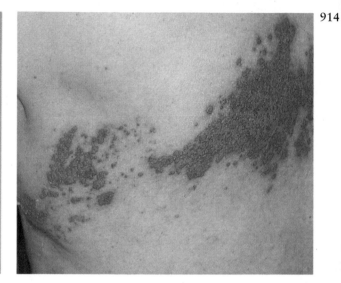

913 **Acanthosis nigricans.** Symmetrical hyperpigmented hyperkeratotic epidermal changes are found in the flexures. The onset in adult life is frequently associated with intra-abdominal adenocarcinomas. This patient developed a pleural effusion, and investigations showed secondary adenocarcinoma infiltrating the pleura.

914 **Herpes zoster** occurs when cell-mediated immunity is impaired and the patient is immunosuppressed by advanced carcinomatosis, reticulosis or lymphatic leukaemia.

Diagnostic investigations

The aim is to confirm the clinical diagnosis and to assess the extent of dissemination.

Radiographic features of bronchial carcinoma
The radiograph is almost invariably abnormal by the time the patient presents with symptoms. The radiographic appearances are variable. Peripheral carcinomas appear as rounded lesions, which may have 'pseudopodia' radiating from the surface. Central tumours are likely to cause collapse or consolidation of a lobe or segment, or involve hilar and mediastinal glands, which enlarge. Effusions are common and diaphragmatic paralysis caused by mediastinal entrapment of the phrenic nerve may occur. Necrosis in a carcinoma mimics the radiographic appearance of a lung abscess.

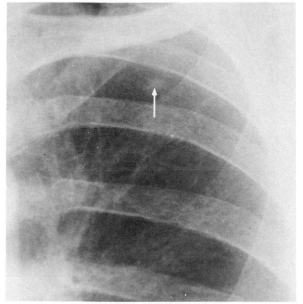

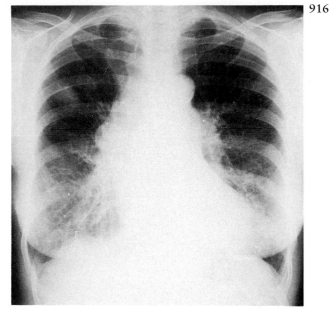

915 Solitary pulmonary nodule (arrowed). Early bronchial carcinomas are usually found by chance. At thoracotomy, a small adenocarcinoma was removed. The average size of a peripheral tumour is 3 cm at the time of diagnosis.

916 Proximal bronchial neoplasm. Prominent right hilum and widened mediastinum due to an advanced small cell carcinoma in the right bronchus intermedius. This posteroanterior film was taken when the patient complained of dyspnoea and presented with superior vena cava obstruction.

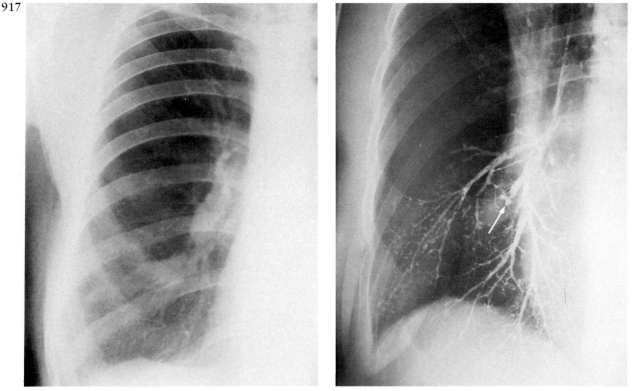

917 Proximal bronchial neoplasm. Recurrent right lower lobe pneumonia.

918 Bronchogram showing occlusion of a segmental basal bronchus by a tumour (arrowed). A squamous cell tumour was successfully resected (same as **917**).

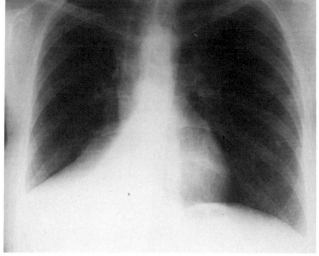

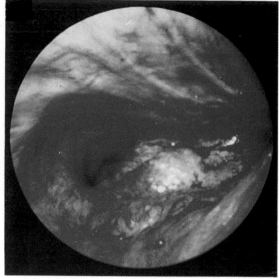

919 **Proximal bronchial neoplasm.** Collapse of right lower lobe by small cell carcinoma.

920 **Proximal bronchial neoplasm.** Bronchoscopic appearance showing occlusion of right main bronchus. (Same patient as shown in **919**.)

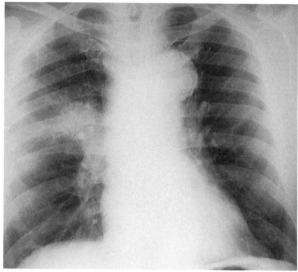

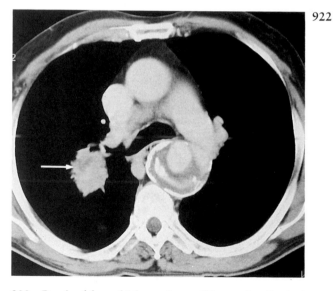

921 **Proximal bronchial neoplasm.** Right hilar mass.

922 **Proximal bronchial neoplasm.** CT scan (mediastinal window) showing 4 cm mass adjacent to right hilum (arrow). An incidental finding was a large aneurysm of the descending aorta.

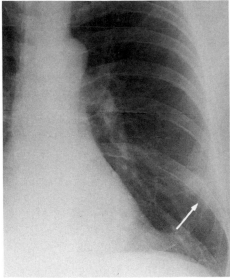

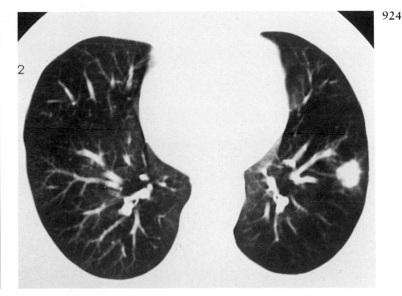

923 **Peripheral bronchial neoplasm.** Solitary peripheral nodule in left lower lobe (arrow).

924 **Peripheral bronchial neoplasm.** An irregular uniformly dense opacity is present. Accurate percutaneous needle biopsy was achieved by CT control in the prone position.

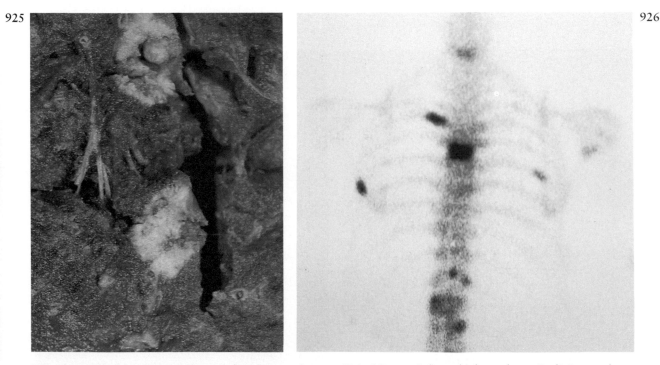

925 **Peripheral bronchial neoplasm.** Lobectomy specimen of a 2 cm squamous cell carcinoma. The tumour has been bisected. Resection may be curative at this early stage. (Same patient as shown in **924**.)

926 **Metastatic bronchial neoplasm.** Radioisotope bone scan showing deposits in the ribs and spine from a small cell carcinoma.

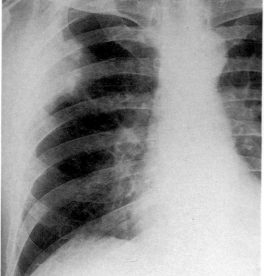

927 **Peripheral bronchial neoplasm.** Rib involvement, with lysis of the second and third ribs.

928 **Peripheral bronchial neoplasm.** CT scan demonstrating peripheral neoplasm invading the adjacent ribs. (Same patient as shown in **927**.)

Squamous cell carcinoma

This is the most common type of lung cancer. It is usually centrally situated in the proximal airways and may undergo central necrosis and cavitation.

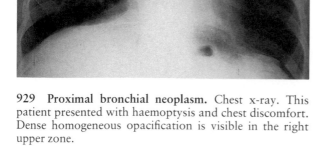

929 **Proximal bronchial neoplasm.** Chest x-ray. This patient presented with haemoptysis and chest discomfort. Dense homogeneous opacification is visible in the right upper zone.

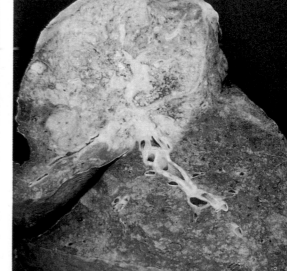

930 **Pneumonectomy specimen with a cavitating necrotic tumour** in a middle-aged coal worker. The yellow granular 'cheesy' appearance is typical of a squamous cell carcinoma. Obstruction either by intraluminal growth or by stenosing tumour encircling the wall may lead to infection and collapse of the lung distal to the lesion.

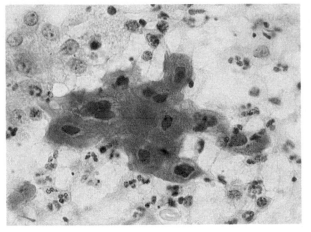

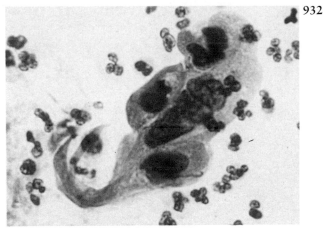

931 Sputum cytology. Layers of polygonal epithelial cells with hyperkeratinised, orange-ophilic well-differentiated malignant squamous cells with angular hyperchromatic coarse textural nuclei. Some contain concentric whorled keratin pearls. (Papanicolaou×175.)

932 Well-differentiated squamous cell carcinoma. Bronchial brush cytological specimen. Keratinised 'tadpole' caudate cells with large 'heads', elongated pseudopodial tails, pyknotic nuclei and dense orange-ophilic cytoplasm. (Papanicolaou×350.)

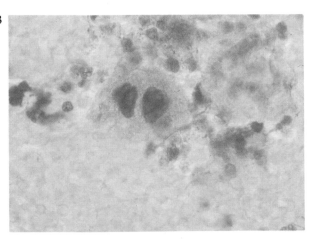

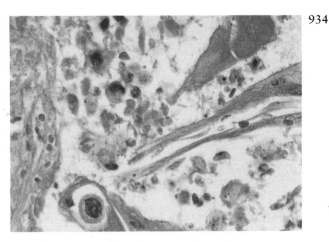

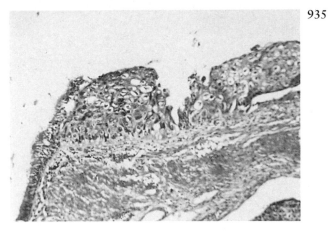

933 Poorly differentiated squamous cell carcinoma. Sputum cytology. Cells, occurring singly and of variable size, with irregular nuclei and eosinophilic cytoplasm. Multinucleated cells may be found. (Papanicolaou×350.)

934 Squamous cell carcinoma. Bronchial biopsy specimen. The bronchial mucosa (not shown) was normal. Exfoliated tumour cells lie in the bronchial lumen, showing keratin pearl formation. (H & E×350.)

935 Squamous cell carcinoma. Operative specimen showing malignant change in the bronchial epithelium. Note the characteristic intercellular bridges, cell nest formation, keratin and whorling arrangement of polygonal neoplastic epithelial cells. (H & E×100.)

936

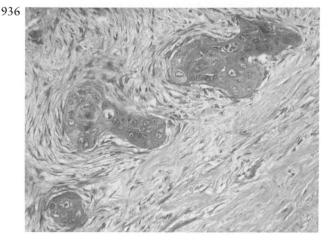

937

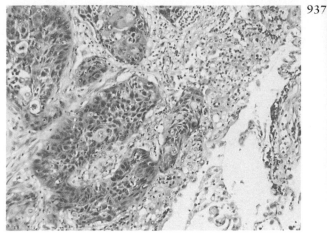

936 Well-differentiated squamous cell carcinoma. Bronchial biopsy. Lung resection specimen. Bands of tumour cells show stratification and keratinisation with the formation of distinctive keratin cells and intracellular cytoplasmic bridges. (H & E × 150.)

937 Well-differentiated squamous cell carcinoma. Lung resection specimen showing keratin pearls.

Small cell carcinoma (oat-cell)

938

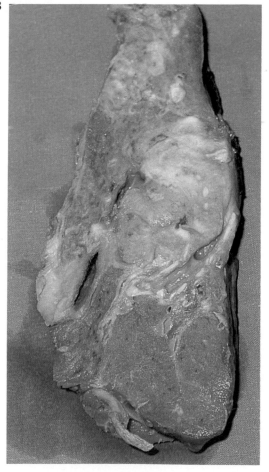

Small cell carcinoma, which accounts for about one-fifth of bronchial carcinomas, commonly arises in the major bronchi and spreads rapidly to the regional lymphatics. The pulmonary vessels are involved at an early stage and widespread haematogenous metastases are frequent at presentation. Most bronchial carcinomas occurring in patients under 40 years of age are of this type. The clinical course is aggressive and the median survival time in untreated cases is about three months.

Surgical resection is seldom a feasible option but small cell carcinoma is highly responsive to radiotherapy and chemotherapy. Modern intensive combination chemotherapy prolongs the median survival time to 10–15 months, particularly in patients with disease limited to the thorax.

938 Small cell carcinoma. Pneumonectomy specimen. Tumour arising in bronchus to apical segment lower lobe, metastasising to the hilar nodes and pleura.

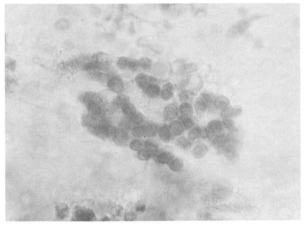

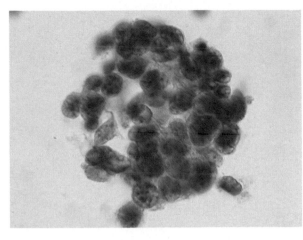

939 Small cell carcinoma. Sputum cytology. Clumps of darkly staining cells. Each nucleus contains one or two inconspicuous nucleoli. The dense nuclear chromatin, scanty cytoplasm and moulding of adjacent nuclei are characteristic. (Papanicolaou×175.)

940 Small cell carcinoma. Bronchial brush cytological specimens. Small (10–12μm) tightly packed, darkly staining cells with scanty cytoplasm and ovoid, spindle- and round-shaped moulded nuclei with diffuse chromatin patterns and inconspicuous nucleoli. The cells are about twice the size of lymphocytes, which they resemble. (Papanicolaou×175.)

941 Bronchial biopsy. The cells are small with deeply staining nuclei and scanty cytoplasm and, although of various shapes, tend to be spherical or ovoid (oat-grain shaped). They arise from the Kulchitsky-like cells lying in both the bronchial epithelium and in mucous glands, and therefore share some features of bronchial carcinoid tumours.

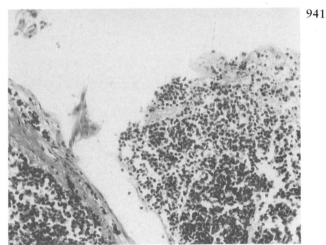

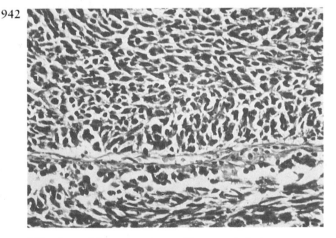

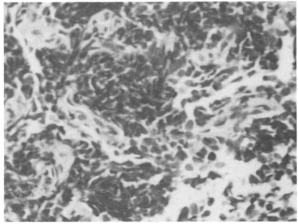

942 Lung biopsy specimen. Characteristic appearances with small round or oval cells with closely packed nuclei and little cytoplasm. (H & E×64.)

943 Small cell carcinoma. Lung biopsy specimen. Intermediate subtype, rather larger cells with angulated nuclei showing moulding and organoid patterns, and 'ribboning' and 'rosettes' in which the tumour cells arrange themselves in circular groups. (H & E×64.)

Large cell carcinoma

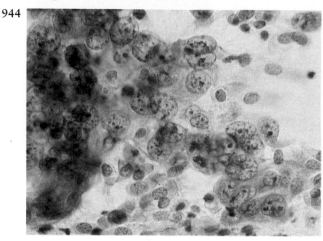

These tumours account for about 15% of lung cancers. They tend to be anaplastic, peripherally placed and, when examined by electron microscopy or special stains, often show features of squamous cell carcinoma or adenocarcinoma. The clinical course is aggressive, with rapid pleural spread and early extrathoracic dissemination.

944 Large cell undifferentiated carcinoma. Bronchial brush cytological specimen. Large malignant cells which are not keratin-positive on staining and have vesicular or hyperchromatic nuclei and prominent nucleoli. (Papanicolaou×175.)

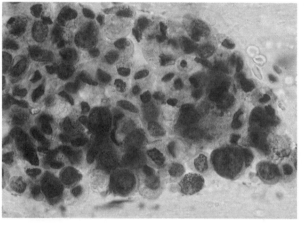

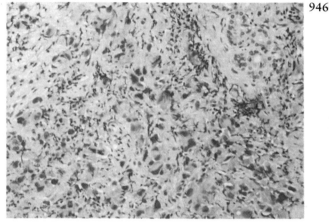

945 **Large cell undifferentiated carcinoma.** Needle aspiration specimen. Large, darkly staining cells.

946 **Large cell undifferentiated carcinoma.** Biopsy specimen. Large tumour cells, some with prominent nucleoli. No evidence of squamous or glandular differentiation, no mucin on special stains and no evidence of stratification.

Adenocarcinoma

These tumours are usually situated in the lung periphery and only involve the proximal bronchi as they spread. Growth is slow and a large size may be reached before symptoms occur. Adenocarcinoma accounts for about one-fifth of bronchial carcinomas. The tumour arises from mucous glands in small bronchi at the lung periphery. About 50% arise at the extreme periphery of the lung, spreading over the pleura in a similar macroscopic fashion to mesothelioma. Tumours arising in lung scars caused by asbestosis, healed tuberculosis or chronic interstitial fibrosis are most often of this type. No clear association between adenocarcinoma and cigarette smoking has been established.

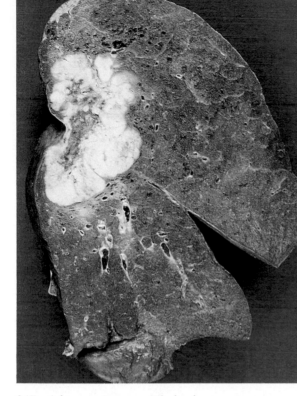

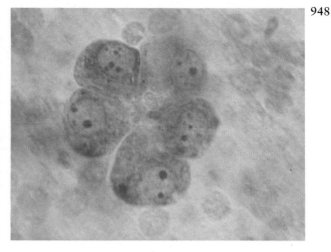

948 Adenocarcinoma. Cytology showing a cluster of malignant cells. The distinctive features are the ample vacuolated cytoplasm and multiple nucleoli. (Papanicolaou ×305.)

947 Adenocarcinoma. Whole lung pneumonectomy specimen. The peripheral position of the tumour is shown.

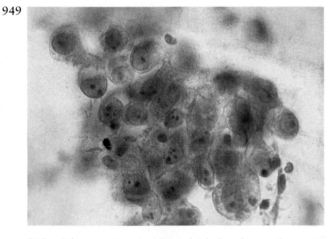

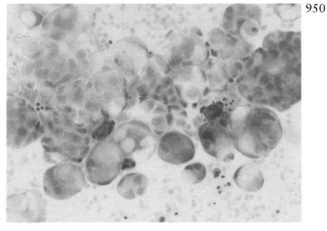

949 Adenocarcinoma. Bronchial brush cytology. A large three-dimensional group of malignant cells with pleomorphic hyperchromatic smoothly contoured nuclei, prominent multiple nucleoli and a moderate amount of cytoplasm staining positive for mucin. (Papanicolaou ×175.)

950 Cytology of pleural fluid showing adenocarcinoma cells. Considerable experience is required to diagnose correctly the presence of malignant cells in pleural fluid.

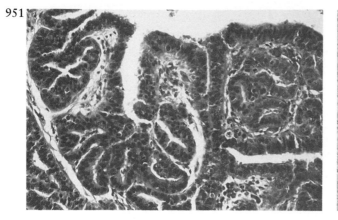

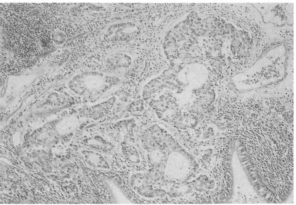

951 Moderately differentiated adenocarcinoma. Lung biopsy specimen, showing glandular differentiation. These tumours may produce epithelial mucins that can be identified by special stain.

952 Adenocarcinoma. Lung biopsy specimen.

Bronchiolo–alveolar cell carcinoma (alveolar cell carcinoma)

Alveolar cell carcinoma accounts for about 5% of all lung cancers (figures quoted range from 1–9%). It is often a diagnosis of exclusion, based on the absence of a primary adenocarcinoma elsewhere, a peripheral location in the lung parenchyma and a histological appearance that is characterised by the growth of malignant cells along alveolar walls.

It may present with chest pain, dyspnoea, weight loss and cough, or as a chance finding of a peripheral asymptomatic opacity on a routine chest radiograph. Massive bronchorrhoea is classically described but rare and, if present, tends to be a late manifestation. A history of chest disease is often present and a high percentage of these tumours arises in areas of scarring or more generalised fibrosis (systemic sclerosis).

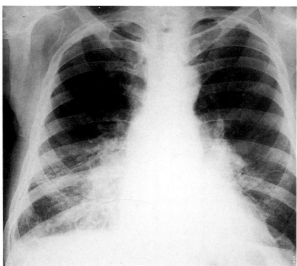

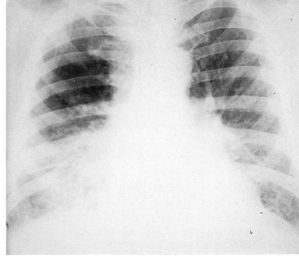

953 Bronchiolo–alveolar cell carcinoma. Bilateral lower zone shadowing was initially attributed to chronic pulmonary oedema in this emphysematous patient.

954 Bronchiolo–alveolar cell carcinoma. Three months later more extensive shadowing is visible. A tissue diagnosis was established by trephine biopsy. Same patient as shown in 953.

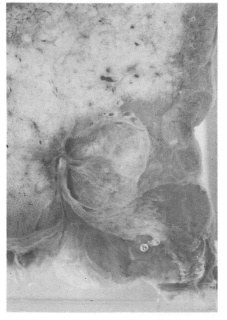

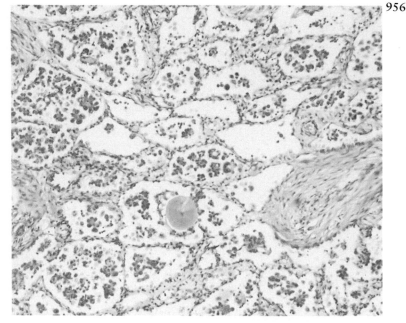

955 Bronchiolo–alveolar cell carcinoma. Macroscopic specimen showing a chronic abscess cavity, with adjacent lung consolidated with greyish-white tumour.

956 Bronchiolo–alveolar cell carcinoma. Lung biopsy. Tumour cells line the alveolar walls, forming papillary structures with shedding of clumps of malignant cells into the alveolar spaces. Spread throughout the lungs is by a combination of direct growth and aspiration of secretions containing tumour cells to form satellite lesions with a gravitationally related distribution.

957

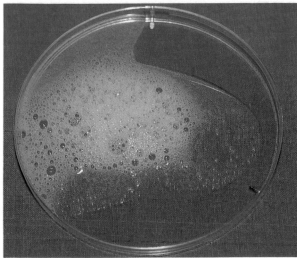

957 Bronchiolo–alveolar cell carcinoma. Bronchorrhoea is a common but not invariable feature. The sputum was copious and frothy.

Secondary tumours in the lung

Pulmonary metastases may be found in around a third of all cases of malignant disease. The most common metastases are from adenocarcinoma of the gastrointestinal tract (30%), the genitourinary tract (25%), the breast (18%) and sarcomas (10%). Spread to the lungs is by the vascular or lymphatic systems.

The common radiographic appearances of pulmonary metastases are:

- Discrete and usually rounded, single or multiple nodules of different sizes.
- Widespread 'snow storm' pattern.
- Coarse linear shadowing caused by lymphatic spread.

Pain from pleural involvement and dyspnoea caused by extensive embolic small vessel occlusion may occur.

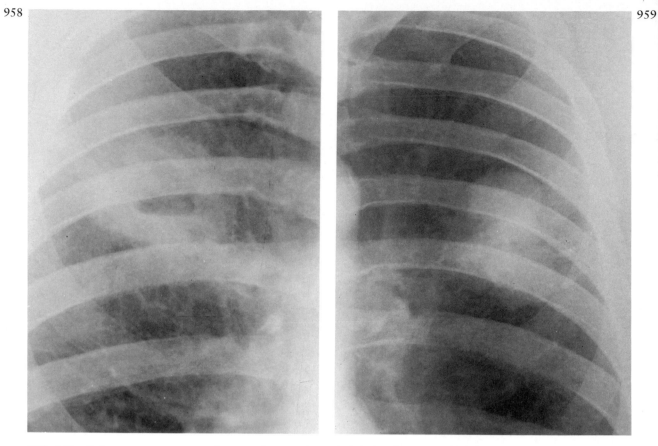

958, 959   Pulmonary metastases – hypernephroma. A single lobulated mass in the left lung and a cavitating thick-walled shadow in the right lung were caused by metastases from hypernephroma. It is unusual for metastases to cavitate, but when they do, hypernephroma is often the cause.

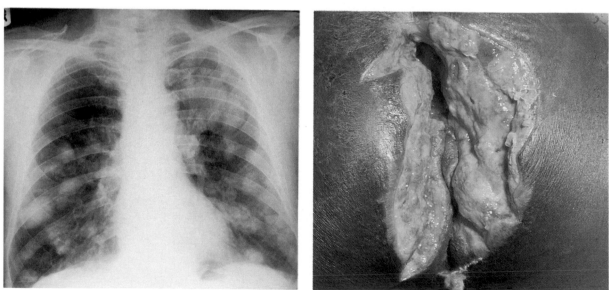

960, 961   Pulmonary metastases. Multiple rounded 'cannon ball' opacities from a large ulcerating rectal carcinoma.

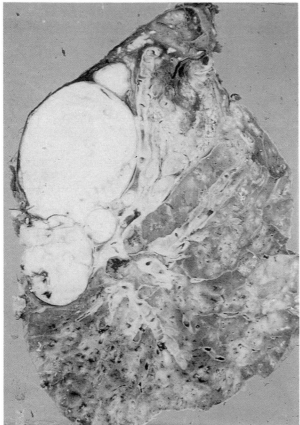

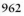

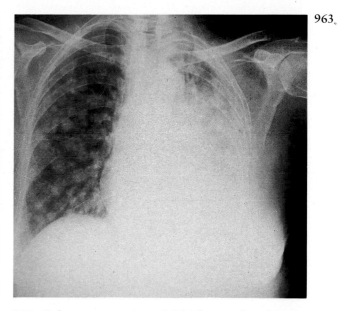

963 Pulmonary metastases. Multiple secondary deposits with left pleural effusion from a seminoma.

962 Multiple secondary deposits from carcinoma of the colon. The lower lobe contains multiple small lymph-angitic deposits, whereas the upper lobe contains large tumour masses. Carcinoembryonic antigen was strongly positive.

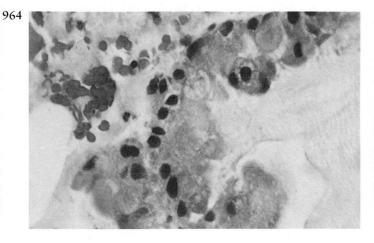

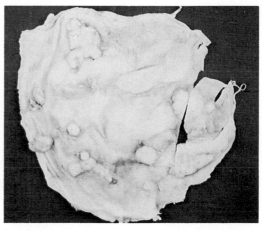

964 Pleural metastases. Pleural biopsy with mucus-secreting cells from metastases.

965 Pleura showing multiple yellow secondary deposits.

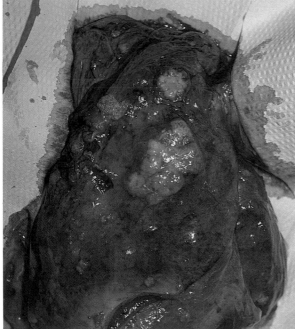

966 Necropsy specimen. Multiple pleural deposits of varying size from metastic adenocarcinoma.

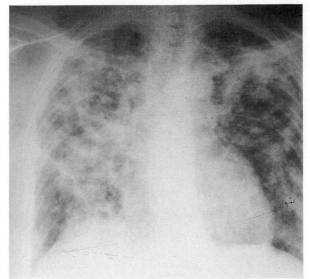

967 Pulmonary metastases – adenocarcinoma. The primary site was not identified in this patient. Most cases arise from gynaecological, prostatic or breast primary tumours. As this group of malignant tumours can be palliated by chemotherapy, a detailed search for the primary site can be worthwhile. Other possible primary sites include occult primary tumours of the pancreas, stomach, colon, liver or lung.

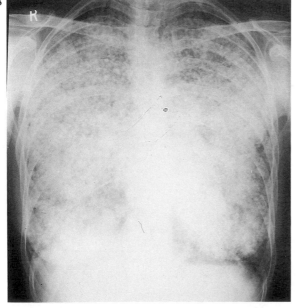

968 Disseminated haematogenous metastases from a follicular thyroid carcinoma. This 'snow storm' of metastatic deposits remained unchanged for many months because of the slow growth of the tumour. The initial radiographic appearance was of a fine micronodular pattern. Similar appearances are seen in pulmonary metastases arising from other highly vascular primary tumours, such as chorioncarcinoma osteosarcoma and renal carcinoma.

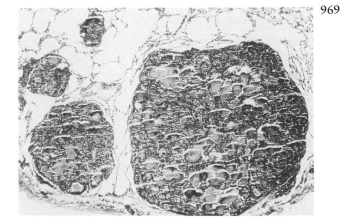

969 Metastatic follicular thyroid carcinoma – pulmonary metastases. Colloid-containing thyroid tissue, together with lung, is seen in this drill biopsy specimen. Same patient as shown in **968**.

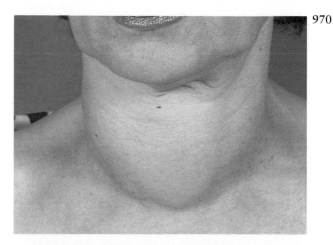

970 **Multinodular goitre** which underwent malignant change. Same patient as shown in 968, 969.

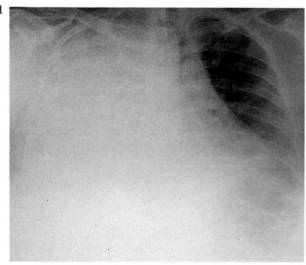

971 **Massive pleural effusion secondary to metastatic ovarian carcinoma.**

972 **Pleural metastases.** Considerable pleural thickening secondary to malignant infiltration from metastatic ovarian carcinoma. Same patient as shown in 971, after aspiration of effusion and chemotherapy.

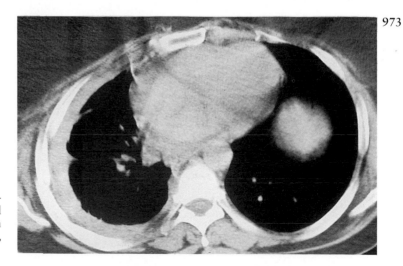

973 **Pleural metastases.** CT scan (mediastinal window) demonstrating unilateral pleural thickening from metastatic ovarian carcinoma. Same patient as shown in 971, 972.

Lymphatic spread of carcinoma in the lung

Lymphangitic spread within the lung parenchyma (lymphangitis carcinomatosa) is virtually exclusive to adenocarcinoma. It is seen in association with primary bronchial adenocarcinoma, when the lymphatic spread is confined to the ipsilateral lung, or as part of the pattern of dissemination of breast, primary gastrointestinal or genitourinary adenocarcinoma. It commences with mediastinal lymphatic involvement spreading to the pulmonary and pleural lymphatic channels and in the later stages invades adjacent lung tissue to give a nodular pattern of pulmonary deposits.

The diagnosis may be suspected from a history of progressive dyspnoea, with or without a productive cough, and diffuse infiltrates on the chest radiograph, often with lymph stasis lines due to engorged lymphatic vessels.

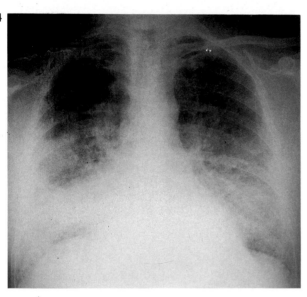

974 **Lymphangitis carcinomatosa.** Posteroanterior chest x-ray. Pulmonary infiltration in a 59-year-old male patient who presented with breathlessness, cough and wheeze. Transbronchial biopsy revealed clumps of malignant cells. The radiographic differential diagnosis includes pulmonary oedema, opportunistic infections and, in patients given previous chemotherapy, cytotoxic drug-induced lung disease. Cyclophosphamide and methotrexate are commonly implicated.

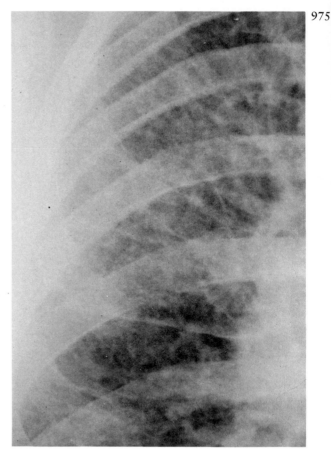

975 **Long hairline shadows in the upper lung fields,** running from the hilum towards the periphery. These lines (Kerley 'A' lines) are lymphatics infiltrated by tumour and are a radiographic manifestation of lymphangitis carcinomatosis.

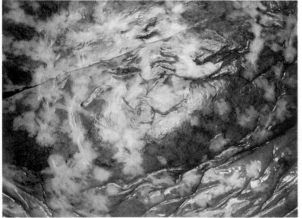

976 Lymphangitis carcinomatosa. Pleural surface macroscopic appearance of a postmortem specimen of lung. Multiple deposits of tumour with prominence of lymphatic channels.

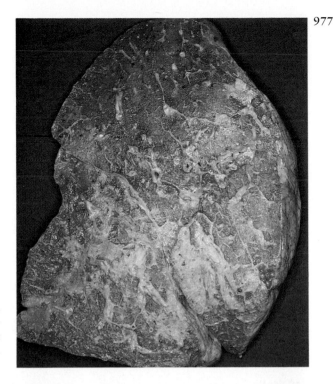

977 Lymphangitis carcinomatosa. Macroscopic appearance of whole lung section showing consolidation by grey-white tumour spreading along vascular and lymphatic channels, and invading laterally to give a nodular pattern of pulmonary and pleural deposits.

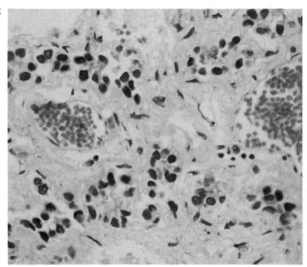

978 Lymphangitis carcinomatosa. Microscopic appearance. Infiltrating metastatic poorly differentiated adenocarcinoma extending within the lymphatics and blood vessels. The primary arose from the lateral lobe of the prostate.

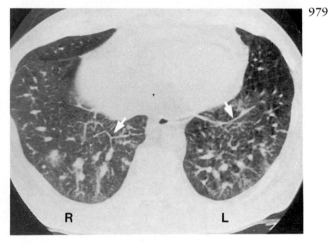

979 Lymphangitis carcinomatosa. CT scan. Irregular branching linear densities are present centrally, just behind the cupola of the diaphragm on both sides. The torn netting appearance on the right (arrowed) and the beaded chain appearance on the left (arrowed) are typical of this condition and are due to tumour infiltration in the interlobar septa. HRCT is much more sensitive than standard radiographs in revealing the presence of tumour infiltration in the lymphatics and septa.

Rare pulmonary tumours– tumours of epithelium
Bronchial carcinoids

These tumours, sometimes described as bronchial adenomas, comprise about 2% of pulmonary neoplasms. Bronchial carcinoids usually present at a much earlier age than carcinomas, often before the fifth decade. Cough and haemoptysis with signs of lobar collapse are common.

Carcinoids are derived from the duct epithelium of bronchial mucous glands. About 90% are typical carcinoid tumours. The remainder resemble salivary gland tumours (adenoid cystic carcinomas).

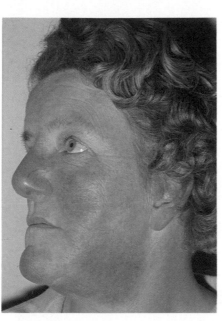

980   Carcinoid facial flushing. This dramatic sign is rare in bronchial carcinoids but common in gut carcinoids. Abdominal cramp, diarrhoea, oedema, wheeze, breathlessness and flushing are caused by the tumours releasing various vasoactive substances. The release of these substances from a primary lung carcinoid may damage valves in the left side of the heart.

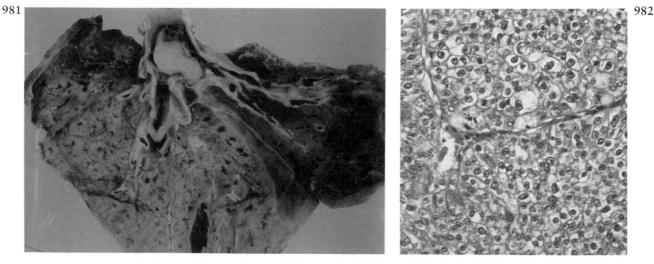

981   Whole lung section of bronchial carcinoid occluding a lobar bronchus. Local excision may be sufficient, although some carcinoids have the potential to metastasise to lymph nodes.

982   Bronchial carcinoid tumour. Histology showing sheets of small regular polygonal cells with small rounded nuclei and pale cytoplasm. Bronchoscopy provides confirmatory histology in 75% of cases. Beware – carcinoid tumour can readily be confused with oat-cell carcinoma. (H&E×300.)

Cylindroma (adenoid cystic carcinoma)
This is a rare tumour, although it is the most common primary malignant tumour of the trachea. The ideal treatment is excision, but if this is not feasible, radiotherapy will often produce prolonged remission.

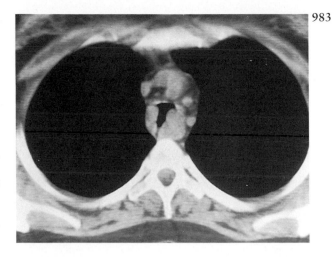

983 Cylindroma of the trachea. CT scan appearance. Irregular tumour masses narrow and distort the lumen of the trachea. There is gross thickening of the wall of the trachea, but no invasion of the surrounding structures.

CT scanning is unique in its ability to display both the lumen and the extramural structures with such clarity.

Tumours of neural tissue

Neural tumours may be classified as: neuro-lemmomas, arising from the Schwann cell; neuro-fibromas from the nerve sheath; ganglioneuromas from the neurone, and their malignant counterparts, neurosarcoma and neuroblastoma.

984 Neurolemmoma. CT scan showing ovoid enlargement of the peripheral nerve adjacent to the spinal column (arrow A), with erosion of the vertebral body and rib (arrow B).

Tumours of mixed cell origin

Hamartoma
Hamartomas are usually regarded as a developmental anomaly rather than as a true neoplasm. They are rare, benign and usually discovered incidentally on routine radiograph.

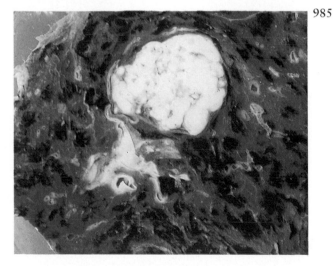

985 Hamartoma. Foci of calcification are present in the solitary well-circumscribed lobulated creamy-white mass. Hamartomas contain the normal tissues of the bronchial wall, but cartilage, mixed connective tissue and gland-like clefts lined by cuboidal epithelium are also present. Hamartoma is often solitary and subpleural, and a chance finding during routine chest x-ray. It may 'bounce off' the end of an aspiration biopsy needle because it is so hard.

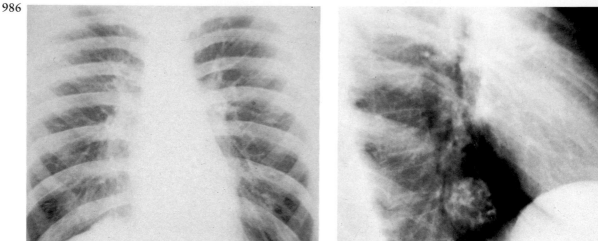

986, 987 Hamartoma. The posteroanterior film (**986**) shows an abnormal contour to the right diaphragm. The lateral film (**987**) shows a solitary sharply demarcated round lesion in which speckles of 'popcorn' calcification are present. This appearance is very characteristic of hamartoma.

Hodgkin's disease

Hodgkin's disease is characterised by painless and progressive lymphadenopathy with cachexia, malaise, pruritus and fever. Mediastinal gland involvement is common. Primary disease of the lung is rare, but it may occasionally arise in bronchial lymph glands and remain localised for months or possibly years.

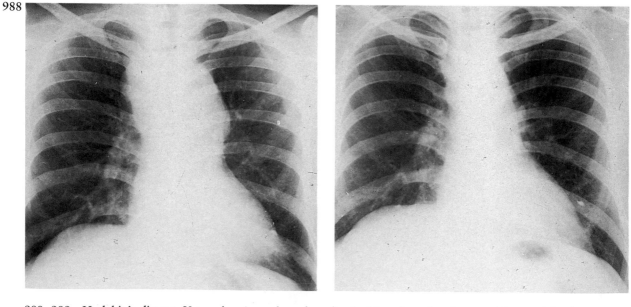

988, 989 Hodgkin's disease. X-ray showing enlarged mediastinal lymph nodes. As no evidence of the disease was present below the diaphragm, it remained a stage 2 disease, suitable for radiotherapy. Radiotherapy caused rapid shrinkage of the mediastinal lymphadenopathy (**989**).

Secondary Hodgkin's disease of the lung is present in 40% of cases during the course of the disease. In about 20% of these, there is no evidence of mediastinal lymph node involvement. The chest radiograph may show hilar gland involvement with direct lung invasion; lobar infiltration, which may cavitate and resemble tuberculosis; fine or coarse unevenly disseminated nodules, which tend to be well defined at first; and the irregular or disseminated round lesions; which may resemble metastatic tumour.

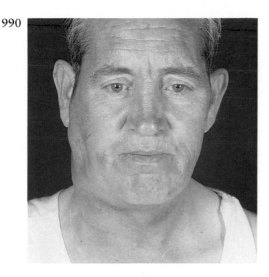

990   **Hodgkin's disease.** Large lymph nodes on both sides of the neck. There was also enlargement of the mediastinal lymph nodes.

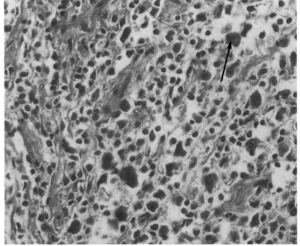

991   **Hodgkin's disease.** Lymph node histology. The tumour is composed of histiocytes, polymorphs and Reed–Sternberg giant cells (arrowed) with 'mirror image' double nuclei.

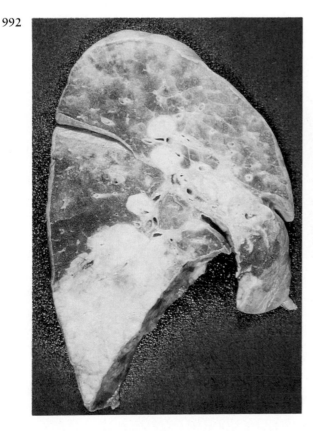

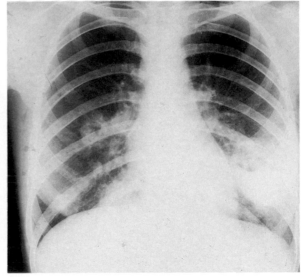

992   **Primary Hodgkin's disease** of the lung may occasionally arise in the lymph nodes related to bronchi. Macroscopically, the surface of the tumour is yellow and lobulated. The lower and middle lobes are involved and separate nodules are present in the upper lobe.

993   **Cavitating Hodgkin's disease.** Coarse, well-defined nodules may cavitate or become confluent.

Thymoma

Thymoma is the most common anterior mediastinal tumour and is due to a neoplastic proliferation of the epithelial skeleton of the thymus gland. It may present at any age, but the peak incidence is in the fifth or sixth decades. Complete surgical excision offers the best prospect of a cure and is necessary to establish the benign or malignant nature of these tumours.

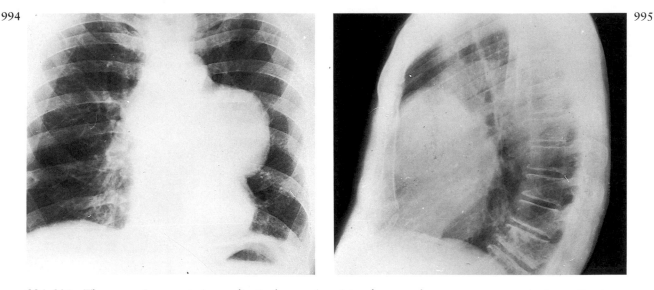

994, 995 Thymoma. Large anterior mediastinal mass. A variety of cysts and tumours may occur in the mediastinum, especially lymphomas, metastatic carcinoma, teratomas and malignancies arising in the thyroid and thymus.

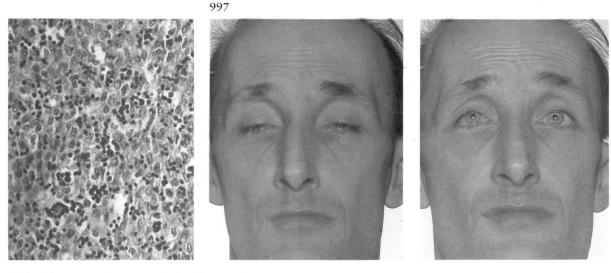

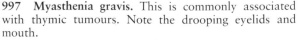

996 Thymoma. Surgery disclosed a solid tumour composed of reticular cells and lymphocytes – appearance typical of a thymoma. These tumours may be locally invasive and require postoperative radiotherapy.

Thymic tumours are found in up to 40% of patients with myasthenia gravis and, rarely, may also be associated with hypogammaglobulinaemia, B cell lymphopenia, systemic lupus erythematosus and polymyositis.

997 Myasthenia gravis. This is commonly associated with thymic tumours. Note the drooping eyelids and mouth.

998 Tensilon test for myasthenia gravis. The prompt relief of weakness supports the diagnosis. This patient was cured by thymectomy.

28 Bronchiectasis and cystic fibrosis

Bronchiectasis is the morphological term used to describe the condition of chronic dilatation of one or more bronchi. A common, disabling and often fatal illness in the pre-antibiotic era, it is now comparatively rare in developed countries. It remains a major cause of morbidity and mortality in some parts of the world, especially in areas with limited medical facilities. The true incidence is almost certainly an underestimate, for simple imaging will identify only gross disease, and the non-specific symptoms are often attributed to chronic bronchitis.

The main types recognised are:

- Follicular (cylindrical).
- Saccular.
- Atelectatic (middle lobe syndrome).

In all three types there is dilatation and inflammation of subsegmental airways, mucopurulent secretions and airways obstruction which may result in fibrosis of small airways. Whatever the initial cause, inflammation damages the bronchial walls, leading to replacement of normal ciliated cuboidal epithelium. The airways become colonised by avirulent bacteria, especially *Haemophilus influenzae*, leading to a sequence of recurrent infections associated with impaired mucociliary clearance and excess mucous secretion.

The principal feature is a chronic cough that is productive of copious, often blood-stained, sputum. The physical signs include cyanosis and coarse crackles with wheeze. In advanced cases, chronic malnutrition, sinusitis, fingernail clubbing (see page 326), cor pulmonale and frequent bronchopulmonary infections may occur. Advanced bronchiectasis is often accompanied by hypertrophy and anastomosis between the bronchial and pulmonary vessels, causing right-to-left shunts which are the site of haemoptysis. Haemoptysis may be severe.

Bronchiectasis is usually acquired in childhood, often after a recognisable respiratory infection complicating measles, pertussis or influenza, or after repeated or prolonged pneumonitis. The majority of patients display a slow progression over many years.

Table 60. Predisposing factors of bronchiectasis.

Congenital anatomical defects	Bronchomalacia
	Tracheobronchomegaly
	Pulmonary sequestration
Mechanical bronchial obstruction	Foreign body
	Inspissated mucus
	Tumour
	Extrinsic compression – nodes
	– tumour
Inflammatory pneumonitis	Aspiration of gastric contents
	Inhalation of caustic chemicals
Immunodeficiency states	Primary selective Ig deficiency
	Panhypogammaglobulinaemia
	Leukocytic dysfunction CGD
Mucociliary clearance defect	Genetic – primary ciliary dyskinesia, cystic fibrosis
	Acquired – Young's syndrome
Chronic obstructive pulmonary disease	
Allergic bronchopulmonary aspergillosis	
Collagen vascular diseases	
Inflammatory bowel disease	
Granulomatous lung disease (including tuberculosis)	

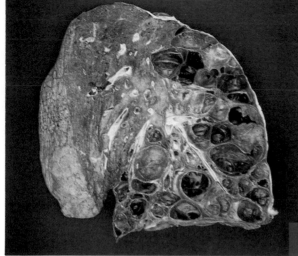

999 Extensive saccular bronchiectasis in the lower lobe. Necropsy specimen, sagittal section. Note the large thin-walled 'cystic' cavities, which are in continuity with the bronchi. The normal ciliated epithelium is destroyed by inflammation and the bronchi and bronchioles are lined by metaplastic squamous epithelium.

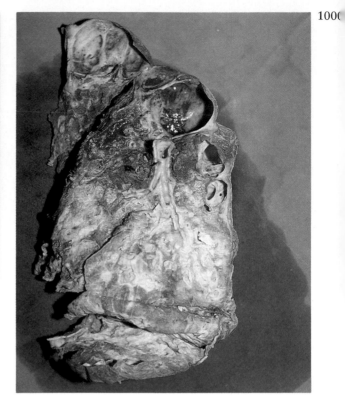

1000 Extensive saccular bronchiectasis. Right lung pneumonectomy specimens showing widespread bronchiectasis with large cystic spaces in the upper lobe, considerable destruction of the lung substance, and a thick mantle of inflammatory tissue surrounding the walls of dilated bronchi in the lower lobe.

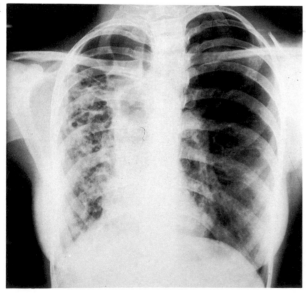

1001 Extensive saccular bronchiectasis. Contracted destroyed right lung with many cystic spaces. The mediastinum is deviated to the affected side and the rib space is narrowed, showing the marked loss of volume. Same patient as shown in **1000**.)

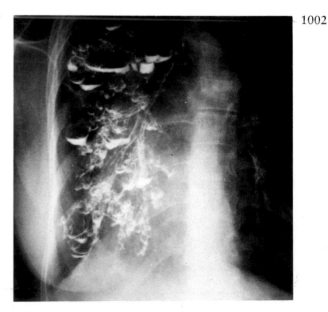

1002 Extensive saccular bronchiectasis. Bronchogram showing large cystic spaces in the right lung.

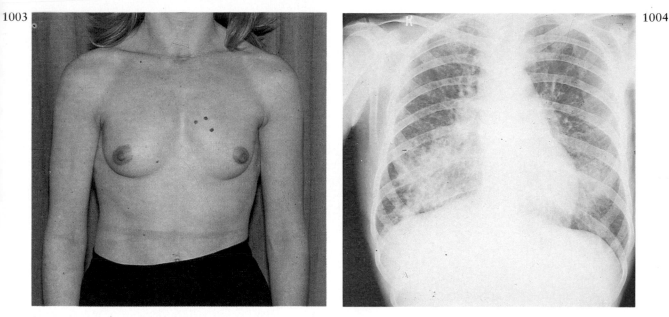

1003, 1004   Generalised follicular bronchiectasis. This 26-year-old woman developed bronchiectasis after severe infantile pertussis. About 50 ml of purulent sputum was expectorated daily. Tracheostomy was performed during a life-threatening infection at 21 years of age, after which cyanosis and finger clubbing had developed. Exercise tolerance was limited to 100 yards on flat ground.

Note the hyperinflated square-shaped chest and powerful intercostal muscles which are a consquence of long-standing airflow obstruction.

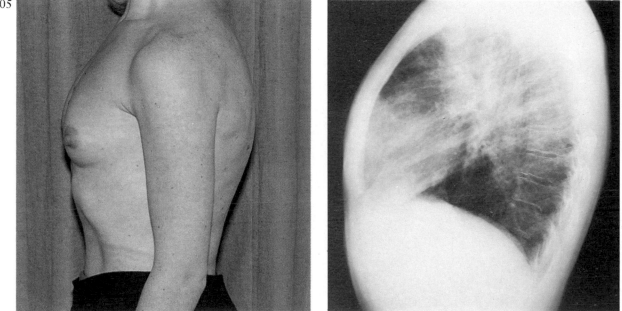

1005, 1006   Generalised follicular bronchiectasis. Hyperinflated chest with deep posteroanterior depth both clinically and radiographically. (Same patient as shown in 1003, 1004.) The posteroanterior and lateral chest x-rays show increased bronchovascular markings and linear fibrotic shadows, especially prominent in the right lower zone where there are parallel 'tram-line' shadows related to bronchial wall thickening and 'honeycombing' due to the presence of follicular (cystic) bronchiectasis.

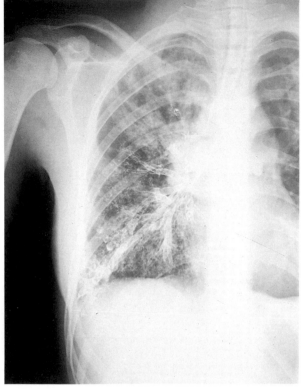

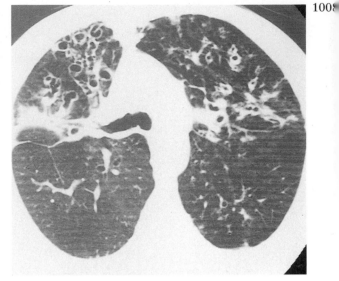

1008 Bronchiectasis. CT scan. Irregular dilated thickened bronchi with marked wall thickening are present in the anterior segments of both upper lobes. The lower lobes show the effect of limited emphysema but no bronchiectasis. High resolution CT is the most accurate non-invasive method available for demonstrating bronchiectasis.

1007 Generalised follicular bronchiectasis. Bronchogram of right lung showing dilated cylindrical bronchi, especially in the right lower lobe. (Same patient as shown in 1003–1006.)

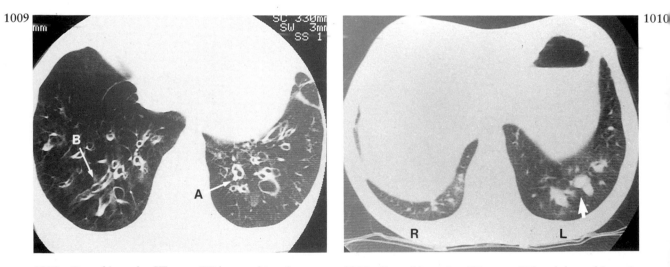

1009 Bronchiectasis. CT scan. Widespread involvement of both lower lobes. In cross section a signet ring appearance (arrow A) confirms that the cavity is a bronchus. The artery accompanying the bronchus forms a rounded projection within or without the ring of the bronchus. Seen in the plane of the scan the abnormal bronchi are demonstrated as thickened parallel lines with a dilated lumen (arrow B).

1010 Bronchiectasis. CT scan. Dilated bronchiectatic cavities filled with mucus confined to the posterior basal segments of the left lower lobe and not visible on the standard posteroanterior and lateral radiographs. This 'gloved finger' appearance on CT is relatively uncommon as an isolated finding (arrow).

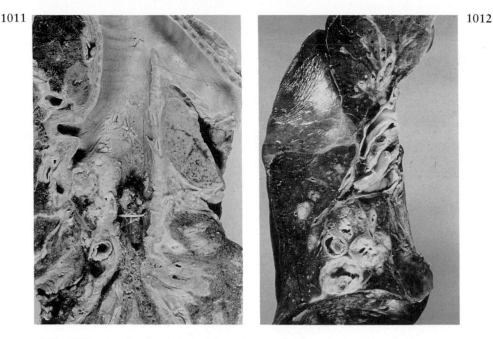

1011, 1012 **Foreign body bronchiectasis** may develop many years after unrecognised aspiration of a foreign body, leading to a postobstructive localised progressive bronchiectasis. These two examples – inhaled denture fragment (**1011**), and rabbit vertebra aspirated when eating (**1012**) – have impacted in dependent airways, leading to saccular bronchiectasis.

Primary ciliary dyskinesia (Kartagener's immotile cilia syndrome)

Primary ciliary dyskinesia, an autosomal recessive condition with incomplete penetrance, occurs with a frequency of between 1:15,000 and 1:30,000. In this condition the ultrastructure of cilia throughout the body is disordered, giving rise to slow and poorly coordinated ciliary beating.

Poor mucociliary transport in the respiratory system results in rhinitis, sinusitis, recurrent bronchitis and bronchiectasis. Immotility of spermatozoa causes male infertility. When the rotation of the embryonic gut is not guided by ciliary movements, the rotation takes place at random, resulting in situs inversus in around half of affected individuals. This syndrome is far more common than we realise. The chest physician should arrange for sperm examination of infertile males with recurrent bronchitis, even in the absence of situs inversus.

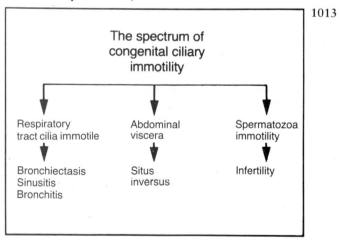

1013 The spectrum of congenital ciliary immotility.

355

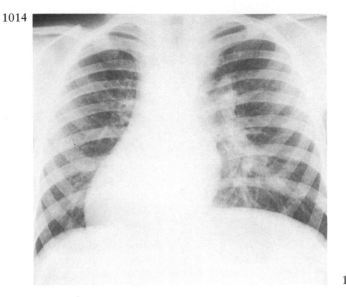

1014 Dextrocardia.

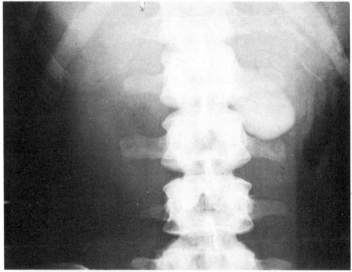

1015 **Cholecystogram** demonstrates a left-sided gall bladder.

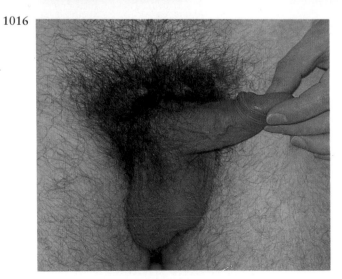

1016 **Dextrocardia – a sign.** The left testis normally hangs lower than the right, but this situation is reversed in situs inversus. This may be regarded as a bizarre physical sign of dextrocardia.

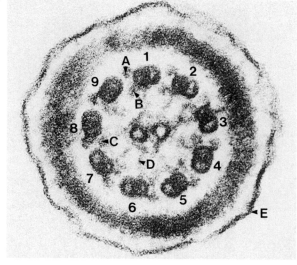

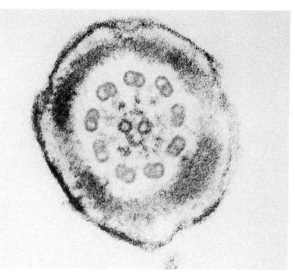

1017 Electron micrograph giving definition of terms used for various components of normal cilium seen in cross section (×320,000). The spermatozoa of men with this syndrome are immotile but living. The sperm tails have flagellar mutants in which sperm axonemes lack dynein arms of spoke heads. (A = outer dynein arm, B = inner dynein arm, C = nexin link, D = radial spoke, E = cell membrane.)

1018 Immotile spermatozoa with absent dynein arms. Dynein is an ATPase protein concerned with the production of energy for ciliary movement. Partial or complete deficiency of inner, outer or both dynein arms may occur.

Cystic fibrosis (CF)

Cystic fibrosis is characterised by chronic bronchopulmonary infection, pancreatic insufficiency with malabsorption and high sweat sodium concentration.

Transmitted as an autosomal recessive disorder, it is due to a single gene abnormality on the long arm of chromosome 7. The estimated frequency in Europeans is 1:2500, whereas in the Chinese the incidence is much lower at about 1:100,000.

Microbiology and lung damage

The lungs of CF patients are usually normal at birth. Lung damage, ultimately fatal, results from repeated bacterial infections and airway blockage by sticky secretions.

Common respiratory pathogens in cystic fibrosis are:

- *Staphylococcus aureus.*
- *Haemophilus influenzae.*
- *Pseudomonas aeruginosa.*

1019

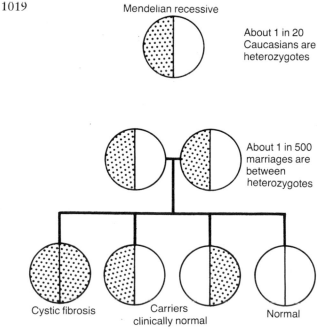

Mendelian recessive

About 1 in 20 Caucasians are heterozygotes

About 1 in 500 marriages are between heterozygotes

Cystic fibrosis

Carriers clinically normal

Normal

About 1 in 2000 children will be homozygotes with cystic fibrosis, i.e. 1 in 4 pregnancies in marriages between heterozygotes

1019 Genetics of cystic fibrosis.

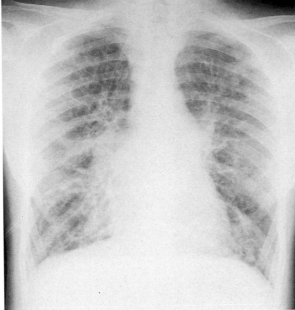

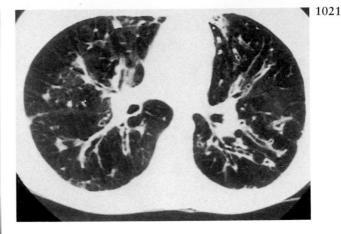

1021 Cystic fibrosis. Characteristic CT scan appearances: thickened dilated bronchi extend from the hila across two-thirds of the lung field. There is usually more bronchial wall thickening and less dilatation than in pyogenic bronchiectasis. The lungs are usually over-inflated, bringing the upper lobe bronchi into the plane of the scan. The upper lobes tend to be more involved than other areas of the lung.

1020 Cystic fibrosis. Chest x-ray of an adult patient. Widespread irregular nodular and patchy shadowing throughout all lobes, several ring shadows, line shadows due to bronchial wall thickening and prominent hila due to pulmonary hypertension. Medical treatment failed, necessitating organ transplantation.

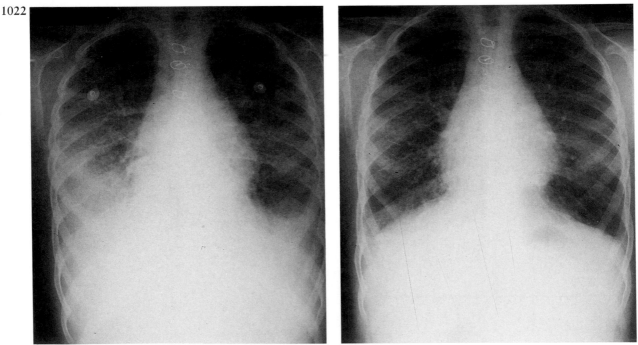

1022, 1023 Cystic fibrosis. Chest x-ray after successful heart/lung transplantation, a treatment which offers some CF patients the prospect of prolonged good quality life. The pulmonary shadowing (**1022**) was caused by an episode of acute rejection, controlled and cleared with five days of high dose immunosuppression (**1023**).

INDEX

Numbers in **bold** type refer to illustrations.